Contemporary Managed Care

Contemporary Managed Care

Readings in Structure, Operations, and Public Policy

Edited by Marsha R. Gold

Health Administration Press
Chicago, Illinois

02 01 00 99 5 4 3 2

Library of Congress Cataloging-in-Publication Data

Contemporary managed care / edited by Marsha R. Gold.

p. cm.

Includes bibliographical references and index.

ISBN 1-56793-078-6

1. Managed care plans (Medical care)—United States. I. Gold, Marsha R.

RA413.5.U5C675 1998

362.1'04258'0973—dc21 98-2665

CIP

The paper used in this publication meets the minimum requirements of American National Standard for Information Sciences—Permanence of Paper for Printed Library Materials, ANSI Z39.48–1984. ∞ ™

Health Administration Press
A division of the Foundation
of the American College of
Healthcare Executives
One North Franklin Street
Chicago, IL 60606-3491
312/424-2800

CONTENTS

ACKNOWLEDGMENTS

ALL THE the contributors to this book and I appreciate the foresightedness and assistance, both financial and intellectual, of the various organizations and entities that have supported and funded the work included here. These include the Physician Payment Review Commission, The Robert Wood Johnson Foundation and its Center for Studying Health System Change, the Health Resources and Services Administration, the Health Care Financing Administration, the Agency for Health Care Policy and Research, the Office of the Assistant Secretary for Health of the United States Department of Health and Human Services, The Commonwealth Fund, and The Henry J. Kaiser Family Foundation.

Mathematica Policy Research, Inc., kindly provided staff support to develop this anthology, and I am indebted to Harold Beebout, Mathematica's Director of Research, for his support on this project, and also to my colleague Judith Wooldridge, who helped review plans for the book and the production process. Joanne Pfleiderer provided advice and guidance on issues of presentation, style, and communication. Patricia McCall, my secretary, was essential in organizing material needed for this anthology.

Personally, I appreciate the support and guidance I received in understanding managed care from a number of individuals I am fortunate to have known. In particular, I want to acknowledge the insights I gained from Merwyn Greenlick, from James Doherty, and from many other managed care executives and clinician leaders. I also am indebted to the staff at Health Administration Press for their competence and enthusiasm in this work.

PUTTING MANAGED CARE AND THIS ANTHOLOGY IN PERSPECTIVE

Marsha Gold, Sc.D.

Many people are searching for a better understanding about the structure and operation of contemporary managed care. The term *managed care* is used to describe not only the forms of coverage that integrate financing and delivery but also the organizations that provide this coverage: health maintenance organizations (HMOs), preferred provider organizations (PPOs), and point-of-service (POS) plans. This anthology draws together insights gained from a large and varied—but very much interrelated—set of studies on the topic. Now more than ever, understanding contemporary managed care is critical, because it is no longer an alternative healthcare delivery system—it is the dominant one for privately insured people and is a growing one for the publicly insured. With this change come opportunities, issues, and challenges that policymakers and other participants in the system must address in order to maximize managed care's potential benefits and minimize its risks.

The studies documented in this volume were funded mainly by the federal government or foundations. Many of these studies have produced findings that figure prominently in today's debate about managed care. All of the articles were peer reviewed, and most appeared in well-established refereed journals in health services research. The research was conducted by staff at Mathematica Policy Research, Inc., often with the active collaboration of other researchers both in academia and in the public and private sectors.

By combining these papers into a single volume organized by topic, we hope to make the research more accessible and the cross-cutting themes and insights more obvious. While the studies are not a comprehensive inventory of all the issues and research relevant to managed care, they represent a large body of the work in this area. We believe they will give policymakers, educators, and others a meaningful foundation for understanding what managed care means or should mean for the healthcare system in the future.

Anthology Road Map

The first two parts of this reader describe managed care. The second two focus on important policy and market issues associated with its growth.

Part 1 addresses the important questions of what managed care is today and how it compares to what existed in the past. This section specifically examines managed care's explosive growth in this country over the past decade, placing it in historical context and summarizing recent work on its current trends and evolution.

Part 2 investigates the seeming "black box" of managed care. The term *managed care* has become a catch-all phrase for a diverse set of products and entities that are rapidly emerging in today's marketplace. The articles in this section develop insight into the structure and operation of managed care plans today, focusing on such issues as the most important features of managed care, how plans differ, and what the great variation in products and plans means for the design and implementation of research.

Part 3 focuses on managed care in two important public programs—Medicare and Medicaid. Together, these programs account for almost half of healthcare spending (Levit et al. 1996). Both are publicly funded, and both serve particularly vulnerable subgroups of the population—two main reasons for the longstanding research interest in their performance.

Part 3 presents findings from several important national studies on Medicare and Medicaid managed care. Of the two programs, Medicare is far easier to study because its structure is more uniform and databases more developed, albeit still limited. More is known about Medicare performance generally and about Medicare managed care specifically than about any other sector of health insurance or managed care. Tapping this knowledge to help guide Medicare managed care as it expands and diversifies is a challenging and important endeavor.

Medicaid, in contrast, has been more difficult to study. Research on the program has historically been limited by the diversity of individuals covered, the wide range of state programs Medicaid comprises, and the rather sparse and often inconsistent data available nationally from states. The Medicaid research documented here has confronted these limitations by exploring the state initiatives in depth, highlighting their still-evolving experience with Medicaid managed care and the importance of implementation and oversight to program performance. This information can provide important insight into the challenges posed by Medicaid managed care as it expands.

Part 4 is broadly focused on the future—particularly on issues emerging with the growth of managed care. This section addresses what the evolution of managed care thus far will mean for its future as well as for the future of the healthcare system as a whole. It also looks at what health system change will mean for the development of relevant measures and data to assess health system performance. The issues raised in this section involve measuring access to care and consumer satisfaction in a managed care environment. Also summarized is the design of the Community Tracking Study, a national longitudinal study to monitor the effects of managed care and health system change on the U.S. population.

Reference

Levit, K. R., H. C. Lazenby, B. R. Brade, C. Cowan, P. McDonnell, L. Sivarajan, J. Stiller, D. Won, C. Donham, A. Long, and M. Stewart. 1996. "Data View: National Health Expenditures, 1995." *Health Care Financing Review* 18 (1): 175–214.

PART

1

THE EVOLUTION OF MANAGED CARE

Introduction: The Changing Shape of Managed Care

Managed care has exploded in the past decade to become the dominant form of coverage for privately insured individuals (Jensen et al. 1997). It is also rapidly beginning to dominate Medicaid, representing more than one-third of recipients in 29 states and the District of Columbia (Rowland and Hansen 1996). While enrollment in Medicare managed care lags behind, it is nevertheless growing quickly, with 14 percent of beneficiaries now enrolled and more expected, given the provisions in the 1997 Balanced Budget Act to expand Medicare+Choice (BNA 1997).

This dramatic growth in managed care has challenged policymakers, consumers, the press, and all those involved in the healthcare industry to understand the proliferation of organizational models and products it has spawned. Furthermore, these products are offered by an increasingly diverse group of sponsors and are authorized under a set of federal and state statutes that grow more complex each year. The first set of three articles establishes the historical context for these changes and offers insight into current trends in, and the evolution of, managed care.

Until recently, HMOs were the prototypical and often the only form of "managed care," setting the stage for such systems as we know them today. The first article, "Understanding the Roots: Health Maintenance Organizations in Historical Context," summarizes the history of HMOs in the United States, identifying the features that have traditionally defined HMOs and suggesting four historical phases through which HMOs have evolved over time. The article also discusses:

- the shift from the initial prepaid group practice form of organization to the independent practice association (IPA) model built on community-based providers;
- the growing commercialization of managed care, paralleling other trends in the health industry; and
- the increasingly competitive and market-based environment in which managed care exists.

The next two articles in this section delve further into the managed care industry today. "Trends Toward a National Health Care Marketplace" examines the extent to which current trends mean that the local marketplace is being increasingly controlled by national firms, while "The Role of Managed Care 'Products' in Managed Care 'Plans'" provides insight on the range of managed care products now offered by health plans nationally.

References

Bureau of National Affairs (BNA). 1997. "Special Supplement: Conference Report, Joint Explanatory Statement on Medicare/Medicaid, and Children's Provisions of H.R. 2015." *H. Report* 5 (31): 105–217.

Jensen, G., M. Morrissey, S. Gaffney, and D. Liston. 1997. "The New Dominance of Managed Care: Insurance Trends in the 1990s." *Health Affairs* 16 (4): 125–36.

Rowland, D., and K. Hansen. 1996. "Medicaid: Moving to Managed Care." *Health Affairs* 15 (3): 150–52.

CHAPTER

1

UNDERSTANDING THE ROOTS: HEALTH MAINTENANCE ORGANIZATIONS IN HISTORICAL CONTEXT

Marsha R. Gold

WHILE MANAGED care has come to refer to an increasingly diverse set of insurance products and organizations, the roots of managed care are based in history and in the evolution of the HMO model. Thus, a historical perspective is relevant to understanding managed care today. In this update to part of an earlier paper, the health maintenance organization (HMO) organizational form is defined and its historical evolution described in terms of four developmental phases. The paper closes with some observations on the HMO form today in managed care and in the U.S. healthcare system.

The HMO Model

What we refer to as HMOs were traditionally defined as organizations with contractual responsibility to provide or assure the delivery of ambulatory and inpatient services to a defined, voluntarily enrolled population for a fixed, prepaid fee, with the HMO assuming at least part

Adapted from "Health Maintenance Organizations: Good or Bad for Canada?" Part I. *Canadian Review of American Studies* 23 (3): 31–55.

of the gain or risk for these services (Wetherille and Norbdy, as cited in Luft 1980).

The central feature that has historically distinguished HMOs from traditional insurance and practice is that HMOs integrate the financing and delivery systems. HMO organizations represent organized medical care systems responsible for providing or arranging for enrollees to receive all medically necessary care included in the contracted benefit package. In general, HMO benefits have been comprehensive, providing first dollar coverage with limited cost sharing at the point of service (Gold 1990). These services have been financed by a prepaid periodic fee that is fixed in advance.

The prepaid fee, or "capitation rate," has been viewed as providing the HMO organization with incentives for efficiency and a population-based focus. The HMO structure differs considerably from traditional fee-for-service practice, where income is linked to individual services with little ability to shift funding across settings of practice and few financial incentives to coordinate care. HMO organizations may benefit if they prevent illness or provide early treatment, decreasing the occurrences of later and more serious illnesses. The savings generated through avoided care reward the plan and may be used to fund additional benefits attractive to consumers, leading them to enroll in the plan. While there is the risk that these incentives will lead to denial of necessary services, research has indicated that, in general, HMOs provide care of equal or better quality, resulting in savings largely through reduced hospitalizations, improved initial access to services, and overall satisfaction levels equivalent to traditional fee-for-service systems (Luft 1981; Miller and Luft 1996; Miller and Luft 1997).

The concept of risk is central to both HMO design and the role that HMOs play in the American health system. The HMO entity typically has been at risk for delivering all needed health services, developing complex risk-sharing arrangements with its associated providers to encourage partnership and cost-effective delivery. Per capita payment also has been perceived as providing HMOs with incentives to encourage prevention, case management, and cost-effective practice.

The HMO's structure modifies the concept of freedom of choice. Those choosing to enroll in the HMO have agreed to receive services from the HMO's provider panel unless referred elsewhere; this relationship has been commonly referred to as a "lock-in," because it means that enrollees seeking care elsewhere must pay for that care at their own expense.[1] The concept of a lock-in has been critical in American HMOs so that as risk-bearing entities, HMOs are in a position to manage care and control utilization and provider behavior. Until most recently, most individuals enrolling in HMOs have done so voluntarily, based on a choice between alternative insurance plans offered by employers (both traditional and HMO systems or, more recently, a continuum of managed care products).

In the United States, there have been two major forms of HMOs. The first, prepaid group practices, comprised virtually all the original HMOs. Organized around a prepaid multispecialty group practice, these plans historically delivered care through integrated medical facilities staffed by physicians and other providers affiliated generally full-time with the plan. There are two HMO models: a staff model (e.g., Group Health Cooperative of Puget Sound), in which physicians are directly employed by the HMO and receive a salary; and a group model (e.g., Kaiser-Permanente), in which the HMO contracts, typically at a capitated rate, with a multispecialty physician group. Although a number of the original prepaid group practices tended to own their own hospitals, most current prepaid group practices do not, with these services provided on a contractual basis through existing community-based facilities.

The other major organizational form that has evolved is the individual practice association (IPA) in which the HMO contracts with multiple providers, most of whom are in solo, single specialty, or small group practice in the community; these providers tend to receive only a small portion of their income from the HMO, retaining an active fee-for-service practice.[2] The first IPA was developed in 1954 as a competitive response by physicians to the growth of prepaid group practices, but IPAs were relatively uncommon until the mid-1970s.

Because IPAs are based on a dispersed delivery system of providers based in the fee-for-service system, they have presented different and far-reaching management challenges from those that face the more tightly organized prepaid group practice with its more tightly defined networks. But IPA models also have been easier to set up as they have lower capitalization requirements. The wider provider networks in IPA HMOs have served to increase HMO enrollment, particularly as individuals enrolling are better able to retain established physician relationships.

Stages of HMO Development

Examined historically, one can distinguish four phases of American HMO development. The composition and role of the HMO industry, the environment, and the expectations of HMOs differed in each phase.

Stage I: Pioneer Phase (late 1920s to early 1970s)

During this initial phase, the term HMO did not yet exist, but the basic principles defining these organizations were developed (Gold 1991; Nelson 1987; Mayer and Mayer 1985). These initial organizations had their roots in the group practice movement and in consumer, labor, and industry efforts to provide more comprehensive and affordable coverage. Early HMO-like organizations were almost exclusively prepaid group practices; Kaiser Foundation Health Plan, Group Health Cooperative of Puget Sound, Group Health (Minneapolis), Health Insurance Plan of Greater New York, Group Health Association (D.C.) and a number of other plans still with a dominant role in the industry were created in this period.

Most of the very early plans were developed for particular industrial or community groups as a means to secure affordable care and access to services in an environment where few alternatives existed. With the development of enlarged insurance alternatives after World War II (Starr 1982) and the expansion of prepaid group practices into metropolitan areas, the concept of "dual choice" based on voluntary enrollment was refined to define how HMOs could relate to the evolving insurance industry.

In 1970, there were 33 HMOs with about 3 million enrollees in the United States with a localized focus heavily based in selected communities, including the West Coast and certain large cities (National Industry Council for HMO Development 1984). While small in number, these plans were sufficiently threatening to the medical community. Thus, HMO physicians were often denied hospital privileges, medical society membership, and access to necessary referral services; a number of states enacted laws restricting "the corporate practice of medicine" and otherwise providing barriers to HMO growth—often successfully challenged in the courts. The later part of the pioneer phase coincided with an era of rapid expansion of the American healthcare system. Cost was less a concern than access, the federal government began to assume an increasingly central role in health policy development, and provider support for change such as the passage of Medicare and Medicaid, in 1965, was garnered by promises not to interfere with the practice of medicine or the freedom of providers to define payment rates (Marmor 1973).

Stage II: Federal Preemption Phase (early 1970s–1980)

During this second phase, the federal government actively sought to encourage the development of HMOs as a mechanism to restructure financing and delivery in the United States to improve capacity and efficiency. This change was viewed as a prelude to national health insurance. Provider resistance continued to be strong, however, and influenced federal action (Brown 1983). The keystone event was the enactment of the Health Maintenance Organization Act in 1973.

A major historical point in the development of HMOs in the United States, this act actually established and defined the term *HMO*, including the structural and design requirement, which federally qualified plans had to meet. The act's requirements (later amended) for HMOs were extensive, leading HMOs to argue they were in an adverse competitive position with respect to traditional insurers. To facilitate growth, the act provided capital support for HMO development: $145 million in federal grants and $219 million in loans were ultimately provided for about 115 operational HMOs (Iglehart 1984). The act also solidified the concept of dual choice by allowing federally qualified plans to mandate employers to offer the HMO option where it was available.[3] IPAs were formally recognized in the act, with growth encouraged by requirements allowing mandates for employers to offer at least one prepaid group practice and one IPA (Dorsey 1975). The act also preempted restrictive state laws.

While HMO growth was slower than anticipated (Brown 1983), there were 236 HMOs with 9.1 million members by 1980, when financial developmental assistance was phased out (Gruber et al. 1988). Of these, 139 were prepaid group practices and 97 were IPAs; eighty-one percent of enrollment was in the former, mostly in group model plans (Kraus et al. 1991). As this phase drew to a close, cost containment increasingly was replacing access as the key health policy concern, support for strong federal leadership in health policy was eroding, and competitive models for healthcare delivery were receiving increased attention (Christianson and McClure 1979).

Stage III: Privatization and Competition Phase (1980s)

Despite the withdrawal of federal financial support in the early 1980s, the HMO industry grew more rapidly during this third phase than before, with the number of plans more than doubling and enrollment increasing fourfold (Gruber et al. 1988; GHAA, *Patterns*, 1991). In the 1980s, the concept of competition grew to play a considerably stronger role in the evolution of the HMO market. The number of HMOs available in major metropolitan markets grew considerably (Christianson et al. 1991), and the number of HMO options available to employees expanded rapidly. Most new entrants were IPAs, with fewer capital requirements. The for-profit sector of the industry grew as a means to secure needed capital (Ermann 1986), and industry growth secured Wall Street attention (Iglehart 1984). HMO sponsors became increasingly diverse, including insurer organizations and publicly traded healthcare firms, with greater involvement of both regionally and nationally owned firms. Stage III also included the development of more options for HMOs to participate in publicly sponsored insurance programs like Medicare and Medicaid (Langwell and Hadley 1989; Freund and Neuschler 1986). However, barriers to participation remained, and HMO penetration was considerably less under these public payor systems than under the pluralistic and dominant employment-based insurance system.

The scope of changes in this era is apparent from looking at data on the HMO industry as it entered Stage IV. In 1991, half of all enrollees were in plans sponsored by corporate entities owning or managing multiple HMOs. Two-thirds of plans serving 47 percent of enrollees were organized on a for-profit basis (GHAA, *Patterns*, 1991). Prepaid group practices by this point represented only a quarter of all plans though 42 percent of all enrollees.

At the close of Stage III, several forces that would influence the HMO industry in the 1990s were developing. HMO growth began to slow down around 1988, and new starts declined as existing plans focused attention on improving revenues and better controlling expenses to overcome the decreasing levels of profitability, which had reached their lowest level in 1987 (GHAA 1990; *Patterns*, 1991). Mergers became more common, and a few well-publicized HMO bankruptcies led to increased regulatory attention at the state level.

With their total health benefits costs often increasing by more than 20 percent per annum (Higgins 1991), employers, many already self-insured (McDonnell et al. 1986), took action to restructure their health benefits. In response to market pressure, traditional indemnity insurers increased their sponsorship of HMOs, often within an integrated managed care strategy. This sponsorship resulted in the increased proliferation of preferred provider, point of service, and other products designed to provide incentives for employees and their dependents to choose presumably more cost-effective providers (Gabel et al. 1989, 1990).

To enhance the ability of HMOs to compete in this environment, the HMO Act was amended in 1988. The amendments allowed federally qualified plans the option to offer a limited open-ended product allowing enrollees to seek care "out-of-network" on a nonreferral basis, generally with considerable cost sharing in the form of deductibles and coinsurance. Additional rating flexibility was provided for adjustment based on anticipated group experience; the equal dollar contribution requirement of employers for the HMO option was eliminated in favor of a "nondiscrimination" test. The amendments called for a sunset of the employer mandate by 1995. Steeped in a market-based philosophy, the Reagan and Bush administrations were less committed to the regulatory oversight implicit in the HMO Act (GHAA, *Patterns*, 1991).

Stage IV: Consolidation, Maturation, and Integration (1990s)

With this fourth phase of HMO development still under way, its final structure is yet to be defined. From the perspective of the employment-based insurance system, the previous separation between financing and delivery has eroded; employees seeking to retain a traditional indemnity plan with unlimited freedom of choice of providers pay substantially for the option, if indeed it is available.

Over the 1990s, growth in managed care skyrocketed. Much of this growth was in new and less tightly managed care products than the traditional HMO product. In 1990, HMOs accounted for 33 percent of the privately insured market (Sullivan and Rice 1991). Two other managed care forms, preferred provider organizations (PPOs) and point-of-service plans (POSs), accounted for 13 percent and 5 percent respectively of the market. The remaining 62 percent were covered by indemnity plans, albeit most of the time in plans using various forms of utilization review. By 1995, just over a quarter (27 percent) of workers were in conventional indemnity plans (Jensen et al. 1997). Twenty-eight percent were in HMOs, 25 percent in PPOs, and 20 percent in POS plans. Particularly in the latter 1990s, managed care entities that had salaried physicians increasingly divested themselves of these entities so they could more flexibly compete against plans less burdened with a fixed capacity of providers. HMOs based on the traditional prepaid group practice concept added other models to attract marketshare and expand their reach (Gold et al. 1996).

Few physicians or providers today can ignore managed care. In 1995, 84 percent of all physicians nationally had a managed care contract (Simon and Emmons 1997). The average physician with a managed care contract earned more than a third of his or her revenue (36.1 percent) from such a contract. About a third of physicians had a managed care contract involving capitation, though on average these physicians received only 19 percent of their income from such contracts.

While it is beyond the scope of this paper to explore fully all these changes and pressures, it is clear that the historically strong differentiation between HMO and fee-for-service systems in the United States is eroding in terms of a continuum of plans defined by the extent and kinds of managed care features (Gold and Hurley 1997; Feldman, Krawlewski, and Dowd 1989).

How managed care will be shaped in the years ahead is uncertain: Some view the future as a continuing set of diverse choices, and others as the gradual transition to more tightly managed systems. Still others argue that in becoming the dominant system, managed care has lost its distinctiveness. How government will influence these trends is also unclear, with managed care becoming much more central to the current policy debate, and a plethora of legislation being considered in the states and Congress. Though the resistance to managed care has some parallels to that in the early pioneer stage of HMO history, a key distinction is that today managed care is the dominant, not an alternative and reasonably distinct, delivery system. Health care also has become increasingly complex and expensive since the 1930s.

The key questions, as managed care moves from an alternative to a dominant healthcare system, are if and how the concept of HMOs as a form remains relevant. Already, today's HMOs depart considerably from the community-based and independent prepaid group practice model from which they emerged. As the managed care scope has expanded, insurance and delivery arguably have become more intertwined. But they are now arguably also moving in the opposite direction, as "intermediate entities," often provider-sponsored networks (either corporate or independent), form and contract on a network basis with managed care plans who delegate some managed care functions. Thus, key questions of the future are how the entities we have called HMOs continue to evolve, and indeed what meaning the concept has in relation to its historical roots.

Notes

1. An increasing number of HMOs also offer an "open-ended product" allowing enrollees to self-refer to "out-of-network" providers. These enrollees face considerable cost sharing in the form of deductibles and coinsurance for out-of-network services.
2. Networks are the fourth model typically defined. Networks are a hybrid between a group and an IPA model. Under the network model, the HMO typically contracts with multiple physician groups. These physicians also tend to retain considerable fee-for-service income or income other than from the HMO. In recent years as the HMO industry has evolved, a large share of HMOs represent mixed models, incorporating a provider network with components of numerous models.
3. While the mandate requirement was not often invoked, its existence led most large- and medium-sized employers to offer one or more HMO options along with their traditional indemnity plan.

Works Cited

Abel-Smith, Brian. 1988. "The Rise and Decline of Early HMOs: Some International Experience," *The Milbank Quarterly* 66: 694–711.

Brown, Larry. 1983. *Politics and Health Care Organization: HMOs as Federal Policy.* Washington, DC: The Brookings Institution.

Christianson, Jon B., and Walter McClure. 1979. "Competition in the Delivery of Medical Care," *New England Journal of Medicine* 301 (11 October): 797–848.

Christianson, Jon B., et al. 1991. "The HMO Industry: Evaluation in Population Demographics and Market Structure," *Medical Care Review* 48 (Spring): 3–45.

Dorsey, Joseph L. 1975. "The Health Maintenance Organization Act of 1973 (P.L. 93-222) and Prepaid Group Practice," *Medical Care* 13 (January): 1–9.

Ermann, Dan. 1986. "Health Maintenance Organizations: The Future of the For-Profit Plan," *Journal of Ambulatory Care Management* 9 (May): 72–84.

Feldman, Roger, John Krawlewski, and Bryan Dowd. 1989. "Health Maintenance Organizations: The Beginning or the End," *Health Services Research* 24 (June): 191–211.

Freund, Deborah, and Edward Neuschler. 1986. "Overview of Medicaid Capitation and Case Management Initiatives," *Health Care Financing Review* (Annual Supplement, December): 21–30.

Gabel, John, et al. 1989. "Employer-Sponsored Health Insurance in America," *Health Affairs* 9 (Summer): 117–28.

———. 1990. "Employer-Sponsored Health Insurance in America 1989," *Health Affairs* 9 (Fall): 161–75.

Gold, Marsha. 1991. "HMOs and Managed Care," *Health Affairs* 10, no. 4 (Winter): 189–206.

Gold, Marsha, and Dennis Hodges. 1989. "Health Maintenance Organizations: Structure, Performance, and Current Issue for Employee Health Benefits Design," *Journal of Occupational Medicine* 33 (March): 286–88.

———. 1991. "HMOs and Managed Care," *Health Affairs* 10, no. 4 (Winter): 189–206.

Gold, Marsha, and Dennis Hodges. 1989. "Health Maintenance Organizations in 1988," *Health Affairs* 8 (Winter): 125–38.

Group Health Association of America. 1989. *HMO Industry Profile, Vol. 1*, Washington, DC.

———. 1990. *HMO Industry Profile, Vol. 2*, Washington, DC.

———. 1991. *HMO Industry Profile, Vol. 3*, Washington, DC.

———. 1991. *Patterns of HMO Enrollment* (June) Washington, DC: GHAA.

———. 1992. *Patterns of HMO Enrollment* (June) Washington, DC: GHAA.

Gruber, Lynn, Maureen Shadle, and Cynthia L. Polich. 1988. "From Movement to Industry: The Growth of HMOs," *Health Affairs* 7 (Summer): 197–208.

Higgins, A. Foster. 1991. *Health Care Benefits Survey, Vol. 1*. New Jersey: Health Care Benefits Survey.

Iglehart, John K. 1984. "HMOs (For Profit and Not-for Profit) on the Move," *New England Journal of Medicine* 18 (3 May): 1203–1208.

Jensen, Gail A., Michael Morrisey, Shannon Gaffney, and Derek K. Liston. 1997. "The New Dominance of Managed Care: Insurance Trends in the 1990s," *Health Affairs*, vol. 16, no. 1 (January/February): 125–36.

Jones, Stanley. 1990. "Multiple Choice Health Insurance: The Lessons and Challenge to Private Insurers," *Inquiry* 27 (Summer): 161–66.

Kraus, Nancy, Michelle Porter, and Patricia Ball. 1991. *Managed Care: A Decade in Review 1980–1990*. Excelsior, MN: Inter Study.

Langwell, Kathryn M., and James P. Hadley. 1989. "Evaluation of the Medicare Competition Demonstration." *Health Care Financing Review* 11 (Winter): 65–80.

Luft, Harold S. 1987. *Health Maintenance Organizations: Dimensions of Performance.* New Brunswick, NJ: Transaction Books.

Marmor, Ted. 1973. *The Politics of Medicare.* Chicago: Aldine Press.

Mayer, T. R. and G. G. Mayer. 1985. "HMOs: Origins and Development," *New England Journal of Medicine* 312: 590–94.

Miller, Robert and Harold Luft. 1997. "Managed Care Performance: Is Quality of Care Better or Worse?" *Health Affairs*, vol. 16, no. 5 (September/October): 7–25.

Miller, Robert and Harold Luft. 1996. "Managed Care Performance Since 1980: A Literature Analysis," *Journal of the American Medical Association*. 1996: 271, 1512–9.

National Industry Council for Health Care Delivery. 1984.

Nelson, A. 1987. "The History and Spirit of the HMO Movement: The Early Years," *HMO Practice* 1: 75–85.

Simon, Carol J. and David W. Emmons. 1997. "Physician Earnings at Risk: An Examination of Capitated Contracts," *Health Affairs*, vol. 16, no. 3 (May/June): 120–26.

Starr, Paul. 1982. *The Social Transformation of American Medicine*. New York: Basic Books.

Sullivan, Cynthia and Thomas Rice. 1991. "The Health Insurance Picture in 1990," *Health Affairs*, vol. 10, no.2: 104–15.

CHAPTER

2

TRENDS TOWARD A NATIONAL HEALTH CARE MARKETPLACE

Janet M. Corrigan, Jill S. Eden,
Marsha R. Gold, and Jeremy D. Pickreign

PRIOR TO the 1970s, acute health care services were provided almost exclusively through locally owned organizations (e.g., hospitals, physician practices, health maintenance organizations), operating within loosely structured community health systems.[1] Most major decisions involving the organization and delivery of services were made at the community and/or state level, through formal and informal mechanisms (e.g., state certificate-of-need processes, representation of leading employers on multiple hospital boards of directors). It is this "localized character" of the health care delivery system that, until quite recently, distinguished the health care industry from most other major industries, which embraced concepts of industrial organization during the first half of the 20th century (Starr 1982).

During the last two decades, the health care industry has experienced growth in organizations that are national in focus—organizations that operate in multiple markets not all clustered in one geographic region. Starting in the mid-1970s, the hospital industry began to experience consolidation through the formation of multihospital organizations at both the national and regional levels, and there continue to be notable examples of growth in national hospital companies (Gray 1991). Between 1988 and 1995, Columbia/HCA grew, through acquisition of several multihospital organizations, to a 330-hospital system operating in 37 states and two European countries (Heineccius 1995). There are also signs of consolidation in the physician group sector. PhyCor, founded in 1988, currently operates 27 multispecialty group clinics with approximately 1,400 physicians in 18 states.[2]

But the most striking growth in national organizations has occurred during the 1990s in the insurance and managed care industries. Although the insurance market traditionally has been characterized by both national insurance companies operating alongside state/regionally based Blue Cross and Blue Shield plans and smaller "niche" players, recent mergers and acquisitions have produced organizations of significant size focusing primarily on the delivery of managed care—products that integrate various aspects of financing and delivery. For example, the recent acquisition of U.S. Healthcare by Aetna Life and Casualty Company creates the nation's largest managed health care company serving 23 million people (Tomsho 1996), and the acquisition of MetraHealth by United HealthCare in mid-1995 brought its total membership to more than 14 million (Cerne 1995).

Although it is often said that "health care, like politics, is local," it is likely the emergence of national managed care companies and national provider organizations will have some impact on how care is delivered in local communities. To the extent that national companies benefit from greater access to capital markets and economies of scale, there is the potential for these companies to improve quality and efficiency through investment in technology (e.g., clinical information systems), the development of specialized systems of care (e.g., disease-state management programs), enhanced management systems (e.g., financial accounting systems, marketing), and access to specialized clinical and managerial expertise.

But concerns have been voiced that national companies, almost all of which are for profit, may seek returns on investment at the expense of access and quality. There are worries that these firms may be less responsive to community needs, such as care of the uninsured and provision of public health services, the benefits of which accrue to society at large. There is also the concern that over time, national companies may engage in predatory pricing to drive out competition, leaving consumers with few choices. The purpose of this paper is threefold:

- To summarize information available from existing data sources on trends in ownership of health care organizations (e.g., health maintenance organizations [HMOs], preferred provider organizations [PPOs], hospitals, physician practices) by national corporations for purposes of assessing the rate of growth and overall significance of this trend.

- To identify factors that encourage or impede the growth of national managed care companies, the sector which has exhibited the most pronounced growth in national companies in recent years, and to discuss how these forces are changing over time.
- To discuss likely future directions and outstanding research issues.

Although this paper's primary focus is the growth in the number and size of national companies, this trend is intertwined with growth in the for-profit health care sector. Virtually all health care organizations that have grown to be national in scope in recent years are for-profit organizations. For the most part, access to equity capital is a prerequisite to the pursuit of a national growth strategy. But it is important to note that there are for-profit organizations that for one reason or another have chosen not to pursue a national growth strategy.

Our focus on national organizations, rather than for-profit firms, is consistent with a desire to better understand whether there are certain long-term, competitive advantages enjoyed by these companies. The existence of such competitive advantages would lead one to conclude that over time, the health care industry will be dominated by a limited number of very large health insuring and/or health care delivery organizations, each having a presence in many or most geographic areas in the United States. Alternatively, the absence of such long-term competitive advantages would imply more diversity in the size and mix of health care organizations both across and within local health care markets.

Trends in the Ownership of Health Care Organizations

In this section, we analyze secondary data on trends and developments in four health care sectors—HMOs, PPOs, hospitals, and medical practices—which as a group represent the majority of organizations/providers involved in the provision of managed care products. By examining and analyzing these four sectors, we are able to gauge the breadth and depth of the trend toward national ownership within the health care industry, and to identify similarities and differences in trends across sectors.

HMO Companies

Accompanying the steady increase in recent years in enrollment in HMO products has been rapid growth in "national" HMO companies, defined here as firms that own HMO plans in two or more nonbordering census divisions with combined enrollment of at least 100,000 HMO members. In 1990, the HMO industry was dominated by non-national plans—345 or 63% of the 544 health plans in the United States were local or regional plans (see Table 1). Similarly, almost 58% of the nation's approximate 35 million HMO members were in non-national plans. But by 1994, while the number of HMO plans had climbed to 571, the proportion of HMOs that were local or regional plans had decreased seven percentage points to 56% and the majority of the nation's nearly 51 million HMO enrollees were now in national firms.

For the United States as a whole, the percentage of the population enrolled in HMOs increased from 14% to nearly 20% between 1990 and

Table 1 HMO Industry: Growth of National and Non-National Companies, 1990–1994

	1990		1994		Percentage Change 1990–1994
	Number	%	Number	%	
HMO companies					
Total U.S.	300	100.0	292	100.0	−2.7
National HMO companies[a]	16	5.3	19	6.8	18.8
Non-national HMO companies	284	94.7	273	93.5	−3.9
Number of licensed HMO plans[b,c]					
Total U.S.	544	—	571	—	5.0
National HMO plans	199	100.0	251	100.0	26.1
Not for profit (Kaiser only)	12	6.0	12	4.8	—
For profit	187	94.0	239	95.2	27.8
Non-national HMO plans	345	100.0	320	100.0	−7.2
Not for profit	161	46.7	153	47.8	−5.0
For profit	184	53.3	167	52.2	−9.2
HMO enrollees (in 1,000s)					
Total U.S.	34,966	—	50,982	—	45.8
National HMO plans	14,807	100.0	27,424	100.0	85.2
Not for profit (Kaiser only)	6,526	44.1	6,599	24.1	1.1
For profit	8,281	55.9	20,825	75.9	151.5
Non-national HMO plans	20,159	100.0	23,558	100.0	16.9
Not for profit	11,690	58.0	14,990	63.6	28.2
For profit	8,469	42.0	8,568	36.4	1.2

Source: Group Health Association of America's 1991 and 1995 National Directories of HMOs (databases on diskette).
Notes: National HMO companies are defined here as firms that own HMO plans in two or more nonbordering census divisions with combined enrollment of at least 100,000 members.
[a]See Table 2 for an enumeration of national HMO companies.
[b]Twenty-five HMO plans in 1990 were excluded due to missing ownership data; 20 were excluded in 1994.
[c]Three HMO plans in 1990 were newly organized with no enrollment; 24 in 1994.

Figure 1 Percentage of Population Enrolled in all HMOs and National HMOs, 1990 and 1994

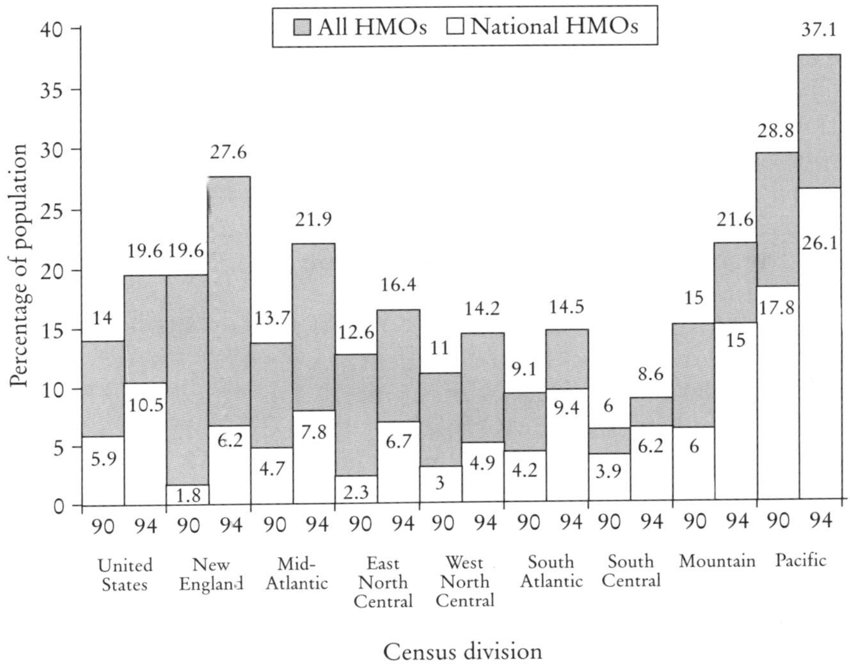

Source: Group Health Association of America's 1991 and 1995 National Directories of HMOs; databases on diskette.

1994, while the percentage of the population in national HMO firms increased from 6% to about 10% (see Figure 1). HMOs, in general, and national HMO firms, in particular, were most successful in capturing a sizable proportion of the health insurance market in the Pacific states.[3] In 1994, about 37% of the population of the Pacific region was enrolled in HMOs, and about seven out of 10 of these individuals were in HMOs owned by national companies. This in part reflects the fact that many of the companies that are national in scope started out as California-based HMOs, including Kaiser Permanente, FHP International, PacifiCare and Foundation Health Plan.

In 1994, national HMO companies captured their largest shares (65% or more) of regional HMO enrollment in the South Central, Pacific, Mountain, and South Atlantic regions. In contrast, national companies account for less than 40% of the HMO market in the other regions. Although national companies have been most successful in capturing

HMO market share in the South Central region where overall HMO market share was lowest—only 8.6% of the population was enrolled in an HMO in 1994—there is no consistent relationship between HMO market share and penetration by national companies when looking across the eight geographic regions.

National HMO plans are much more likely to be for-profit organizations than are non-national plans (see Table 1). In 1994, 95% of plans owned by national companies were for profit—only those plans owned by Kaiser Permanente were not. By comparison, only 52% of plans owned by non-national organizations were for profit. Interestingly, there was little change in the distribution of health plans of each of these types by profit status between 1990 and 1994.

Table 2 lists the national HMO companies and details their striking expansion from 1990 to 1994. Enrollment growth was greatest in United Healthcare during this time, with its membership increasing by more than 500% and its total HMO market share expanding from 1.2% to almost 5%. In fact, nearly all for-profit, national HMOs dramatically expanded their enrollment and captured a greater share of the HMO market. CIGNA, Prudential, Humana, and PacifiCare Health Systems all doubled their HMO enrollment. Physician Corporation of America expanded from 109,000 members to more than one-half million. Five of 1994's national HMOs—FHP International, Health Systems International, Foundation Health Corporation, Healthsource, and HealthWise of America—were either too small to qualify as a "national" HMO or didn't exist in 1990.

Although it is not possible from existing secondary data sources to identify the proportion of growth in national HMO enrollment resulting from the acquisition of non-national HMO firms by national firms (i.e., purchase of existing HMO covered lives) versus that resulting from expansion in the HMO share of the insurance market (i.e., the conversion of indemnity and PPO insureds to HMO product lines), the latter was probably more significant. Between 1990 and 1994, the number of U.S. residents enrolled in HMOs increased by about 16 million people, while the number of enrollees in national HMO firms increased by about 12.6 million, or 85% (see Table 1). During the same time period, non-national firms experienced a net increase in enrollment of only about 3.4 million covered lives, or 17%.

But it is important to note that there is much variation across national firms in terms of growth strategy. National companies that represent traditional insurers, such as CIGNA, Prudential, Aetna Health Plan, and Sanus/New York Life (see list of national firms in Table 2), in all likelihood derived a sizable share of their new HMO enrollment

Table 2 Enrollment and Growth of National HMO Companies, 1990 to 1994

	National HMO Company		Number of HMO Plans		Number of Enrollees (in 1000s)		Growth in Enrollment (%)	HMO Market Share[a] (%)	
HMO Company	1990	1994	1990	1994	1990	1994	1990–1994	1990	1994
All national HMOs	NA	NA	199	251	14,807	27,424	85.2	42.5	53.8
Kaiser Foundation Health Plan	Yes	Yes	12	12	6,526	6,599	1.1	18.7	12.9
CIGNA	Yes	Yes	42	35	1,573	3,309	110.4	4.5	6.5
United Healthcare	Yes	Yes	8	17	405	2,462	507.9	1.2	4.8
Prudential	Yes	Yes	27	35	874	1,898	117.2	2.5	3.7
U.S. Healthcare	Yes	Yes	8	11	1,105	1,768	60.0	3.2	3.5
FHP International[b]	No[b]	Yes	6	11	865	1,719	98.7	2.5	3.4
Humana	Yes	Yes	13	19	759	1,590	109.5	2.2	3.1
PacifiCare Health Systems	Yes	Yes	5	6	686	1,417	106.6	2.0	2.8
Health Systems International	No[b]	Yes	0	7	0	1,335	NA	—	2.6
Aetna Health Plans	Yes	Yes	18	16	702	1,104	55.5	2.0	2.2
Foundation Health[b]	No[b]	Yes	1	8	295	984	233.6	.8	1.9
Sanus/New York Life	Yes	Yes	4	5	533	710	33.2	1.5	1.4
Physician Corporation of America	Yes	Yes	3	4	109	522	378.9	.3	1.0
Coventry	Yes	Yes	3	4	266	447	68.0	.8	.9
Healthsource[b]	No[b]	Yes	2	11	49	440	798.0	.1	.9
MetraHealth Companies[c]	—[c]	Yes	—	22	—	371	NA	—	.7
Principal Health Care	Yes	Yes	8	17	192	333	73.4	.5	.7
Maxicare Health Plans	Yes	Yes	8	7	302	296	−2.0	.9	.6
HealthWise of America[b]	No[b]	Yes	1	4	37	120	224.3	.1	.2
Lincoln National[d]	Yes	—[d]	13	—	435	—	NA	1.2	—
Metlife[c]	Yes	—[c]	15	—	236	—	NA	.7	—
Travelers[c]	Yes	—[c]	10	—	103	—	NA	.3	—

Source: Group Health Association of America's 1991 and 1995 National Directories of HMOs (databases on diskette).

Notes: National HMOs own HMO plans in two or more nonbordering census divisions with total enrollment of at least 100,000 members. NA = not applicable.

[a]Calculated as a percentage of total HMO enrollees in the United States, which in 1990 and 1994 amounted to almost 35 million and 51 million, repectively.

[b]Although these companies existed in 1990, they did not yet meet the definition of a national HMO company.

[c]MetraHealth was created by the merger of Metlife and Travelers in 1994.

[d]Lincoln National sold its HMO plans between 1990 and 1994. Most were acquired by TakeCare, Corp., which was later acquired by FHP International.

from the successful migration of their non-HMO insureds into HMO product lines. Other health plans, for example U.S. Healthcare, expanded by bringing their HMO products to new markets and using effective marketing and provider relations strategies to attract insureds away from other companies.[4] Still others grew through the acquisition of existing HMO lives or a combination of approaches.[5]

The rapid growth of a limited number of national organizations may have implications for the competitive market within the HMO industry. In 1990, the 10 largest, for-profit national companies accounted for 21% of HMO membership (see Figure 2). But by 1994, the market share of the 10 largest for-profit companies had climbed to 34%, and eight of these companies were also in the top 10 listing for 1990. Accompanying this trend has been the gradual decline in market share of Kaiser Permanente, one of the nation's oldest and largest HMOs.

Survey data are not yet available to determine whether these trends have continued into 1995 and 1996. Anecdotal information does provide evidence of continued consolidation within the HMO industry. For example, a recent report by InterStudy lists 21 HMO acquisitions and mergers that took place in 1995 (InterStudy 1996b). Twelve of these

Figure 2 HMO Market Shares of the 10 Largest For-Profit Companies and Kaiser Permanente, 1990 and 1994

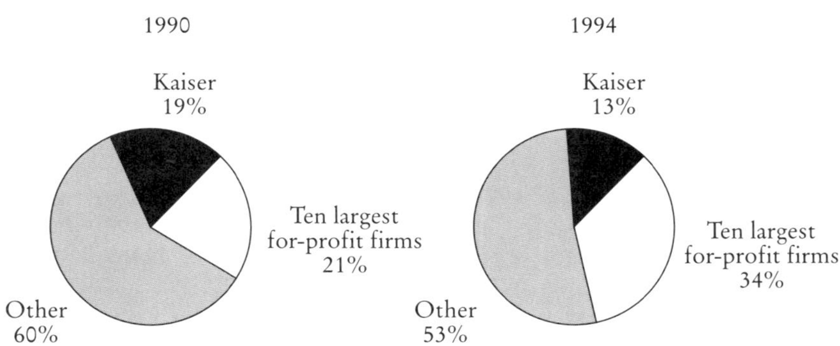

Source: In 1990, the 10 largest for-profit national firms were CIGNA, United HealthCare, Prudential, U.S. Healthcare, FHP International, Humana, PacifiCare Health Systems, Aetna Health Plans, SANUS/New York Life, and Lincoln National. They accounted for 7.4 million of the nearly 35 million HMO enrollees nationwide. In 1994, the 10 largest for-profit national firms were: CIGNA, United HealthCare, Prudential, U.S. Healthcare, FHP International, Humana, PacifiCare Health Systems, Health Systems International, Aetna Health Plans, and Foundation Health. They enrolled nearly 17.6 million of the nation's approximate 51 million HMO members.

acquisitions and mergers involved one or more of the national organizations listed in Table 2.

Preferred Provider Organizations

More Americans belong to PPOs than any other type of managed care entity. The American Association of Preferred Provider Organizations reports that at year end 1994, there were 802 PPOs covering more than 79 million people (see Table 3).[6] While PPOs were not widely available in each state in 1994, PPO networks served at least some region of every state (AAPPO 1996).

As Table 3 indicates, about three-fourths of all eligible enrollees in PPOs were in networks owned by insurance companies or independent investors. Included in these two ownership categories are at least 20 national companies, that is, firms that own PPO networks in two or more nonbordering census divisions.[7] Ten of the 20 national PPO companies also offered HMO products, and as a group their market share totaled 26% of HMO members in 1994.[8]

In view of the overlap in national HMO and PPO companies, it is not surprising that national PPO and national HMO companies appear to be most prevalent in the same geographic regions. For example, South Atlantic and South Central states rank first and second among all U.S. census divisions in both the number of nationally owned PPO plans as

Table 3 Number and Percentage of PPOs and PPO Enrollees by Type of Owner, 1994

	Operational PPOs		Eligible Enrollees[a]	
Type of Owner	Number	%	Number (in 1,000s)	%
Insurance company	371	46.3	18,489	23.4
Independent investor	164	20.4	43,677	55.3
Physician/hospital joint venture	43	5.4	NA	NA
Hospital alliance	39	4.9	2,573	3.3
Other	150	18.7	10,155	12.8
Multiownership	35	4.4	4,148	5.2
Total, all types	802	100	79,042	100

Source: American Association of Preferred Provider Organizations. 1996, 1995 PPO Industry Profile.
Note: NA = not available.
[a]The number of eligible enrollees was estimated applying the multiple 2.3 to the number of eligible employees.

well as nationally owned HMO plans (GHAA 1995b; AMCRA 1995). New England and Mid-Atlantic states are likewise the least penetrated regions for both national PPO and HMO plans.

Hospitals

From 1990 to 1994, there was little change in either the shares of general, acute care hospitals, or hospital beds owned by national firms, or the proportions of inpatient days or admissions accounted for by national firms.[9] Overall, about 14% of all U.S. general, acute care hospitals and 16% of all general, acute care hospital beds were owned by national firms in both 1990 and 1994, and these firms accounted for about 15% of admissions and 14% of inpatient days in both years (see Table 4).

As with managed care plans, penetration by national hospital companies varies considerably by region (see Table 5). In 1994, national companies' shares of total hospital beds and inpatient days exceeded 20% in the Mountain, South Central, and South Atlantic regions, but were

Table 4 Trends in National Companies' Shares of Acute Care Hospitals, Beds, Admissions and Inpatient Days

Assets or Services	1990	1994	Change
Hospitals			
Total	5,170	4,956	−214
National	697	690	−7
Percentage national	13.5	13.9	.4
Beds			
Total	845,122	794,892	−50,230
National	131,303	126,483	−4,820
Percentage national	15.5	15.9	.4
Admissions (in 1,000s)			
Total	30,244	29,505	−739
National	4,555	4,392	−163
Percentage national	15.1	14.9	−.2
Inpatient days (in 1,000s)			
Total	200,758	175,332	−25,426
National	28,441	24,769	−3,672
Percentage national	14.2	14.1	−.1

Source: American Hospital Association's 1990 and 1994 Annual Surveys of Hospitals (on diskette).
Note: Hospitals are defined as "national" if they are *owned* by a multihospital system that owns registered general, acute care hospitals in two or more nonbordering census divisions with at least 1,000 beds. Hospitals that are contract-managed by large multihospital systems are not considered "national."

Table 5 Trends in National and Other General, Acute Care Hospitals, 1990–1994

	Number of Hospital Beds			Number of Inpatient Days (in 1,000s)		
Census Division	1990	1994	Change from 1990	1990	1994	Change from 1990
United States						
Total	845,122	794,892	−50,230	200,758	175,332	−25,426
National	131,303	126,483	4,820	28,441	24,769	−3,672
Percentage national	15.5	15.9	.4	14.2	14.1	−.1
New England						
Total	41,867	36,711	−5,156	11,269	9,151	−2,118
National	1,084	870	−214	305	259	−46
Percentage national	2.6	2.4	−.2	2.7	2.8	.1
Mid-Atlantic						
Total	143,027	138,178	−4,849	41,521	37,589	−3,932
National	7,786	7,465	−321	2,182	1,931	−251
Percentage national	5.4	5.4	0.0	5.3	5.1	−.2
East North Central						
Total	147,415	133,601	−13,814	34,053	28,370	−5,683
National	12,013	11,941	−72	2,897	2,491	−406
Percentage national	8.1	8.9	.8	8.5	8.8	.3
West North Central						
Total	75,353	68,536	−6,817	15,546	12,799	−2,747
National	7,990	9,164	1,174	1,668	1,784	116
Percentage national	10.6	13.4	2.8	10.7	13.9	3.2
South Atlantic						
Total	147,152	142,433	−4,719	35,526	31,660	−3,866
National	30,614	32,833	2,219	6,620	6,412	−208
Percentage national	20.8	23.1	2.3	18.6	20.3	1.7
South Central						
Total	158,874	151,484	−7,390	33,860	30,456	−3,404
National	37,819	39,259	1,440	7,573	7,200	−373
Percentage national	23.8	25.9	2.1	22.4	23.6	1.2
Mountain						
Total	36,084	34,741	−1,343	7,420	6,653	−767
National	11,100	10,080	−1,020	2,275	1,927	−348
Percentage national	30.8	29.0	−1.8	30.7	29.0	−1.7
Pacific[a]						
Total	95,350	89,208	−6,142	21,563	18,654	−2,909
National	22,897	14,871	−8,026	4,920	2,765	−2,155
Percentage national	24.0	16.7	−7.3	22.8	14.8	−8.0

Source: American Hospital Association's 1990 and 1994 Annual Surveys of Hospitals (on diskette).
Note: Hospitals are defined as "national" if they are *owned* by a multihospital system that owns registered general, acute care hospitals in two or more nonbordering census divisions with at least 1,000 beds. Hospitals that are contract-managed by large multihospital systems are not considered "national."
[a]Kaiser Foundation Hospitals are national in 1990 and local in 1994. When Kaiser is removed from the analysis, trends in the Pacific mirror the rest of the nation.

less than 9% in the Mid-Atlantic, East North Central and New England census divisions. In the Pacific states, the proportions of general, acute care hospital beds and inpatient days accounted for by national companies dropped by seven and eight percentage points, respectively. But this drop is the result of Kaiser Permanente having divested itself of a hospital in Cleveland, and as a result, no longer meeting our definition of a national hospital company.

Although the tax status of general, acute care hospitals remained stable from 1990 to 1994 (in both years, around 13% were for-profit facilities), hospitals affiliated with a national system were much more likely to be for profit and the proportion of nationally owned hospitals that are for profit has been increasing over time (see Table 6). In 1990, 63% of nationally owned hospitals were for profit as compared with almost 6% of other hospitals. By 1994, the number of nationally owned hospitals that were for profit rose slightly to 66%, while the proportion of non-national hospitals that were for profit declined slightly.

Trend data for 1990 to 1994 document widespread consolidation of multihospital systems—consolidation both within the pool of nationally owned systems and within the pool of local or regionally owned systems (Table 7). In 1990, there were 279 multihospital systems in the United States; 32 were owned by national firms. By 1994, there were 248 multihospital systems, only 26 nationally owned.

Substantial consolidation is especially apparent among the largest, national multihospital systems (Table 8). In 1990, eight national hospital corporations each owned 25 or more general, acute care hospitals—accounting for 394 hospitals overall. By 1994, only four such national

Table 6 Tax Status of General, Acute Care Hospitals, 1990-1994

	1990		1994	
	Number	%	Number	%
Total U.S. hospitals	5,170	100.0	4,956	100.0
Not for profit	4,476	86.6	4,309	86.9
For profit	694	13.4	647	13.1
National	697	100.0	690	100.0
Not for profit	258	37.0	234	33.9
For profit	439	63.0	456	66.1
Non-national	4,473	100.0	4,266	100.0
Not for profit	4,218	94.3	4,075	95.5
For profit	255	5.7	191	4.5

Source: American Hospital Association's 1990 and 1994 Annual Surveys of Hospitals (on diskette).

Table 7 Consolidation of Multihospital Systems, 1990-1994

	1990		1994		Percentage Change 1990–1994	
	Number of Systems	Number of Hospitals	Number of Systems	Number of Hospitals	Number of Systems	Number of Hospitals
Multihospital systems	279	1,567	248	1,558	−11.1	−.6
National[a]	32	697	26	690	−18.8	−1.0
Non-national	247	870	222	868	−10.1	−.2

Source: American Hospital Association's 1990 and 1994 Annual Survey of Hospitals (on diskette).
[a]Multihospital systems are defined as "national" if they include general, acute care hospitals in two or more nonbordering census divisions with at least 1,000 beds. Contract-managed hospitals are not included.

firms were on this scale, owning 422 hospitals. The largest, Columbia/HCA, was formed when Columbia Hospital Corporation merged with or acquired the hospitals of four large national firms (Hospital Corporation of America, Healthtrust, Humana, and the Epic Healthcare Group), as well as many other smaller systems and hospitals.

In summary, the period of 1990 to 1994 appears to have been characterized by steady contraction of the total hospital market and organizational consolidation, both among national and non-national firms. The proportions of hospitals, beds, hospital days, and admissions accounted for by national companies remained roughly the same. It is too early to ascertain whether these trends continued into 1995 and 1996, but anecdotal information points toward continued consolidation, at least among locally and regionally owned hospitals. For example, Modern Healthcare reports that in 1995, 735 hospitals were involved in mergers and acquisitions, and that most of the contracts were between individual hospitals rather than national chains (Lutz 1995).

Physician Practices

The number and proportion of physicians practicing in medical groups and the number of medical groups themselves have been steadily increasing for many years (AMA 1996a, 1996b).[10] In 1994, about 32% of physicians were practicing in 19,478 medical groups—up from 28% practicing in 15,485 groups 10 years earlier.[11] Although most medical groups are small—95% had 25 or fewer doctors in 1994—nearly 47% of all group physicians actually practice in large groups of 26 doctors and more.

Despite considerable press attention to the "corporatization of medical care" and the era of the "free agent" doctor, American Medical

Table 8 Leading National General, Acute Care Hospital Companies, 1990 and 1994

National Hospital Company[a]	National Hospital Systems 1990	National Hospital Systems 1994	Number of Hospitals 1990	Number of Hospitals 1994	Number of Hospital Beds 1990	Number of Hospital Beds 1994	Percentage Growth in Beds 1990–1994
Columbia/HCA Healthcare Corporation[b]	No	Yes	—	281	—	48,854	NA
Hospital Corporation of America	Yes	No	73	—	15,641	—	NA
Humana, Inc.	Yes	No	75	—	15,366	—	NA
Healthtrust Inc.—The Hospital Company	Yes	No	81	—	9,644	—	NA
Epic Healthcare Group	Yes	No	33	—	3,066	—	NA
Columbia Hospital Corporation	Yes	No	9	—	1,683	—	NA
Tenet Healthcare Corporation[b]	No	Yes	—	63	—	12,640	NA
American Medical International	Yes	No	40	—	8,149	—	NA
National Medical Enterprises	Yes	No	30	—	5,326	—	NA
Daughters of Charity National Health	Yes	Yes	35	36	11,819	11,029	−6.7
Republic Health Corporation/OrNda Healthcorp[b]	Yes	Yes	14	42	2,821	5,827	106.6
American Healthcare Management	Yes	No	17	—	1,945	—	NA
Summit Health	Yes	No	12	—	1,483	—	NA
Kaiser Foundation Hospitals[c]	Yes	No	27	28	5,717	5,619	−1.7
Sisters of Charity Health Care Systems	Yes	Yes	11	15	3,667	3,457	5.7
Eastern Mercy Health System	Yes	Yes	12	12	3,657	3,380	−7.6
Sisters of Charity of the Incarnate Word Health Care System	Yes	Yes	12	10	3,710	3,463	−6.7
Sisters of the Sorrowful Mother-U.S. Health System, Inc.	Yes	Yes	10	9	2,968	3,091	4.1
Mercy Health System	Yes	Yes	17	16	3,689	3,056	17.2
Total national[d]	NA	NA	697	690	131,303	126,483	−3.7

Source: American Hospital Association's 1990 and 1994 Annual Surveys of Hospitals (on diskette).
Note: National hospital companies are defined as multihospital systems that own general, acute care hospitals in two or more nonbordering census divisions with at least 1,000 beds. The leading firms presented here owned a minimum of 3,000 beds in 1994. NA = not applicable.
[a]Listed in descending order of number of beds in 1994.
[b]This firm was created by the merger or acquisition of the hospital companies in the below indented list.
[c]In 1990, Kaiser Foundation Hospitals owned hospitals in Ohio and in the Pacific Region, thus satisfying our definition of a national firm. But by 1994, it had sold its hospital in Ohio and no longer owned hospitals in nonbordrng census divisions.
[d]Includes the firms listed here plus all other national hospital companies (i.e., those with 1,000 or more beds).

Association (AMA) data show that only 2% of medical groups were "investor owned" in 1994, as compared with 1% in 1990 (Tomsho 1996; AMA 1996b). In both years, the majority of medical groups were professional corporations that were owned solely by physicians. On average, investor-owned groups are a bit larger than other groups—in 1994, 10% of investor-owned groups consisted of more than 25 physicians, as compared with about 4% for all groups consisting of more than 25 physicians (AMA 1996a).

Unfortunately, available survey data do not capture an important development in medical group practice—the rapid growth and proliferation of physician practice management (PPM) companies. While in most instances PPMs do not own physician groups outright, they typically acquire a clinic's operating assets, enter into an exclusive long-term management contract with the group, and manage all aspects of the clinic other than the provision of medical services (PhyCor 1996; Harris and Johnson 1995). No one organization appears to be carefully tracking developments in this industry, but the press and investment community frequently cite PhyCor, MedPartners/Mullikin, Caremark International, Coastal Healthcare Group, and InPhyNet Medical Management as national leaders with ambitions to capitalize on the vast medical group market. PhyCor, for example, had 18 clinics and 674 affiliated physicians in 1993. As of March 1996, it was operating 33 clinics with more than 2,100 physicians in 20 states and 500,000 capitated lives (PhyCor 1996).

Discussion

Clearly, the depth and quality of available information describing the owners of health care organizations varies considerably. The Group Health Association of America (GHAA) and the American Hospital Association (AHA) data sets are relatively rich resources for studying trends in HMO ownership and hospital ownership, respectively. But comprehensive, reliable information on PPOs is far from adequate, and ownership and contract management data for medical practices is not currently available.

The previous analysis of ownership across sectors has revealed two findings. First, in the two sectors where trend data are most reliable, namely the HMO and hospital sectors, national companies exhibited somewhat different growth patterns from 1990 to 1994. In the HMO industry, which experienced steady expansion during this period, national HMO companies grew dramatically in terms of number of HMOs; these firms probably also benefited greatly by attracting a disproportionate share of new HMO enrollees during a period of rapid expansion in the HMO share of the insurance market. In the hospital industry, which experienced a steady decline in numbers of hospitals, beds, inpatient days, and admissions, there was little change in the proportions accounted for by national companies.

Second, for both the HMO and hospital sectors, the prominence of national companies varies greatly by geographic region, with both sectors exhibiting remarkably similar geographic patterns. In both sectors, national companies have been most successful in capturing market share within their sector in the Southern, Pacific and Mountain regions, and least successful in the Mid-Atlantic, Central and Northeast regions.

National Managed Care Companies: Factors That Encourage or Impede Their Growth

As discussed in the prior section, the greatest growth in national health care companies between 1990 and 1994 was in managed care organizations offering HMO and PPO products. In this section, we turn our attention to a discussion of factors that have contributed to the rapid growth of these national managed care companies. We are especially interested in identifying long-term competitive advantages from which national managed care companies might benefit, as well as factors that may threaten or impede their continued growth.

Factors that influence the growth of national managed care companies may be categorized into three groups: access to capital; economies of scale; and legal and regulatory structures. For the most part, the first two—access to capital and economies of scale—provide national companies with a competitive advantage, although we will argue that this advantage will be somewhat less important in the future than it has been in the recent past. Legal and regulatory structures have a mixed impact—federal initiatives are more likely to favor national companies or to at least create a level playing field, while state-level initiatives more often than not favor local organizations.

Access to Capital

In this section, we discuss why access to sizable amounts of capital has been particularly important to managed care organizations in recent years, and the characteristics of national managed care organizations that facilitate access to capital.

The need for capital

Ready access to capital has been important in recent years for two reasons. First, market conditions have been particularly favorable for the expansion of managed care products. Thus many in the managed care industry have viewed this as an opportune time to gain a foothold in as many communities as possible to capture the largest share of the expanding managed care market. Second, the infrastructure required for success in the managed care marketplace has become more technologically sophisticated and information driven, necessitating investment in information systems and specialized services and expertise. For most managed care organizations, internally generated capital has fallen far short of that required to support desired growth rates in market share and the number of geographic markets served. It also has been insufficient to build the necessary infrastructure to compete effectively.

Although managed care products have been available in most metropolitan areas for two or more decades and have achieved considerable market share in a few regions (e.g., California), it was not until the early 1980s that many private purchasers turned to managed care. Steady annual growth in premiums exceeding increases in the gross national product, combined with a recessionary economy, provided strong incentive to explore various managed care options. Between 1988 and 1993, the percentage of full-time employees in medium and large private establishments enrolled in HMOs increased from 19% to 23%, and in PPOs from 7% to 26% (Employee Benefits Research Institute 1995).

The managed care organizations in the strongest position to benefit from this "sea change" in private purchaser demand from managed care products were ones with access to sizable amounts of capital. Capital was needed to rapidly increase capacity in existing markets, as well as to expand into new geographic markets. Companies that pursued rapid expansion into numerous geographic markets probably suffered in the short run from small market shares in many of these communities, thus limiting their ability to negotiate with providers and purchasers, and to realize scale economies (Ginsburg and Grossman 1995). But this strategy has allowed many national companies to gain a foothold in local markets from which to benefit from future expansion in the managed care market. The broad geographic areas served by national managed care companies also has afforded them an advantage in seeking contracts with certain Fortune 500 companies that seek to maximize purchasing power (i.e., negotiating deeper discounts) and minimize transaction costs by contracting with a limited number of managed care organizations to serve employees in various geographic sites (Darling 1991).[12]

In addition to responding to increased demand, managed care organizations also have needed capital to build more sophisticated technological infrastructures. The recent expansion in managed care has taken place within an increasingly competitive marketplace in which employers demand information on the cost and quality of alternative products to negotiate the best value. As the rate of premium increases has abated, it is also likely that pressures on managed care organizations to increase efficiency and target the use of scarce resources have intensified.

Capital investments have been, and likely will continue to be, quite substantial in automated information systems, and performance monitoring and improvement systems. In a 1995 survey of 252 HMOs,

InterStudy found that, on average, HMOs employed 40 full-time equivalent (FTE) personnel in information systems support, for a ratio of one FTE information systems staffer for every 3,297 enrollees (InterStudy 1996b). Group model HMOs averaged about $2.50 in per-member-per-month (PMPM) costs of information systems, while other model types average about $1.50 PMPM. When asked about planned capital investment in information systems for the period of 1996–98, group and mixed model HMOs indicated they plan to spend about $20 million and $15 million, respectively, as compared with about $3.75 million, on average, for staff, independent practice association (IPA), and network models.

It is likely that the capital requirements to build an information infrastructure will decrease over time as more software products become available through secondary markets. Due to the rapid evolution and diversity of managed care organizations and products over the last 10 years, off-the-shelf products of information system vendors have been unable to keep pace with user requirements, so many managed care plans invested in building their own in-house systems tailored to meet specific needs.[13] But in recent years, the size and sophistication of the health information industry has increased dramatically, opening up many opportunities for managed care organizations to pursue leasing, outsourcing, and partnership arrangements (Hester and Harris 1995).

Managed care companies also have invested capital in building performance monitoring and improvement tools and systems (e.g., quality monitoring, provider profiling, practice guidelines, utilization review) to manage risk, and assess quality and resource use (Heinen et al. 1993; Leatherman et al. 1991; Murray et al. 1996). Although capital investments in this area are probably quite variable across managed care plans, a 1994 survey of HMOs and PPOs found that 74% had provider profiling capabilities, 83% conducted clinically focused studies on a regular basis, and 32% had established written practice guidelines (Gold et al. 1995).

As with the case of information systems, many of these products should be more readily available in the future with less upfront capital investment, for two reasons. First, through the efforts of the public sector and private sector oversight organizations, there are now more quality and utilization management tools available in the public domain (see for example, AHCPR 1996). Second, many quality and utilization management tools and software systems now can be leased or purchased through secondary markets (Hester and Harris 1995).

Characteristics that facilitate access to capital

In general, national managed care companies are ones that have benefited from one or more of the following: 1) the option of obtaining capital through equity markets; 2) lower per unit costs of equity capital due to the reduced risk associated with diversification across multiple geographic markets and health insurance products, and the ability to spread the fixed costs of underwriting across larger issues; and 3) the freeing up of insurance reserves to be used as investment capital.

As a result of their predominantly for-profit status, national companies enjoy ready access to equity financing, an additional source of capital not available to not-for-profit organizations.[14] Access to equity capital allows for-profit organizations to raise larger amounts of capital, and at a faster pace, than not-for-profit organizations. Although many believe that the cost of equity capital is cheap relative to debt financing, analyses indicate that over the long term, equity financing may be more expensive than is debt financing (Reinhardt 1986).

There is also reason to believe that national managed care companies face somewhat lower per unit costs of equity and debt financing than local companies. This has been the case in the hospital industry. Analyses of multihospital systems versus independent hospitals have shown that systems are perceived as sounder risks because of their larger revenue, assets, and equity bases, as well as their greater ability to spread the risk of borrowing and to time debt acquisitions to swings in the market (Ermann and Gabel 1986). Since the typical stock or bond issue of a national company is greater than that of a typical local company, it is also likely that national companies benefit from economies of scale associated with the fixed costs of underwriting.

Lastly, the national managed care companies with roots in the indemnity insurance business have experienced a "freeing up" of insurance reserves, thus making capital available to be used for other investment purposes. Since the inception of the Employee Retirement Income Security Act of 1974 (ERISA) and subsequent amendments, the proportion of private employers sponsoring self-insured health coverage products has increased steadily—in 1992, 67% of employers indicated that they were self-insured for their most prevalent traditional indemnity or preferred provider organization medical plan (Employee Benefits Research Institute 1995). National insurance companies, facing a dwindling health insurance business, have used the capital formerly tied up in state required insurance reserve accounts, as well as other sources, to accelerate efforts to develop replacement products (mainly third-party administrative services or PPO products). It is likely that the reduction in required insurance reserves from the increase in self-insured employers has been offset in part by the slow but steady increase in HMO products during the last two decades. By definition, HMO products include both the insurance and care delivery functions, however, about one-third of HMO plans are now contracting with self-insured employers to provide nonrisk

"HMO-like" products (i.e., ones that use the same provider network, quality and utilization management systems as HMO products) (InterStudy 1995).

Do National Companies Have Cost Advantages?

National HMOs tend to be very large organizations representing sizable numbers of enrollees. As discussed earlier, in 1994 there were 19 national companies. Nearly all had enrollments of about 300,000 or more, and about one-half had over one million enrollees.

Although there is little empirical evidence available on economies of scale associated with the provision of managed care products, by unbundling the products and examining specific functions, we can draw some tentative conclusions about areas where scale economies are likely to be most significant.

In general, managed care products consist of insurance, administrative (e.g., marketing, information systems, performance monitoring and improvement), and care delivery (e.g., physician and hospital services) functions. For some product administrative functions, the scale economies probably have been quite significant, while those associated with the insurance and care delivery functions likely have been less substantial.

Insurance functions

There are some economies of scale associated with the provision of insurance, but how far these economies extend beyond growth in insureds within a given state is less clear. It is important to note that national insurance companies have existed side by side with local and regional insurance companies for many decades, thus suggesting that national companies do not experience significant long-term competitive advantages.

Larger companies have a greater capital base over which to spread insurance risk and are generally in a stronger position to satisfy state reserve requirements than smaller companies. Smaller companies do have the option of purchasing reinsurance to protect against very large losses, but at some cost. Many believe that state reserve requirements have impeded efforts of various locally based, provider-sponsored managed care organizations (e.g., provider-sponsored networks) to develop full-risk managed care products and compete directly with larger organizations, both national and local (McIlrath 1996).

Although there are some scale economies associated with the insurance function, state-specific insurance regulations limit the ability of national companies to reap benefits beyond those experienced by large local companies. For example, state reserve requirements typically provide certain unit cost economies as the total number of insureds covered by an insurance or managed care company increases, but only those insureds that reside within the state are recognized in the calculations.

Product administrative functions

National companies benefit from scale economies to some degree in performing most product administrative functions, including: marketing, information systems, performance monitoring and improvement, and provider network development and administration.

In marketing managed care products, national companies see benefits in the design and development of marketing materials and in advertising campaigns. Local companies may enjoy certain intangible advantages, such as name recognition and established relationships with purchasers and consumers, but over time national companies likely will enjoy these as well.

There are probably substantial scale economies associated with information systems. First, because of the extent to which national companies pursue high volume and sole source purchasing of hardware and software, they benefit from price discounts. Second, national companies may be able to provide greater access to specialized expertise and tailored, ongoing employee training programs. Third, through ownership and control of local organizations, national companies may be better able to standardize information systems across operating units and sites in ways that voluntary cooperative efforts do not. The standardization (e.g., unique enrollee and provider identification numbers, common clinical coding and classification systems, standard definitions, and conventions for collecting and coding resource data) produces immediate advantages in terms of reduced average operating costs across sites. It also results in less tangible benefits that may be particularly important over the long term, such as the ability to integrate data across various levels of care (e.g., hospital, physician practices, non-acute care providers) to support shared clinical decision making.

There are also some scale economies in establishing performance improvement and monitoring systems. Many national companies have acquired specialized expertise (e.g., practice protocols, comparative data) to assist their health plans in implementing performance improvement programs. For example, the Prudential Insurance Company's Center for Health Care Research in Atlanta employs research scientists with backgrounds in statistics, epidemiology, survey research, medicine, public health, business and systems, to serve as a source of expert advice and assistance to Prudential plans across the country (Gazmararian and Lewis 1996). United Healthcare's "Benchmarking Program" provides a mechanism for individual health plans to compare their performance on a variety of quality measures with that of other United Healthcare plans (Heinen et al. 1993).

But the scale economies experienced by national companies likely are being offset to some degree by increased availability of normative data through voluntary cooperative efforts that allow all types of health plans, both local and national, to benefit from the learning experiences of others and to share data (see, for example, Nerenz, Zajac, and Rosman 1993). Normative data also are increasingly available through the efforts of oversight organizations, purchaser coalitions, proprietary organizations, and the media (see, for example, Minnesota Health Data Institute 1995; National Committee for Quality Assurance 1995).

Lastly, in the area of provider network development, local plans owned by national companies may benefit from greater access to specialized expertise, such as legal and contracting services. But national companies probably have little advantage if any over local organizations in negotiating with hospitals or physicians, since bargaining power is determined more by market share in a given community than market share nationally.

Care delivery systems

There are two types of scale economies applicable to care delivery functions: ones that apply to consolidation within a geographic market, and those that apply to consolidation either within or across geographic markets. Thus far, most care delivery economies of scale fall in the former category.

Most apply to consolidation within local markets because, for the most part, the delivery of health care services takes place at the local level. Although individuals may travel long distances for highly specialized services, and telemedicine opens the possibility of establishing specialty consultation networks that extend beyond community-level geographic boundaries, these types of services have been the exception rather than the rule.

Because of the localized, labor-intensive nature of health care, economies of scale associated with health care delivery are believed to be quite modest. For example, physician practices have benefited from some economies of scale by sharing facilities and coordinating administrative services (Pope and Burge 1992). Similarly, consolidation of hospital services at the local level yields economies of scale up to about 300 to 325 beds, but results are inconclusive as to the existence of further unit cost economies at still higher scales (Cowing, Holtman, and Powers 1983; Vita et al. 1991; Mobley and Frech 1994). Analyses of independent hospitals versus those belonging to multihospital systems have failed to demonstrate production efficiencies associated with system membership (Dranove, Durkac, and Shanley 1996).

There are a few selected care delivery functions for which the economies of scale are probably quite significant and apply to consolidation of organizations located in different geographic areas. These include bulk purchasing of medical supplies, equipment, and pharmaceuticals, and malpractice insurance coverage. Many local organizations enjoy some of these economies through voluntary participation in purchasing programs, but some national health care organizations pursuing sole source purchasing claim additional discounts up to 12% (Wilson 1987; Heineccius 1995).

Although the economies of scale associated with care delivery likely have been quite modest to date, it is widely recognized that many of the potential benefits of organized delivery systems are tied to "clinical integration"—the coordination of patient care services across the various functions, activities, and operating units of a system (Gillies et al. 1993). To achieve greater levels of clinical integration, it is likely that sizable sums of capital will be invested in the design of specialized systems of care (e.g., disease state management systems) and automated medical records. But to date, capital investments in these areas appear to have been more limited.

Legal and Regulatory Policy

The legal and regulatory policies established by state and federal governments have been, and likely will continue to be, an important determinant in the rate of growth of national companies and the geographic markets they serve. More often than not, state-level laws and regulations have the intended or unintended consequence of erecting certain barriers to national companies, while federal policies have been more favorable.

Variability in states' insurance laws and regulations that apply to health insuring and provider organizations hampers the efforts of national companies to benefit from economies of scale through standardization of operations (e.g., quality and utilization management, information systems and reporting). During the last two years, most states have undertaken processes aimed at tightening oversight of managed care organizations, and there now are numerous examples of state legislation that address detailed clinical and operational issues, such as the minimum hospital length of stay for normal deliveries, the definition of what constitutes emergency care, and the contents of provider contracts (Somerville

1996; State Health Watch 1996; American Health Line 1995). The impact of these state regulatory initiatives is lessened by federal statutes that prohibit states from imposing insurance regulation on self-funded employee benefit plans (HIAA America 1996). Variability across states in regulatory and oversight structures is minimized further by efforts of the National Association of Insurance Commissioners to develop and promote model legislation, and national accrediting organizations to encourage states to rely on private sector oversight programs in carrying out licensing responsibilities.

In addition to state insurance laws and regulations, states also have the potential to shape their local markets by preempting federal antitrust laws. So far, little antitrust action has been taken against insurance companies, managed care plans, or national hospital chains engaged in mergers and acquisitions, although the Federal Trade Commission and Department of Justice have reviewed many of these cases (National Health Policy Forum 1995; GAO 1994). But states have the authority to override federal antitrust laws under certain circumstances (i.e., if a state explicitly chooses to displace competition with regulation and establishes regulatory structures to supervise and control the anticompetitive conduct), and during the last few years, many states have exercised this authority. As of late 1995, 20 states had enacted some form of law excepting health care from antitrust regulation (National Health Policy Forum 1995). It is too early to tell whether the additional regulatory structures established by these states will tend to open or close local markets to entry of national companies.

Discussion of Findings and Future Research Issues

Our analysis suggests that growth in national managed care companies likely will continue for some time. Due to their access to capital, national companies have a distinct advantage in responding to rapid increases in market demand, and have benefited greatly from the sense of urgency on the part of private purchasers to contain costs through managed care. There likely will be another surge in managed care enrollment as Medicare and Medicaid programs provide greater options for beneficiaries. But many anticipate the transition to managed care will be more gradual for Medicare, and that variations in state Medicaid programs and regulations will lessen the competitive advantages that national companies derive from scale economies.

Although we anticipate that the factors discussed will continue to lead to growth of national managed care companies, it is too early to conclude that national organizations have long-term, competitive advantages over local or regional organizations in providing managed care products. Indeed, there are some reasons to believe that in the future, the competitive advantage that national managed care companies have enjoyed may narrow. As more local and regional managed care companies convert to for-profit status, they also have the option of raising equity capital. In addition, the maturation of secondary markets for information systems and performance monitoring offer health plans the choice of leasing systems and tools, thus reducing the upfront capital requirements necessary to build the organizational infrastructure to provide managed care products, and allowing these organizations to reap some of the benefits of economies of scale.

It is too soon to assess the potential diseconomies of scale that national managed care companies may experience. Robinson (1996) discusses three factors that are believed to have contributed to limits on firm size in other industries: incentive attenuation, influence costs, and organizational insularity. Incentive attenuation refers to lessening the linkage between financial incentives to employees and the company's profits and losses. Influence costs arise when managers, employees, and suppliers compete over the use of the firm's resources, rather than cooperate to increase productivity and output. Insularity occurs when a firm loses touch with its consumers' preferences and its competitors' strengths and weakness, and becomes wedded to the status quo to the detriment of innovation.

There is also the potential for state policies and regulatory structures to alter the rules of the competitive marketplace. The rapid pace of change, exacerbated by a recent loss of public support for public sector initiatives, has made it difficult for both federal and state governments to redefine their roles within a competitive marketplace. However, there now are many developments underway at the state level that may shape the future growth of national companies. These include the promulgation of new insurance and regulatory structures applicable to various types of managed care organizations, and enactment of state antitrust exception law. It will be some time before the ultimate impact of these developments is known.

In looking forward, there are some areas that would benefit from further work:

- **Arrangements between local and national organizations.** In conducting the analysis of trends in ownership, it became apparent that there are many different types of arrangements between local and national organizations that fall short of ownership, but represent much more than a service contract. For example, in describing relationships between individual hospitals and other organizations, the American Hospital Association (AHA) uses terms such as ownership, sponsorship, affiliation, shared services corporation, and subsidiary. Arrangements between physician practices and physician practice management companies transfer varying degrees of control to management companies. What is needed is a clearly defined topology of relationships that captures the degree to which governance and key strategic and management decisions are transferred to national organizations; this topology should be made applicable across health care sectors.

- **Impact on communities.** The growth in national health care companies may have implications for communities—both community health care systems and the broader, economic infrastructure of communities. Although national health care companies differ in the degree to which they pursue centralized management, some centralized decision making and consolidation of services at the regional or national levels is necessary to capture economies of scale. It is unclear whether this shift in decision making and functional responsibility will lessen the ability of individual communities to provide support (through cross-subsidization) for uncompensated care, public health, and graduate medical education. Analyses of these issues will be particularly challenging in light of the need to evaluate the effects of several important changes underway in the health system, including the trend toward national ownership, the change in health care organizations' tax status from not for profit to for profit, the growth in managed care, and the increase in competitive markets.

Notes

1. Although there have been a few hospital and HMO chains that extended beyond community and state boundaries (e.g., Kaiser Permanente, Sisters of Mercy Hospitals Corporation), they have been limited in market share and tended to be not-for-profit organizations with decentralized governance and management approaches.
2. PhyCor generally acquires the operating assets (i.e., receivables, inventory and equipment) of existing multispecialty medical clinics and then operates these clinics under long-term service agreements with affiliated physicians' groups that agree to practice exclusively through the company's clinics (Harris and Johnson 1995).
3. The New England region consists of Connecticut, Maine, Massachusetts, New Hampshire, Rhode Island and Vermont. Mid-Atlantic includes New Jersey, New York and Pennsylvania. East North Central includes Illinois, Indiana, Michigan, Ohio and Wisconsin. West North Central includes Iowa, Kansas, Minnesota, Missouri, Nebraska, North Dakota and South Dakota. South Atlantic includes Delaware, District of Columbia, Florida, Georgia, Maryland, North Carolina, South Carolina, Virginia and West Virginia. South Central includes Alabama, Kentucky, Mississippi, Tennessee, Arkansas, Louisiana, Oklahoma and Texas. Mountain

includes Arizona, Colorado, Idaho, Montana, Nevada, New Mexico, Utah and Wyoming. Pacific includes Alaska, California, Hawaii, Oregon and Washington.

4. During this period, U.S. Healthcare obtained HMO licenses and began offering HMO products in numerous Northeastern and Southern states.
5. Two examples are FHP and Coventry. FHP, a regional West Coast health plan in 1990, grew to national stature by 1994 by acquiring plans owned by TakeCare Corporation, which had itself recently acquired plans formerly owned by Lincoln National. Between 1990 and 1994, Coventry Corporation increased its enrollment from 265,500 to 446,842, or by 68%, with three-fourths resulting from growth in enrollment in the three plans it owned in 1990 and one-fourth from the acquisition of a fourth HMO, Southern Health Services (Group Health Association of America 1991ab, 1995ab).
6. Tallying PPOs and PPO networks has been consistently problematic since their beginning. Recent reports reflect effort to avoid double counting of networks and eligible employees (estimated at 2.28 dependents per employee). Due to our concerns about the reliability of earlier survey data, we have chosen not to make historical comparisons.
7. Due to limitations in secondary data sources (i.e., incomplete data, inconsistent definitions of ownership), we were not able to identify with certainty all PPO companies that satisfy our definition of national (i.e., ones that operate PPO networks in at least two nonbordering census divisions). The national firms we have identified include: Aetna Health Plans, Anthem Health Systems, CIGNA, CNA Managed Care, Community Care Network, Ethix, FHP, John Hancock, Health Economics, Healthstar Managed Care, Healthsource, Humana, Medview Services, MetraHealth, Principal Health Care, Private Healthcare Systems, Prudential, Sanus/New York Life, USA Health Network, and U.S. Healthcare.
8. These firms included: Aetna Health Plans, CIGNA, FHP, Healthsource, Humana, MetraHealth, Principal Health Care, Prudential, Sanus/New York Life and U.S. Healthcare. As a group, they enrolled more than 13.2 million of the nation's almost 51 million HMO enrollees.
9. National hospital companies were identified as firms that own general, acute care registered hospitals in two or more nonbordering census divisions with a total of 1,000 beds or more.
10. The American Medical Association (AMA) defines a medical group practice as: "The provision of health care services by three or more physicians who are formally organized as a legal entity in which business and clinical facilities, records, and personnel are shared. Income from medical services provided by the group are treated as receipts of the group and distributed according to some prearranged plan." This definition is reviewed by the AMA periodically, but has changed little since it was developed in 1964 (AMA 1996a, p. 1).
11. Although the AMA's census of medical groups is the most comprehensive available, the response to this survey has dropped markedly in recent years from 88% in 1988 to 60% in 1991 and further to only 40% in 1995. These aggregate data were estimated by the AMA based on survey responses and historical experience (AMA 1993, 1996a).
12. Over time, some of the competitive advantages enjoyed by national managed care companies in serving national employer accounts have eroded as local/regional plans have found ways to collaborate to provide broad geographic coverage and a full

menu of products. For example, the HMO Group, an association of group and staff model HMOs, oversees a network of health plans that serve Xerox (Darling 1991).

13. In the survey of HMOs conducted by InterStudy, it was found that most health plans have developed in-house information system capabilities to support claims processing, reporting data to purchasers and providers, and facility management functions (InterStudy 1996b). For the claims processing, reporting, and facility management functions, the proportions of these plans with completely or mostly internally customized systems were about 40%, 68%, and 52%, respectively.
14. Most national managed care organizations are publicly traded and raise equity from shareholders; some with roots in the indemnity insurance industry are mutual companies that raise equity from policyholders.

References

Agency for Health Care Policy and Research (AHCPR). 1996. AHCPR Releases Conquest 1.0 Database. Research Activities No. 192, U.S. Department of Health and Human Services, Washington, D.C.

American Association of Preferred Provider Organizations (AAPPO). 1996. 1995 PPO Industry Profile.

American Managed Care and Review Association (AMCRA). 1995. GHAA AMCRA 1995–96 Managed Health Care Directory. Washington, D.C.: AMCRA Foundation.

American Health Line. 1995. 50-State Report on Health Care Reform Activities. Alexandria, VA.: American Political Network Publications.

———. 1996. Daily News Briefing 4(236). Alexandria, Va.: American Political Network Publications.

American Hospital Association (AHA). 1991a. 1990 AHA Annual Survey of Hospitals. Database on diskette. Chicago.

———. 1991b. AHA Guide to the Health Care Field, 1991 Edition. Chicago.

———. 1995a. 1994 AHA Annual Survey of Hospitals. Database on diskette. Chicago.

———. 1995b. AHA Guide to the Health Care Field, 1995–96 Edition. Chicago.

American Medical Association (AMA). 1993. Medical Groups in the U.S.: A Survey of Practice Characteristics, 1993 Edition. Chicago.

———. 1996a. Medical Groups in the U.S.: A Survey of Practice Characteristics, 1993 Edition. Chicago.

———. 1996b. Census of Medical Group Practices, unpublished 1991–92 and 1994–95 data. Division of Survey and Data Resources, Department of Data Survey and Planning. Chicago.

Cerne, F. 1995. Can United Healthcare Make a Silk Purse out of a Sow's Ear? *Hospitals and Health Networks*. Sept. 5.

Cowing, T. G., A. G. Holtmann, and S. Powers. 1993. Hospital Cost Analysis: A Survey and Evaluation of Recent Studies. In *Advances in Health Economics and Health Services Research*, vol. 4, R. M. Scheffler and L. Rossiter, eds. Greenwich, Conn.: JAI Press.

Darling, H. 1991. Employers and Managed Care: What Are the Early Returns? *Health Affairs* (Winter) 147–60.

Dranove, D., A. Durkac, and M. Shanley. 1996. Are Multihospital Systems More Efficient? *Health Affairs* 15 (1): 100–104.

Employee Benefits Research Institute. 1995. *Databook on Employee Benefits*. Third Edition. Washington D.C.

Ermann, D., and J. Gabel. 1986. Investor-Owned Multihospital Systems: A Synthesis of Research Findings. In *For-Profit Enterprise in Health Care*, Institute of Medicine, National Academy of Sciences.

Gazmararian, J. A., and N. Lewis. 1996. Health Services Research in the Prudential Health Care System. *Medical Care Research and Review* 53: S82–S91.

General Accounting Office (GAO). 1994. Health Care: Antitrust Enforcement under Maryland's Hospital All-Payer System. Washington, D.C.

Gillies, R. R., S. M. Shortell, D. A. Anderson, and K. L. Morgan. 1993. Conceptualizing and Measuring Integration: Findings from the Health Systems Integration Study. *Hospital and Health Services Administration* 38: 467–89.

Ginsburg, P. B., and J. M. Grossman. 1995. Health System Change: The View from Wall Street. *Health Affairs* 14 (4): 159–63.

Gold, M., R. Hurley, T. Lake, T. Ensor, and R. Berenson. 1995. Arrangements Between Managed Care Plans and Physicians: Results From a 1994 Survey of Managed Care Plans. Report prepared for the Physician Payment Review Commission. Washington, D.C.

Gray, B. H. 1991. *The Profit Motive and Patient Care: The Changing Accountability of Doctors and Hospitals*. Cambridge, Mass.: Harvard University Press.

Group Health Association of America (GHAA). 1991a. 1991 National Directory of HMOs. Washington, D.C.

———. 1991b. 1991 National Directory of HMOs. Database on diskette. Washington, D.C.

———. 1995a. 1995 National Directory of HMOs. Washington, D.C.

———. 1995b. 1995 National Directory of HMOs. Database on diskette. Washington, D.C.

Harris, G. E., and R. Johnson. 1995. PhyCor, Inc. Smith Barney, New York.

Health Care Strategy Associates. 1996. Unpublished data. Washington, D.C.

Health Insurance Association of America (HIAA). 1996. *Managed Care: Integrating the Delivery and Financing of Health Care*. Washington, D.C.

Heineccius, L. 1995. Columbia/HCA: A National Profile. Washington State Hospital Association. Seattle.

Heinen, L., E. Peterson, K. Pion, and S. Leatherman. 1993. Quality Evaluation in a Managed Care System: Comparative Data to Assess Health Plan Performance. *Managed Care Quarterly* 1: 62–76.

Hester, P. C., and G. E. Harris. 1995. Overview of the Health Care Information Technology Sector: Entering the Age of Information in Health Care. Smith Barney, New York.

InterStudy Publications. 1996a. *The InterStudy Competitive Edge 6.1: Part I—HMO Directory*. Decision Resources Inc., St. Paul, Minn.

———. 1996b. *The InterStudy Competitive Edge 6.1: Part II—Industry Report*. Decision Resources Inc., St. Paul, Minn.

———. 1995. *The InterStudy Competitive Edge 6.1: Part II—Industry Report*. Decision Resources Inc., St. Paul, Minn.

Leatherman S., E. Peterson, L. Heinen, and L. Quam. 1991. Quality Screening and Management Using Claims Data in a Managed Care Setting. *Quality Review Bulletin* 17: 349–59.

Lutz, S. 1995. A Record Year for Hospital Deals. *Modern Healthcare*. Dec. 18–25; 43.

McIlrath, S. 1996. Who Will Regulate Provider-Run Plans? *American Medical News* April 1; 3.

Minnesota Health Data Institute. 1995. You and Your Health Plan: 1995 Statewide Survey of Minnesota Consumers. Minneapolis.

Mobley, L. R., and H. E. Frech III. 1994. Firm Growth and Failure in Increasingly Competitive Markets: Theory and Application to Hospital Markets. *Journal of the Economics of Business* 1: 77–93.

Murray, J. F., N. A. Hanchak, and N. Schlackman. 1996. Health Services Research at U.S. Quality Algorithms, Inc. *Medical Care Research and Review* 53: S104–S117.

National Committee For Quality Assurance. 1995. Report Card Pilot Project: Technical Report. Washington, D.C.

National Health Policy Forum. 1995. Consolidation in the Health Care Marketplace and Antitrust Policy. Issue Brief #660. Washington, D.C.: The George Washington University.

Nerenz, D. R., B. M. Zajac, and H. S. Rosman. 1993. Consortium Research on Indicators of System Performance (CRISP) *Joint Commission Journal on Quality Improvement* 30 (12): 577–85.

PhyCor, Inc. 1995. Form 10-K. Submitted to the U.S. Securities and Exchange Commission (Commission File No. 0-19786). Nashville, Tenn.

———. 1996. 1995 Annual Report. Nashville, Tenn.

Pope, G. C., and R. J. Burge. 1992. Inefficiencies in Physician Practice. In *Advances in Health Economics and Health Services Research*, vol. 13, R. M. Scheffler and L. F. Rossiter, eds. Greenwich, Conn.: JAI Press.

Reinhardt, U. 1986. The Nature of Equity Financing. In *For-Profit Enterprise in Health Care*, Institute of Medicine, National Academy of Sciences.

Robinson, J. C. 1996. The Dynamics and Limits of Corporate Growth in Health Care. *Health Affairs* 15 (2): 155–67.

Somerville, J. 1996. HMOs Face State Legislative Efforts to Rein Them In. *American Medical News* April 22/29; 5–6.

Starr, P. 1982. *The Social Transformation of American Medicine*. New York: Basic Books.

State Health Watch. 1996. SHW Publications Inc., Yardley, Pa.

Tomsho, R. 1996. "Free Agent" Doctors are Selling Practices, Signing Job Contracts. *Wall Street Journal*. March 12; A1.

Vita, M. G., J. Langenfeld, P. Pautler, and L. Miller. 1991. Economic Analysis in Health Care Antitrust. *Journal of Contemporary Health Law and Policy* 7: 73–115.

Wilson, P. 1987. Maximizing Sales to Hospital National Accounts—The Multi-Hospital Phenomenon. *Health Industry Today* October.

CHAPTER

3

THE ROLE OF MANAGED CARE "PRODUCTS" IN MANAGED CARE "PLANS"

Marsha Gold and Robert Hurley

MANAGED CARE has grown explosively in the past decade and is now the dominant form of health plan coverage for privately insured individuals (Gabel et al. 1994). Though still less common in Medicare and Medicaid, it continues to grow rapidly (Zarabozo, Taylor, and Hicks 1996; Rowland and Hansen 1996). By managed care, we mean forms of coverage that integrate financing and delivery, as well as the organizations that provide this coverage—health maintenance organizations (HMOs), preferred provider organizations (PPOs), and point-of-service (POS) plans.

To date, most research has emphasized traditional arrangements involving HMOs, particularly the prepaid group practice model, with much less research focusing on PPOs and newer hybrid models like POS plans (Gold, Nelson et al. 1995). In addition, relatively little attention has been paid to the internal heterogeneity in plans, that is, how arrangements within the same plan may vary across products, although multiple products are increasingly common in today's managed care market (Gabel et al. 1997). By products, we mean different types of

HMO, PPO, and POS coverage (as defined later) offered by a single HMO or PPO organization.

In this paper, we provide a new analysis of these issues, drawing on information collected as part of a national survey of managed care plans and their arrangements with physicians. Earlier reports have highlighted differences in existing arrangements in group/staff HMOs, network/independent practice association (IPA) HMOs, and PPOs (Gold et al. 1995 a, b). Our analysis extends that work by exploring in more depth the range and characteristics of managed care products offered by each of these types of organizations. In so doing, we hope to provide insight on the changing shape of managed care. We also hope to contribute to efforts to reconceptualize managed care "plans" and their "products" for future research and policy development.

Data Sources and Methods

This study is based on a 1994 survey that we conducted by telephone with a stratified random sample of group/staff HMOs, network/IPA HMOs, and PPOs in 20 markets nationwide. We selected the markets from the 54 largest metropolitan areas (where 86% of HMO enrollees reside), stratified by size (under one million people or one million or more) and managed care penetration (under 30%, 30% to 49%, or 50% or more). Proceeding in two stages, we first selected markets, and then plans of each of the three types within those markets using methods previously described (Gold et al. 1995 a, b). The number of group/staff HMOs and network/IPA HMOs was proportional to their respective share of nationwide HMO market (39% and 61%, respectively). Although national data suggest that HMOs and PPOs then enrolled about the same number of individuals, we restricted the PPO sample to 30% of the total because we expected PPOs to be less diverse and to have fewer managed care features.

In total, 108 plans responded to the survey, reflecting an overall response rate of 78% of eligible plans. These 108 plans enrolled 33.5 million people; 15.2 million were in HMOs, representing 35% of the national HMO enrollment at the time the sample was selected. Most plans had 100,000 or more members and many had more than 250,000. Smaller plans are underrepresented relative to the universe of plans nationwide, but not relative to their share of enrollment nationwide. Nearly all plans had been established before 1990 and many before 1980. For-profit plans accounted for 59% of the sample and for about three-quarters of the network or IPA HMOs and PPOs.

We conducted the survey between June and September 1994. All plan representatives were interviewed using the same instrument, which contained more than 300 items. Respondents were senior clinical managers and health plan executives designated by the plan's chief executive officer. Because of the length of the questionnaire, we allowed up to three respondents whose areas of expertise corresponded to the three major areas surveyed (plan and network design, payment and financial incentives, quality and utilization monitoring).

To provide perspective on the role of plan products in shaping plan features, we structured the instrument to provide information on the multiple products offered by each sampled plan. The products were defined as follows:

- **Traditional HMO:** a network of providers affiliated with an HMO that delivers health care services to enrolled individuals. Other than for some specialized services or emergencies, services provided to enrollees from providers outside the network generally are not covered.
- **Open-ended HMO:** similar to a traditional HMO but with coverage for self-referred, out-of-network care that involves more extensive patient cost sharing.
- **PPO without a primary care gatekeeper:** enrollees are given a financial incentive to use a "preferred" network of providers, usually through differences in coinsurance or deductibles. Enrollees can receive services without referral from a primary care physician.
- **PPO with a primary care gatekeeper:** similar to non-gatekeeper PPOs, except that enrollees must get prior approval from a primary care physician for most specialty physician, ancillary, or hospital services.
- **Exclusive provider organization (EPO):** enrollees are covered only for services provided by EPO network providers. Out-of-network use is covered in rare circumstances such as emergencies. Unlike traditional HMOs, EPOs usually do not incur financial risk.
- **Point-of-service plan:** enrollees select network or non-network physicians at the "point of service," usually with significant differences between network and non-network care in terms of coinsurance or deductibles. One example is a "triple option" product in which enrollees can choose to use HMO, PPO, or non-network providers with no, little, or large coinsurance payments, respectively.

We designed the survey to capture information on the range of products offered by each plan and to distinguish between arrangements used in various products. To account for critical characteristics that could vary greatly by product (e.g., basic physician payment), we asked about each product offered. For less critical characteristics, we asked about the typical arrangement and whether it applied to all products. Where it did not, we used various approaches (depending on the detail desired) to identify the differences in arrangements across products.

Our results are limited in that they are based on what the respondents said, rather than on an audit of what they do, how well they do it, and how strongly the plans' arrangements influence physician practice. However, as part of a follow-up to the original study, we conducted site visits in 1995 to seven of the surveyed plans (Hurley et al. 1996). For five of the plans, we convened focus groups of affiliated physicians familiar with and experienced in plan practices. Though these visited plans are not necessarily representative of the sample, the insights from the visits support the validity of the survey findings. We found that survey data on such items as payment methods, physician selection criteria, and product enrollment levels were complete in visited plans and accurate for the time period covered, though changes may have been made since. The changes we observed confirmed our general survey findings, though specific survey point estimates may not be constant. In interpreting the survey findings, we draw at times on insights from the site visits, noting in the text where we have done so.

Findings

Extent of Multiple Products

Multiple product offerings are more common than single product offerings in the plans we surveyed: 71% of the plans offered two or more products (Table 1). Network/IPA plans are more likely to offer multiple products and to have enrollment distributed across them. On average, traditional HMO products account for only 67% of the total enrollment in these plans. In contrast, the traditional HMO product accounts for 89% of the enrollment, on average, in group/staff HMOs. Traditional PPO products account for 87% of the enrollment in PPO plans. (Estimates of multiple products may be somewhat understated among PPOs since we excluded from the eligible PPO sample five plans already in the study as part of the HMO sample.)

Most plans with multiple products offer at least three options. Traditional HMOs, traditional PPOs (i.e., without a gatekeeper), and open-ended HMOs are by far the most common products. The network/IPA segment of the industry shows the most diversity. Among multiple product network/IPA plans, the traditional HMO still had the largest share of new enrollees in 1994, but other products (especially open-ended HMOs) were almost as likely to be the fastest growing. The largest plans are more likely to offer multiple, rather than single, products (57%

Table 1 Product Offerings by Plan Type, 1994

Product or Measure	All Plans (%)	Group/Staff (%)	Network/IPA (%)	PPO (%)
Traditional HMO	78	100	100	17
Open-ended HMO	44	38	68	10
PPO without gatekeeper	59	24	58	97
PPO with gatekeeper	25	21	22	34
EPO[a]	16	10	16	21
Other	21	24	26	10
With multiple products	71	59	88	85
With three products	26	24	40	14
With four + products	19	14	26	10
Mean enrollment in HMO	56	89	67	4
Mean enrollment in PPO	34	4	20	87

Source: Mathematica Policy Research/Medical College of Virginia survey sponsored by Physician Payment Review Commission.
[a]EPO = exclusive provider organization.

of plans offering multiple products versus 26% of plans offering single products had 250,000 or more members).

Group/staff model plans were by far the least diversified in 1994. Of those we surveyed, 39% offered only one product, and the HMO product accounted for 89% of the total enrollment among the rest. PPO products with or without a gatekeeper were offered by only 38% of the sampled group/staff plans.

Rationale for Offering Multiple Products

Multiple products tend to be offered for one of two reasons: to expand choice in response to customer interest or to ease consumers' transition to more traditional managed care arrangements. The customers include both purchasers and individual consumers. Among plans offering multiple products, 44% gave an open-ended response that fell in the first category and 24% gave one that fell in the second category, with the remainder offering other, mixed, or no reasons. Group/staff HMO plans were more likely than other plans to cite transitioning as a reason for offering multiple products (45%), although they, too, cited choice more often (55%). This might be expected since group/staff HMOs are structured specifically to offer the traditional HMO product, and they also may have a more traditional view of the preferred managed care model. Expanding choice was the most commonly cited reason across markets at all levels of managed care penetration, though it was the more dominant reason in low-penetration markets. This may indicate that establishing a presence in a low-penetration market requires plans to make their products more acceptable to people whose experience with products that restrict choice is limited.

How Plans Vary Arrangements Across Associated Products

Plans are more likely than not to use the same provider network for all their products. Among those offering multiple products, two-thirds use the same provider networks for all of them. This is true even for group/staff plans, despite the often distinctive characteristics of provider networks in such plans. (Whether this is influenced by the fact that more than half of group/staff plans—52%—are mixed models is unclear.)

Plans vary in the responsibilities they give their primary care physicians for patients covered by different products (Table 2). The differences are logical, since products in part are defined by the form and responsibilities of the network physicians. Network/IPA plans almost always require patients to choose an individual primary care physician in their HMO products, but rarely do in their PPO products except for those based on a gatekeeper model. Group/staff plans make similar distinctions, though they are more likely than network/IPAs to be based on multispecialty group practices and less likely to require patients to select an *individual* physician. Both kinds of HMOs typically hold primary care physicians responsible for referrals; for PPO products, primary care physician referrals are required only in gatekeeper PPOs. PPOs offering HMO products structure responsibilities for these products similar to the way HMOs structure them. (The lack of complete congruence in practices for a given plan and product type probably illustrates a level of complexity and nuance that is hard to capture in any standard question.)

The dominance of product over plan type in arrangements with physicians does not carry over as clearly into payment policies. Our previous findings show that payment through any other means than traditional fee-for-service (FFS) is rare in PPO products but typical of HMOs (Gold et al. 1995b). We find here that all of the group/staff HMOs, and all but two of the 29 PPOs pay primary care physicians on a pure FFS basis in their PPO products. However, 17 of the 35 network/IPAs with PPO products pay primary care physicians in some way other than pure FFS in at least some of their PPO products. (Comparable data for specialists were not uniformly provided by plans.) These plans use FFS with bonus/withholds and capitation in about equal proportions. In all except four cases, network/IPAs that pay physicians some way other than pure FFS use the same means for all products.

Managed care features, such as focused studies and physician profiling, are generally less likely to be used in PPO products even if plans employ them otherwise (Table 3). Because of the small sample size, we had difficulty identifying differences across types of PPO products. However, as expected, features such as focused studies appear more often in gatekeeper PPOs than in other PPO products. Network/IPA plans appear more likely than PPOs to use the managed care features we examined in the PPO products these plans offer, a finding not fully explained by differences in the mix of PPO products across the two types of plans.

Insight Into Particular Products and Their Role in the Marketplace

PPO products

Though the majority of plans we surveyed offer some form of PPO product (traditional PPO, gatekeeper PPO, or EPO), group/staff HMOs are

Table 2 Responsibility of Primary Care Physicians in Products Offered by Plan Type, 1994

Measure	All Plans	Group/Staff	Network/IPA	PPO
Number offering product				
Traditional HMO	84	29	50	5
Open-ended HMO	46	11	32	3
PPO without gatekeeper	63	7	28	28
PPO with gatekeeper	27	6	11	10
Percentage requiring patient to choose individual primary care physician[a]				
Traditional HMO	82	61	92	100
Open-ended HMO	76	58	81	—[b]
PPO without gatekeeper	8	14	7	7
PPO with gatekeeper	67	33	73	80
Percentage generally holding primary care physicians responsible for referrals[a]				
Traditional HMO	94	86	92	100
Open-ended HMO	76	90	69	100
PPO without gatekeeper	13	14	11	14
PPO with gatekeeper	81	100	64	90

Source: Mathematica Policy Research/Medical College of Virginia survey sponsored by Physician Payment Review Commission.
[a]Of those offering product.
[b]Too few plans.

Table 3 Use of Selected Managed Care Features in PPO Products by Plan Strata, 1994

Plan/Product Type	Percentage Using Managed Care Feature				
	Focused Studies	Profiling	Practice Guidelines[a]	Medical Record Access	Sample Size[b]
Total					
Percentage of all plans that use it	83	74	63	95	108
Percentage of all PPO offerers that use it	77	77	63	95	75
Percentage with product that use it in:					
PPO	42	42	—[e]	89	64
G-PPO[c]	70	42	—	92	27
EPO[d]	47	35	—	94	17
Group/staff					
All plans	100	76	76	93	29
All PPO offerers	100	91	91	91	11
Percentage with product that use it in:					
PPO	57	43	—	86	7
G-PPO[c]	80	20	—	83	6
EPO[d]	—	—	—	—	3
Network/IPA					
All plans	96	86	76	98	50
All PPO offerers	97	94	83	97	35
Percentage with product that use it in:					
PPO	48	45	—	83	29
G-PPO[c]	73	45	—	100	11
EPO[d]	63	63	—	100	8
PPO					
All plans	45	52	28	93	29
All PPO offerers	45	52	28	93	29
Percentage with product that use it in:					
PPO	32	39	—	96	28
G-PPO[c]	60	50	—	89	10
EPO[d]	17	0	—	83	6

Source: Mathematica Policy Research/Medical College of Virginia survey sponsored by Physician Payment Review Commission.

[a]Respondents were not asked to distinguish among the products where practice guidelines were present.

[b]Several percentages were calculated using one plan fewer than the sample size indicates due to missing data.

[c]G-PPO = gatekeeper PPO.

[d]EPO = exclusive provider organizaiton.

[e]Too few plans or data not available.

less likely than network/IPAs to do so (38% vs. 70%, respectively). And when group/staff HMOs do offer PPOs, the total share of enrollment in these products is smaller than it is in network/IPAs (14% vs. 31%). Group/staff plans offering PPOs, like other plans offering PPOs, tend to have most of their enrollment in traditional PPOs; unlike other plans, they are almost as likely to offer gatekeeper as traditional PPOs.

In most cases, the differences in characteristics of plans offering PPOs, compared with those that do not, appear to reflect differences in the composition of plans in each strata rather than any unique attributes (data not presented but available in Hurley et al. 1996). However, among group/staff models, nonprofit plans are less likely than for-profits to offer PPO products, and those not offering PPOs are less likely to be owned by insurers or national managed care organizations. Within each type of plan, those owned by commercial insurers are more likely than those owned by Blue Cross-Blue Shield to offer PPOs, a finding consistent with other national data (see Gabel, forthcoming).

Point-of-service products

To explore the prevalence of POS products and the characteristics of plans offering them, we combined three products into a single "any POS product" category: open-ended HMO, gatekeeper PPO, and "other" POS. This approach is limited, since we could not capture enough information to detail how similar these products are, but each qualifies as a POS product by the commonly accepted industry definition. Using this definition, 66% of the plans (71 of 108) reported offering a POS product (Table 4). Network/IPA plans are more likely to offer such a product (86% as compared with 52% of group/staff plans and 45% of PPOs). This is consistent with previous findings, but likely to be changing with greater pressure from buyers to broaden the product array and from consumers to expand provider choice. POS products are much more common in markets perceived as very competitive, and in markets where managed care is said to be well-accepted by physicians. They appear equally common in plans that give choice as their rationale for offering multiple products as in those that cite ease of transition. One explanation for these findings is that in mature managed care markets, POS products aim to bring in the remaining population; in less-developed markets, POS products aim to establish a beachhead.

Creating the "any POS category" made it possible to determine which plan type is most likely to offer a "triple option" set of products (Table 4). During our site visits, plans reported that this capacity is important to purchasers who want a single carrier as well as a spectrum

Table 4 Market Perceptions for Plans Offering Selected Product Options, 1994

	Number of Plans	Percentage of Plans Offering POS Product[a]	Percentage of Plans Offering Triple-Option Capacity[b]
Total	107[c]	66	43
Model			
Group/staff	29	52	34
Network/IPA	50	86	64
PPO	29	45	17
How well established is managed care in market area?			
Very	55	69	49
Moderately	36	61	33
Not very	16	63	44
How competitive is managed care in service area?			
Very	90	71	47
Moderately	16	38	25
Not very	1	—	—
Over next three years, competition prediction			
Increase a lot	79	65	38
Increase moderately	20	70	55
Stay same	6	67	67
Decrease moderately	2	—	—
How well is managed care accepted by physicians in the area?			
Very	34	74	53
Moderately	60	65	40
Not very	13	46	31
Rationale for multiple-product offering ($N = 75$)[d]	75	92	61
Choice	33	94	61
Transition to traditional product	18	94	61
None or other	24	88	63

Source: Mathematica Policy Research/Medical College of Virginia survey sponsored by Physician Payment Review Commission.

Note: Percentages do not add to 100 because of rounding. Percentages are excluded if fewer than five plans responded.

[a]Open-ended HMO, gatekeeper PPO, or "other POS product."

[b]HMO, PPO, and any POS product.

[c]One plan is missing data on market perceptions.

[d]Includes only plans that offer multiple products.

of products (an HMO, a PPO, and a POS offering). Failure to meet this need can mean the loss of existing accounts and constrained future business opportunities. The findings regarding triple-option capacity parallel those about POS plans: network/IPA plans are most likely to have this capacity and PPOs least likely. Notably, there does not appear to be a relationship between market size or penetration and triple-option capacity. As for POS products, triple-option capacity is associated with markets that are perceived as highly competitive and where managed care is well accepted by physicians. In a multivariate analysis, we further examined both the decision to offer a POS product and the availability of triple-option capacity to assess the independent effects of plan characteristics on these two areas. The results (not presented) were generally consistent with those reported here.

During our site visits, plans reported that they are becoming more comfortable with pricing POS products and are able to document that most care is rendered by network providers (more than 90% in mature POS products). Thus, they see the psychological value of offering the option to use out-of-network services as the principal advantage of a POS product. However, POS products did create some difficulties with network physicians, who did not always understand well—and thus did not communicate well to patients—the complexities of requirements such as referral patterns and payments. Another sensitive issue is that some plans charge out-of-network use against a primary care physician's capitation or referral account. Primary care physicians argued in focus groups that this inappropriately penalizes them for failing to persuade a member to stay in the network when, in fact, the member has the right to use out-of-network services.

Product strategies

The people interviewed during our site visits emphasized that decisions about product offerings are market driven. A number of respondents noted that it is complicated and cumbersome to add products when current ones need substantial refinement. Adding open-ended products in group/staff plans often is especially costly when the only existing network is an exclusive HMO network; that results in a need to establish contracts and payments with a broader network or to contract for a "PPO wraparound." Furthermore, the frequent addition of new products destabilizes enrollment levels in different products, making it difficult to firmly establish the relative profitability of any given product. Plans fear "cannibalization"—that the growth in new products will come at the expense of existing ones.

Attitudes about product proliferation, assessed in the site visits, are mixed and not fully consistent even within plans. Some HMOs (both network/IPA and group/staff types) frankly state concerns that offering the highly popular POS product will undermine their ability to manage care effectively or to be accountable for the health of members who might use out-of-network providers. Others regret having to offer PPOs and indemnity products in response to customer demands. Still others believe that new entrants to markets offer intentionally loose, inclusive networks to gain a foothold, leaving plans already in the market no recourse but to follow suit. Opinions of marketing directors can differ from those of the clinical staff, with the marketing side seeing these developments as inevitable and reflective of legitimate efforts to identify and respond to evolving consumer preferences. They also perceive that "choice sells," and products with tight networks or restricted choice always will struggle for a price advantage that will make them attractive. The site visits confirmed the survey findings that network/IPA plans believe most strongly in giving purchasers multiple options. The site visits also suggest that some plans, including some large Blue Cross-Blue Shield sponsored plans, are more interested in responding to, rather than leading, the market. That is, they would rather have another plan go first in introducing change. These plans tend to have broad, inclusive provider networks, using pricing leverage more often than care management to control costs. They neither necessarily promote one product over another, nor try to "push" consumers toward tighter products.

Discussion

Our findings confirm the growth of multiple product offerings within managed care plans. Given the volatility of markets, the disparate expectations and preferences of buyers and consumers, and the variability across managed care plans, the patterns we describe undoubtedly have grown even more extensive and complex since our study. Thus, the finding that group/staff HMOs are more wedded to traditional products and more interested in "transitional" strategies is likely to remain relevant to understanding these plans. The specific characteristics of the products offered by group/staff plans, however, likely will have evolved by now.

There is little evidence from our study that PPO plans are moving toward HMO products, but most HMOs, especially network/IPA models, offer PPOs to round out their product array. However, these issues are not dealt with sufficiently in a cross-sectional survey such as ours that samples plans by type. In adding to their products, plans also modify or expand the number of sampling frames from which they can be selected. Yet, studying the evolution of plans through national data over time is complicated by the absence of good lists for managed care entities other than HMOs, difficulties in tracking plans across diverse lists, and historical differences in how different products are regulated. Unless managed care entities are regulated with more consistency across products and states, and across state-controlled (insurance) and federal (preempted by the Employee Retirement Security Act) lines of business, it will be difficult to develop better data for tracking change in the managed care industry, its entities, and the products they offer. (State lists are now used widely to cross-validate HMO lists. The license requirement makes it easier to define managed care organizations and their service areas. Further, the federal HMO act historically encouraged relative standardization of the HMO product, a feature not applicable to PPOs and now less relevant to HMOs, though National Committee for Quality Assurance [NCQA] accreditation could serve a similar function.)

In stark contrast to the confusing plethora of labels used for plans (the "alphabet soup") both in the literature and in marketing materials, our findings suggest that most current offerings are distinguished by a few key variations. In fact, virtually all the products we found fell under the limited number of categories we provided, most in only three of them. Thus, it probably is as important to focus on the similarities across products, regardless of their names, as the differences. It also suggests there may be value in identifying a set of core characteristics that can be used to describe and compare products, rather than to focus on developing better and mutually exclusive typologies either of plans or products.

Our results indicate that both the type of plan and type of product are influential in shaping the offerings and their characteristics. The plan type appears most influential in areas like product offerings and strategy; plan also dominates when logistical concerns can be addressed feasibly by standardization across products, as with provider networks. Depending on a firm's structure and philosophy, these decisions may be made at the market, regional, or national level. The product type appears most influential in determining the essential product features that need to be reflected in the arrangements with physicians. For example, measurement and care management techniques that require accountability for defined populations typically are not operationally feasible for products structured to promote free choice among providers at point of service. However, where feasible, plans seem to prefer standardization across products to reduce confusion and administrative burden. Thus, the appropriate unit of analysis in future research will vary with the questions. It often will be necessary to use a nested strategy to accommodate questions that cannot be addressed without benefit of information on the plan, possibly its parent, and the product as well. This will complicate the already complex task of researching managed care, particularly as there is even less standardization in the product names than in the way the plans or entities offering them are named and classified.

Finally, our findings offer an intriguing opportunity to speculate on where the managed care industry is headed and what this might mean. Plans find managing multiple products cumbersome, yet unavoidable, given market demands. As multiple product offerings grow, one likely result for HMO plans is the loss of identity as an "HMO company." Instead, these organizations will develop into multiple product, managed care organizations, or perhaps offerers of both managed care and indemnity products, possibly with nonrisk-based payment for HMO products that can be paid for on a self-insured basis. At the same time, provider-sponsored entities are emerging. Though relatively undeveloped despite the publicity they have received, provider entities are absorbing directly, and especially through managed care organizations, more risk and responsibility for managed care (Robinson and Casalino 1996; Shortell, Gilles, and Anderson 1994). As this occurs, the distinction between managed care organizations and what historically were insurance companies may become more blurred, particularly if risk is shared with purchasers or shifted to intermediate provider entities. If market forces lead provider entities to truly make changes rather than just defend their current positions, some may come to resemble the original HMO structures. That current trends reflect the end of managed care as an alternative delivery system and its challenging emergence as the dominant model is yet another interpretation.

References

Gabel, J., H. Whitmore, C. Bergsten, and L.P. Grimm. 1997. Growing Diversification in HMOs, 1988–1994. *Medical Care Research and Review* 54 (1): 101–17.

Gabel, J., J. Liston, G. Jensen, and J. Marsteller. 1994. The Health Insurance Picture in 1993: Some Rare Good News. *Health Affairs* 13 (1): 327–36.

Gold, M. R., R. Hurley, T. Lake, T. Ensor, and R. Berenson. 1995a. *Arrangements Between Managed Care Plans and Physicians.* Selected External Research Series No. 3. Washington, D.C.: Physician Payment Review Commission.

———. 1995b. A National Survey of the Arrangements Managed Care Plans Make with Physicians. *New England Journal of Medicine* 333 (25): 1678–1683.

Gold, M., L. Nelson, T. Lake, R. Hurley, and R. Berenson. 1995. Behind the Curve: A Critical Assessment of How Little is Known about the Managed Care Arrangements with Physicians. *Medical Care Research and Review* 52: 307–41.

Hurley, R., T. Lake, M. Gold, and D. Almond. 1996. *Arrangements between Managed Care Plans and Physicians II: A Follow-Up Analysis of 1994 Survey Data and Site Visit*

Information. Selected External Research Series No. 6. Washington, D.C.: Physician Payment Review Commission.

Robinson, J., and L. Casalino. 1996. Vertical Integration and Organizational Networks in Health Care. *Health Affairs* 15 (2): 62–76.

Rowland, D., and K. Hanson. 1996. Medicaid: Moving to Managed Care. *Health Affairs* 15 (3): 150–152.

Shortell, S., R. Gilles, and D. A. Anderson. 1994. New World of Managed Care: Creating Organized Delivery Systems. *Health Affairs* 13 (5): 46–64.

Zarabozo, C., C. Taylor, and J. Hicks. 1996. Data View: Medicare Managed Care: Numbers and Trends. *Health Care Financing Review* 17 (3): 243–62.

PART

2

INSIDE THE BLACK BOX OF MANAGED CARE

Introduction: The Importance and Challenge of Understanding Managed Care

As has been mentioned, *managed care* has become a catch phrase for the broad variety of rapidly emerging healthcare products and entities in the current marketplace. The entities serving as managed care plans or offering managed care products are complex organizations. They typically bundle together—through contract affiliations or ownership—physicians, hospitals, and other providers to deliver care to consumers according to the contract between the managed care entity and a purchaser (who is usually not the consumer). Managed care organizations also create an infrastructure that, in different ways and to different degrees, influences provider incentives and practice patterns as well as how patients access providers. These complex relationships have affected the entire healthcare system and all those participating in it. The power of managed care's reach has generated considerable interest in better understanding the structure of managed care organizations. It also has fueled a great deal of debate over what evolving structures in managed care might mean for patient care.

In this second set of four articles, we offer insight into how managed care organizations are structured. The first article, "Behind the Curve: A Critical Assessment of How Little Is Known About Arrangements Between Managed Care Plans and Physicians," reviews the literature through the mid-1990s, critically assessing what is known about the arrangements managed care plans make with their physicians. The article then also proposes a conceptual framework for understanding how managed care organizations are structured in the context of the broader health system, which comprises purchasers, consumers, providers, and regulators. The article then summarizes key questions and current knowledge about the structure of provider networks, the physician payment systems and their associated incentives, and the processes managed care organizations use to influence the use and quality of care. To no one's surprise, the authors conclude that the structure of managed care organizations has developed far more rapidly than information about these changes and what they mean.

The next two articles seek, in different ways, to address gaps in the available information on managed care and to document more fully the processes defining managed care organizations and how they work. In "A National Survey of the Arrangements Managed-Care Plans Make with Physicians," the authors report on a 1994 national survey of HMOs and PPOs and their arrangements with physicians. This article highlights important similarities and differences across the various forms of managed care in terms of provider networks, payment arrangements, and the process of managing care. Also addressed is the considerable structural complexity that is characteristic of these organizations. Arrangements differ within and across organizations, and processes with seemingly similar names may, in fact, differ greatly. In "How HMOs Structure Primary Care Delivery," the authors provide more perspective on the diverse nature of managed care and how this diversity is reflected in the way HMOs structure primary care.

The brisk progression of managed care raises questions about its effect on access, quality, and costs. In particular, information is needed about its infrastructure's effect on physician payment and practice patterns, changes it has brought about in the choices of plans available to consumers, and differences in how consumers need to seek care. On the one hand, managed care has the potential to enhance access and quality by creating more organized systems of coordinated, patient-centered care focused on prevention. On the other hand, managed care's risk-based capitated incentives may prompt plans to skimp on needed care, and poorly organized systems may inhibit, rather than improve, access. Unfortunately, current research has informed this debate in only a limited way (Miller and Luft 1994; 1997); one can also argue that current research fails to support either of these two positions. This uncertainty drives interest in research to identify features of managed care that promote good outcomes, but it is difficult to conduct definitive studies on this topic, because managed care organizations do not "stand still" long enough to be examined. They also differ from each other in important ways that are difficult to capture, particularly with a relatively small number of organizations and little data. These challenges have led to studies with the potential to describe "best practices" and encourage their use. The last article in this section, "Delivering Women's Preventive Services Under Managed Care: Opportunity and Promise," describes results of a study that sought to work collaboratively with health plans to identify how best to provide preventive healthcare services to women.

References

Miller, R., and H. Luft. 1994. "Managed Care Performance Since 1980: A Literature Analysis." *Journal of the American Medical Association* 271 (19): 1512–19.

———. 1997. "Does Managed Care Lead to Better or Worse Quality of Care?" *Health Affairs* 16 (5): 7–25.

CHAPTER

4

BEHIND THE CURVE: A CRITICAL ASSESSMENT OF HOW LITTLE IS KNOWN ABOUT ARRANGEMENTS BETWEEN MANAGED CARE PLANS AND PHYSICIANS

Marsha Gold, Lyle Nelson, Timothy Lake,
Robert Hurley, and Robert Berenson

THE GROWTH of managed care has been explosive in the past decade, resulting in fundamental change in the way in which physicians practice and relate to payers and insurers. According to recent employer surveys, network-based plans account for 54 percent of the market share of privately insured employees (Sullivan et al. 1992). HMO and PPO products accounted for less than 1 percent of group health premium revenues for commercial insurers in 1984, but by 1990, this figure had grown to 25 percent (Hoy, Curtis, and Rice 1991). In 1991, managed care plans provided 22 percent of the typical physician's gross income, an increase of 30 percent over the preceding two years (Murray 1992). The same study reported that more than half of all physicians in the United States participated in at least one HMO network, and the same proportion belong to at least one PPO network. More than 75 percent of

From *Medical Care Research and Review* 52 (3): 307–341.

hospitals in the United States have either HMO or PPO contracts or both (DeLoitte and Touche 1992). In response to the growing competitiveness of the market, providers are forming integrated delivery systems (Shortell, Gillies, and Anderson 1994), and insurers are developing a plethora of managed care products and organizational arrangements with providers. Given the anticipated growth in managed care, it is imperative that we know more about the arrangements between managed care plans and physicians, their variability across plans and their trends over time, and how they may change the way physicians practice. A better understanding of these issues is essential to designing studies of the effects of managed care arrangements on cost, quality, access, and patient and physician satisfaction.

In this article, we provide a framework for examining the arrangements between managed care plans and physicians, and we synthesize current research to identify what we know and do not know about such arrangements. The synthesis focuses on the following questions:

- How do managed care plans select physicians for their networks, integrate them within the plan, and decide which physicians to retain?
- How do plans pay physicians? What types of risk-sharing, bonus arrangements, or both are included in physician compensation packages to encourage cost-conscious behavior and other valued objectives?
- How do plans monitor the care provided by their physicians, and what other methods (in addition to financial incentives) do plans use to influence the practice patterns of physicians in their networks?

We focus on these questions because they define the critical nexus between health plans and the physicians who deliver care in their systems. For each question, we seek information on variations across types of managed care plans and trends over time. We also seek information on the relationships between and among these issues.

To determine what is known about these issues, we reviewed a broad range of materials, including research studies in peer-reviewed journals, conference proceedings, industry publications of descriptive data, and materials published in the health industry trade literature. Because of the dynamic nature of the managed care industry, we focused primarily on materials published within the past five years. We used earlier publications to obtain baseline data for drawing inferences about historical trends. We also contacted key researchers in the field of managed care to identify current research projects relevant to our objective and to determine when the results will become available. Much of the information in the trade literature is anecdotal or opinion, so we did not give it the same weight as published research studies that have been peer reviewed. The trade literature was useful, however, in identifying both developments in the industry and issues that have not yet been studied in the research literature. The review covers the literature through 1993 with selective updates to early 1995.

For purposes of this article, we define managed care as plans and products involving the integration of health care financing and delivery systems. At a minimum, we assume some form of network-based health benefits arrangement—whether insured or self-insured. At one extreme, the degree to which financing and delivery are integrated may be limited to differential health benefits or cost sharing for in-network versus out-of-network care as many basic PPOs are structured. At the other extreme, integration may involve insurers or purchasers committing to arrange or deliver care exclusively through a dedicated network owned or under exclusive contract with the plan as traditional prepaid group practice HMOs have been structured and a few employers are copying (e.g., Southern California Edison).

The most striking finding in our review of the literature is its weakness. The existing literature provides few answers to the range of important questions about how managed care plans relate to physicians. Except for some research on physician payment and incentives within HMOs, most information tends to be anecdotal or unsubstantiated assertions. Both the Group Health Association of America (GHAA) and InterStudy (InterStudy 1994) field surveys of HMOs, which provide some industry-wide estimates of practices for HMOs. SMG (with funds from Marion Merrill Dow) also provides information on HMOs and PPOs. However, only recently have these surveys included items on the arrangements between plans and physicians, and these items tend to be relatively limited. They may also inadvertently bias responses by appearing to indicate that certain practices are socially desirable or preferable (e.g., selecting physicians based on their "quality"). The literature also tends to focus almost exclusively on HMOs rather than PPOs and newer forms of managed care models. And for HMOs, the literature emphasizes traditional arrangements more heavily than newer forms of managed care products. In addition, relatively little attention is given to how arrangements within the *same* plan may vary across managed care products even though the offering of multiple products is becoming increasingly common. Knowledge is also constrained because some surveys, such as those conducted by management consulting firms, are largely proprietary, and results may therefore not be publicly available. In other cases, some plans may be hesitant to respond because of the proprietary nature of the topics covered. Thus, although this article provides an important reference to existing studies, we believe it is clearly most useful in identifying areas and questions that should be the focus of future research.

New Contribution

The major contribution of this article derives from its scope and focus. Specifically, we have sought to integrate findings from both standard sources typically used in academic research and the less traditionally used trade press. The latter tends to be less authoritative but also more current and operationally focused. Unlike most articles reviewing managed care generally, ours is focused. Specifically it is focused on one key nexus that influences the performance of managed care, the structured arrangements between health plans and their medical providers, specifically physicians. With this focus, we aim to identify both the key questions of interest and the current state of knowledge on these questions. We do so within a systems-exchange framework, presented at the outset, that aims to define how our focus (on the plan-physician interaction) fits within the larger system defining health plans and the parties with whom they relate. The framework also illustrates why the three broad questions of concern in this study are important to understanding managed care plans and their potential effects. Our work goes beyond existing efforts (e.g., Welch, Hillman, and Pauly 1990; Weiner and deLissovoy 1993) in including a broader range of variables and their interrelationships. Our work, therefore, provides both a unique synthesis of what is known on the issues we consider and a guide and framework for future research.

Framework

Figure 1 depicts managed care organizations in the context of four key actors in the environment with whom they are dependent: the purchasers, the consumers, the providers, and the regulators. We discuss first the context in which health-plan-physician arrangements exist and then the key specific features that define those arrangements negotiated.

Purchasers, subject to regulatory constraints, define the products that are offered based on contractual arrangements negotiated with various managed care plans. These agreements determine how financial risk is shared if at all between purchaser and the health plan, the benefits that are covered and the premium, and the form of care in products offered (e.g., whether or not patients are "locked in" to the network, required to enroll in specific kinds of plans, and so on). Purchasers also may influence how provider networks are designed. Historically, the purchasers' role in

Figure 1 Systems Framework: Managed Care Organizations

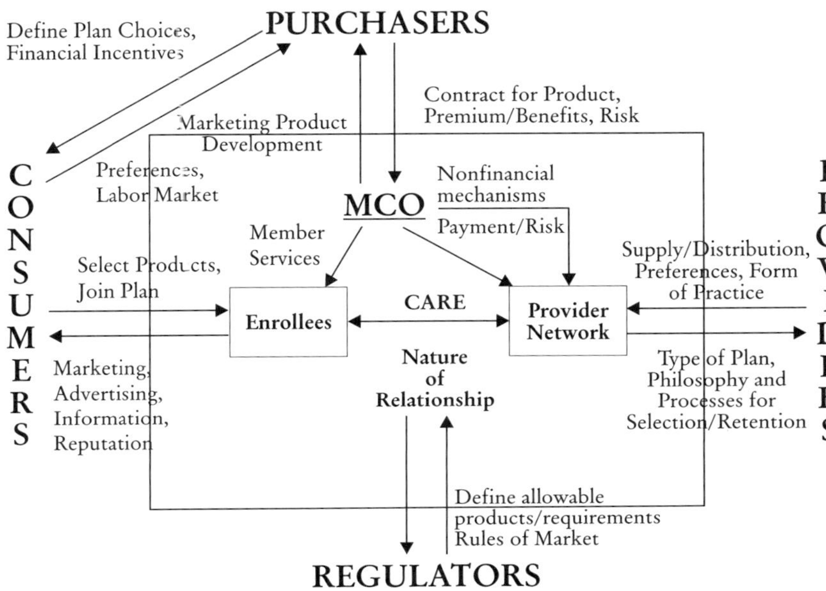

this has been limited to their preferences among managed care model types. However, more recently some purchasers may be exerting a larger influence both over the size of the network or its composition in the interests of offering products that will be attractive to employees and also encourage choices that respond to fiscal concerns of the purchaser. Employers also consider how their health benefits affect their ability to compete in the labor market.

Table 1 shows how diverse managed care products can be defined through variables in purchasers' negotiations with health plans on such issues as risk, provider integration, and patient lock-in. Looking at products this way explains why products offered by organizations classified as HMOs and PPOs are not clearly distinct from one another. It also illustrates why there is confusion about definitions for point-of-service plans and products (Miller and Luft 1991), because these may be offered by HMOs as an open-ended product, by PPOs that are gatekeeper PPOs, or as a triple option plan in which enrollees have a choice between an HMO, PPO, or indemnity benefits (Lutes and Hastings 1993).

Because of third-party coverage, consumer choices are defined by others. Because most private health insurance is obtained through employment based coverage, employers play a key role in determining what

Table 1 Typology of Managed Care Plans

Are Providers Affiliated Full-Time in a Group Setting with the Managed Care Plan?	Is Managed Care Plan at Financial Risk and Are Patients Locked In?			
	Plan at Risk		Plan Not at Risk	
	Lock In	No Lock In	Lock In	No Lock In
Yes	Traditional prepaid group practices (e.g., staff, group)	Open-ended HMO product	EPO (or self-insured HMO arrangement)	PPO (or HMO network used for PPO)
(Yes and No)	Mixed model HMO	Open-ended HMO product	EPO (or self-insured HMO arrangement)	PPO (or HMO network used for PPO)
No	Other HMO (e.g., IPA)	Open-ended HMO product	EPO (or self-insured HMO arrangement)	PPO (or HMO network used for PPO)

health plans are available for selection and what the incentives are for choosing among them. Government purchasers perform similar functions for Medicare and Medicaid beneficiaries. The choices offered and the financial incentives influencing selection then factor heavily, within any given market, in determining the demand and enrollment levels in particular managed care plans and the individual products they offer. In turn these define how closely consumers and physicians are linked. POS products, for example, provide the potential for more "leakage" than traditional HMO providers.

The environment and processes we have discussed all influence the arrangements between managed care plans and physicians. Managed care organizations integrate financing and delivery. Hence, unlike traditional insurance, these organizations involve obligations to deliver or arrange for care, not just pay for it. Plans develop their provider systems taking into account history and health plan philosophy, the previously discussed influences on demand from purchasers and consumers, and the nature of the provider community in any market. The latter is influenced by the supply, geographic and specialty distribution that influence capacity, the form of practice organization dominant in the market (e.g., multispecialty groups or solo practice), and the general attitude of market physicians on managed care and their willingness to contract with it. The latter, of course, is not totally independent but influenced by all the other forces in the environment. Recently, for example, physician perspectives have been eclipsed by those of dominant purchasers in some markets.

Within this context, the arrangements between managed care plans and physicians are then determined by how three types of relationships are defined: (1) the nature of the provider selection, retention, and acculturation process; (2) the nature of financial incentives inherent in the payment form; and (3) the nature of the nonfinancial systems to monitor physicians and influence their practice patterns. These in turn are constrained by the nature of the product, as this determines how physicians relate to patients; and by the arrangements the health plan has made with other providers (e.g., hospitals).

This framework assumes that the extent and type of managed care is defined by how plans approach each of the arrangements they need to negotiate. Through these arrangements, plans define both the cohesiveness of the clinical enterprise and its form. Unfortunately these characteristics are poorly captured by traditional managed care model type definitions and managed care product labels (Table 1). Perhaps this explains why these traditional definitions and labels have become increasingly less useful in today's managed care environment.

Arrangements Between Managed Care Plans and Physicians

The nature of the arrangements between managed care plans and physicians may be expected to vary with a variety of factors, including the following key features of managed care plans and products:

1. *Whether the managed care entity itself bears risk.* This differentiates most HMO products from PPOs. It is important because being at risk may affect arrangements with providers by increasing plan interest in influencing their practice.
2. *The form of physician practice organization and the exclusivity of its relationship to the managed care plan.* In terms of the managed care and physician relationship, fully committed physicians practicing in large multi-specialty arrangements (traditional prepaid group practices) probably differ fundamentally from one or more types of looser arrangements based on physicians in private practice who see managed care and other patients. However, with some insurers purchasing medical group practices, this distinction among models could become somewhat less clear.
3. *Whether patients are "locked in" to the network.* For HMOs, this differentiates traditional from open-ended or point-of-service products. For PPOs, this differentiates traditional from exclusive provider organization (EPO) arrangements;[1] it also could define self-insured arrangements by HMOs. This feature modifies the plan-patient relationship. It may also modify the plan-physician

relationship because it complicates the task of holding physicians accountable for patient management and may inhibit plans from being able to promise or guarantee patient volume to the contractual provider.

Plans' arrangements with physicians are also expected to vary with plans' management philosophy and strategic objectives, and various characteristics of the plan's market area—including the degree of competitiveness, the maturity of the managed care market, physician receptivity to managed care and the accepting of financial risk, and the regulatory environment.

Each plan presumably chooses a set of approaches to its arrangements with physicians that, in combination, maximize its probability of achieving its strategic objectives, subject to any constraints imposed by market characteristics or other factors. For example, plans that capitate primary care physicians and place them at risk for specialty referrals and inpatient care through a withholding account may be expected to place particular emphasis on monitoring physicians to ensure that the financial incentives do not result in underservice. On the other hand, plans operating in areas where physicians are resistant to accepting much financial risk may rely particularly heavily on nonfinancial mechanisms such as utilization management to influence practice patterns. A plan's overall management philosophy concerning its relationship with physicians may also play an important role in these decisions, because managers may have strong beliefs based on prior experience or other factors on the types of arrangements with physicians that would best meet their strategic objectives.

Plans also differ in their strategic objectives, which can significantly influence their arrangements with physicians. Some plans may be content to maintain a given niche in the market, while others may seek to expand their market share significantly and expand into new markets. In addition, in positioning their products in the market, plans differ in the extent to which they emphasize the traditional benefits of managed care (low cost, high quality, coordinated care) versus freedom of choice of providers.

Most of the existing literature has examined the nature of plans' arrangements with physicians for plans classified by model type. However, given the variation across plans of a given model type in such factors as number and type of managed care products offered, strategic objectives and management philosophy, and market characteristics, plans of a given model type may exhibit significant variation in the nature of their arrangements with physicians.

Physician Selection and Retention

Little is known about the network development strategies of managed care plans or about how effectively these strategies create and sustain a network of cost-conscious, high-quality providers—if indeed this is the goal. In synthesizing the literature on these issues, we organize the discussion around the following five key questions:

- What criteria do plans use to select physicians and how do they implement these criteria?
- How do plans integrate and promote the acculturation of physicians into their systems?
- How frequently do plans terminate their relationships with physicians, and what criteria are used to reach such decisions?
- What overall philosophy and strategy guide the efforts of plans in developing networks?
- To what extent do legal and regulatory requirements affect plans' network development strategies?

In examining these issues, it is important to distinguish between two-tiered and three-tiered plans. A three-tiered plan has less ability to select or remove individual physicians from its network but may be better positioned to garner physician cooperation or shift control and risk to physicians.

Selection Criteria and Process

Surveys of HMOs and PPOs typically reveal that they seek "high quality" physicians with "cost-effective" practice patterns for their networks (GHAA 1993a; Langwell, Carlton, and Swearingen 1989). There is little solid evidence in the literature on how they achieve this objective, however, or even whether this objective is really important for plans or merely one that they feel is important to report in surveys. It is important to know what criteria managed care plans use to measure quality and cost-effectiveness, and how, if at all, they implement those criteria in initial hiring/contracting decisions and in their decisions on renewals. The trade and research literature has addressed some of these questions, but most conclusions in the literature are based on anecdotal evidence or dated research (e.g., Fisher, Howard, and Pasternak 1993; Jacobs and Mott 1987; Ballard and Terze 1993; Zalta 1993).

Large insurers have claims data from their traditional indemnity products that could potentially be used to select physicians on the basis of cost-effectiveness, billing practices, and other criteria when they develop or expand managed care networks in new areas. It is not known how many insurers use such data (or precisely *how* they use such data) to select physicians, however. One case that has been widely reported in the media involves the Blue Cross and Blue Shield Association serving the Washington, DC metropolitan area, which recently developed a PPO product and invited about two-thirds of the physicians who were participating in the plan's traditional insurance products to join the PPO network. The determination of which physicians to include in the PPO network was based primarily on a proprietary computer-based profiling system that measured and compared physicians' practice patterns (Iglehart 1994b). The District of Columbia Medical Society has filed suit seeking to prevent the plan from continuing with this method of selecting physicians.

In general, screening new physicians on the basis of practice profiles generated from fee-for-service claims data could be expensive and prone to error. Large amounts of data are required for each physician, and some method of controlling for case mix differences is necessary (or it is at least necessary to investigate whether there is some justification in terms of patient mix for the high costs generated by some physicians). On the other hand, the data may be limited, permitting less assessment of cost-effectiveness than the weeding out of physicians who have a history of "bad" billings.[2]

The credentialing of physicians by managed care plans has assumed increased importance in recent years. Employers are increasingly demanding that managed care plans use effective credentialing systems, and recent court rulings have held that HMOs have a duty to reasonably investigate the competence of their physicians (Kopit and Lutes 1993). The National Committee on Quality Assurance (NCQA), the main accrediting body for HMOs, requires HMOs to have a credentialing process that includes verification of such items as licensure, malpractice history, hospital privileges, and DEA certification (O'Kane 1993). Although accreditation by NCQA is voluntary, increasing numbers of employers are demanding that their HMOs receive NCQA accreditation ("More Employees Demand HMOs Get NCQA" 1993). State regulators generally require HMOs to have a credentialing process in place for selecting physicians, but they typically do not specify the elements to be included in this process (Kopit and Lutes 1993). State laws governing PPOs typically do not include credentialing requirements.

A key development in plans' ability to credential physicians is the establishment of the National Practitioner Data Bank (NPDB), created by the Health Care Quality Improvement Act of 1986. The act requires that providers, insurers, and licensing boards report to the NPDB malpractice suits and other incidents that indicate quality of care problems for physicians (Kongstvedt 1993). HMOs can query the data bank while credentialing their network physicians, but because PPOs lack "health care entity" status as defined in the act, they are not allowed access to the NPDB, at least not without physician approval (Brasher and Sweeris 1991). The extent to which plans use the NPDB to credential physicians is not known.

Many managed care plans delegate responsibility for credentialing physicians to a middle tier such as a medical group or an IPA, which in turn may rely on the credentialing done by another entity such as a hospital. In such cases, the HMO is responsible for ensuring that the ultimate credentialing system meets NCQA standards, and it remains legally responsible for the competence of its network physicians (Kopit and Lutes 1993). It is therefore in the interest of HMOs contracting with a middle tier to retain the right to approve, suspend, or terminate individual physicians, although it is not known how many plans explicitly retain this right in their contracts with middle tiers.

Physician Integration and Acculturation

We know very little about how, or even whether, plans socialize or promote the acculturation of physicians into their systems and, if relevant, their parent corporations. Specific steps to achieve initial orientation and integration are not documented. In addition, the extent to which plans rely on socialization rather than initial selection and pruning to achieve their goals is not clear. It seems plausible that group/staff model HMOs place greater emphasis on socialization than network/IPA model HMOs or PPOs, since the effectiveness and rewards of such efforts are likely to be greatest for physicians in large group practices devoted full-time to the plan. On the other hand, however, some network/IPA model plans and PPOs might place considerable emphasis on socialization efforts in an attempt to offset the lesser degree of integration expected among physicians contracting with the plan for only a portion of their practice. Such efforts are expected to be more successful among physicians for whom plan members comprise a large percentage of their caseloads, as discussed below.

Termination of Physicians

There is little information on the extent of physician turnover in managed care networks, regardless of whether it is plan- or physician-initiated turnover. Thus, it is not clear how stable or long-term the plan-physician relationship is. Plan-initiated termination of physicians may occur for many reasons. For example, plans might terminate physicians if they no longer use a network hospital, if they provide poor-quality care, if they refuse to comply with plan policies or administrative procedures, or if the plan wants to reduce the network size to gain control.

Little is known about the approaches plans use to identify "problem" (i.e., incompetent or high-cost) physicians nor about how plans terminate such physicians. For example, after plans identify problem physicians, it is not clear how much opportunity they give them to modify their behavior. Nor can we be sure about how reliable plans' assessments of physicians are. For specialists, who are in oversupply in some parts of the country, plans can be very selective about whom they keep in their network. In such areas, plans may not invest in trying to modify the behavior of physicians they have identified as problematic or high-cost—they may simply terminate their contracts with such physicians.

Berenson (1991) has argued that many plans have not been as effective as they could be in identifying and removing incompetent physicians. Although many plans are technically able to identify these physicians, Berenson argues that they lack the will to remove them from their networks. However, recent anecdotal evidence suggests that some plans have become aggressive about not renewing contracts with physicians, particularly specialists, in some parts of the country. A group of physicians in Houston who say they were recently dropped without warning from the networks of plans sponsored by two major commercial insurers has filed a lawsuit against the insurers (Winslow and Felsenthal 1993). Although their contracts with the plans gave each side the right to end the affiliation "without cause," the Houston physicians, joined by the county and state medical society, are arguing that to protect physician-patient relationships, insurers should not be allowed to drop physicians from networks without warning. They also argue that Texas law provides them with "due process" rights. However, case law pretty well establishes the right of managed care plans to terminate physicians if they follow a reasonable process (Kopit and Lutes 1993).

Anecdotal evidence suggests that the termination of large numbers of physicians from managed care networks is occurring in a number of metropolitan areas along with network reconfiguration. Sid Stolz, a principal at the consulting firm Towers Perrin, has observed that health plan networks throughout the country are changing to increase cost-effectiveness and that plans not making these changes will be left behind by the competition (Winslow and Felsenthal 1993). On the other hand, there are important market protections against plan actions to arbitrarily and frequently reconfigure their networks. Plans do not want to develop reputations for treating physicians unfairly or for interfering with established physician-patient relationships.

Network Philosophy and Strategy

The logic behind a plan's choice of arrangements with physicians is not well understood. Histories and descriptions of well-established plans such as Kaiser-Permanente (Somers 1971, Smillie 1991), Group Health Association (Berkowitz and Wolff 1988), and others (Friedson 1975) show how the relationship between health plans and their medical staffs have evolved. What current strategies are, whether they even exist, how they may differ between companies, or how they may be evolving, however, is information that is lacking. It may be difficult to determine whether a plan's arrangements with its physicians reflect a preferred strategy or merely an interim measure to accommodate the provider community or to establish a "beachhead" in a market. A better understanding of the tensions and processes could assist in projecting from current practices to the future.

It is important to better understand the strategies that plans follow in constructing physician networks. One strategy is to carefully screen physicians from the outset to obtain a cohesive, relatively small network of providers that the plan can control effectively, and then gradually add physicians over time as necessary to satisfy enrollment demands. An alternative strategy is to use broad initial selection criteria to create a relatively large network, and then "prune" the network over time to eliminate "problem" physicians. This second approach allows plans to achieve faster growth in enrollments, because large networks help satisfy purchasers that members will have adequate access to care, with minimal need to switch physicians. The second strategy may also be justified if plans have inadequate data to carefully screen physicians initially. However, this strategy may be disruptive if the plans prune significant numbers of physicians, requiring enrollees to switch physicians to remain with the plan. In practice, plans may attempt to achieve a balance between these two alternative strategies, although there is little evidence on this issue. The only available evidence pertains to plans sponsored by commercial insurers, who reportedly rely primarily on the broad initial selection strategy (Hoy, Curtis, and Rice 1991).

Recent evidence indicates that HMOs determine the number of primary care physicians required in their networks by considering three factors: (1) actual and projected growth in enrollment, (2) measures of enrollees' access to care, and (3) desires and requirements of employers (Felt, Frazer, and Gold 1994). Almost all group/staff model HMOs use staffing ratios as a tool to adjust their network size to account for enrollment changes. Network/IPA model plans do not use staffing ratios, however, because the physicians with whom they contract treat varying numbers of patients not in the plan. Even in group/staff model plans, staffing ratios play a relatively modest role in decisions about staffing needs, which are determined largely on the basis of experience, strategy, and judgment.

Little information is available on the obligations plans require from physicians concerning the proportion of their patient load comprising plan members.[3] On one hand, plans may prefer to contract with physicians who have a relatively high percentage of plan members in their patient load, because the plans' financial incentives are likely to be more effective, and the physicians may be more receptive to cooperating with the plans and complying with their requirements. On the other hand, some plans may not be seeking to influence physician practice patterns and may prefer to contract for a smaller share of a physician's practice, with the expectation that they may therefore receive a bigger discount by effectively paying marginal cost for excess capacity. This attitude was common in the past but may be becoming less common as managed care plans evolve.

There is little solid evidence in the literature on whether or how plans attempt to influence the proportion of plan members in the patient load of network physicians. U.S. Healthcare, an IPA-model HMO that capitates its primary care physicians (PCPs), offers its PCPs financial incentives to take on a high proportion of plan members as patients (Schlackman 1993). Specifically, PCPs receive an increase over the base capitation rate if they have more than a specified number of plan members as patients or if the number of plan members in their practice increases by more than 10 percent per year. It is not known whether other plans offer similar incentives or use other strategies to achieve this objective.

There is little, if any, information in the literature on how plans negotiate with physicians. For instance, it is not known whether any plans use competitive bidding for specialty care. And for three-tiered HMOs, it is not clear how much (if any) power the plans have to remove individual physicians from the middle tier (i.e., from a medical group or IPA). Various strategies for negotiation have been discussed and recommended in the trade literature, but the actual prevalence of these approaches is unknown (see, for example, Montague 1993, Ellenberger 1993, Korenchuk 1991, and Shouldice 1987).

The middle level of a managed care organization in three-tiered arrangements is an important feature that is not well understood. Studies of financial incentives in HMOs (e.g., Hillman, Welch, and Pauly 1992) tell us something about the distribution of HMOs among two- and three-tiered models and a little about the interrelationships with other organizational features, such as how risk is shared and the nature and size of the risk pool. However, few studies detail the organizational form of the middle level, its functions, and how it modifies both the directness of the relationship between managed care plans and physicians. Also unexplored is how physicians feel about this relationship—including their attitude toward requirements set by the plan and toward the middle entity, over which they may or may not feel they have control.

The renting of physician networks is a strategy commonly employed by commercial insurers offering PPO products (Hoy, Curtis, and Rice 1991). Renting a network is faster and less expensive than developing one by contracting directly with providers. To rent a network, the insurer pays an access fee based on its volume. Hoy, Curtis, and Rice also report that some commercial insurers have developed consortia in which they jointly develop and administer a network in a given geographic area. This gives the insurers greater ability to select and retain providers than they would have if they rented a network, and the market share of the consortium increases its power to negotiate with providers.

The marketplace in which managed care plans and physicians operate has been changing rapidly in the past few years. A number of investor-owned physician management companies have developed and begun buying medical group practices and marketing their services to managed care plans (Day 1993, Freudenheim 1993), and at least one insurer (Aetna) has begun buying such practices directly ("Aetna Goes Doc Hunting" 1993). In addition, physicians, hospitals, and other providers are developing integrated delivery systems that contract with managed care plans (and in some cases, directly with employers) to provide a coordinated continuum of care to plan members (Shortell, Gillies, and Anderson 1994; Burns and Thorpe 1993; Ogden 1993). Such developments are poorly documented, and we know little about how they may be changing the relationship between physicians and managed care plans.

Legal and Regulatory Requirements

Federal and state laws that constrain provider arrangements in managed care plans are reasonably well documented (Lutes and Hastings 1993). However, there is less information on how constraining these requirements are in practice when seen in light of gaps in regulatory authority or enforcement, preemptions under the ERISA statute, or innovative product designs. Questions about the extent to which legal requirements affect the behavior of plans in developing their networks remain unanswered. We know the general legal and regulatory environment in which plans operate, but we do not have a clear understanding from the literature about how certain variations in requirements across states or plan type affect plan behavior in developing networks. The federal HMO Act defines the requirements plans must meet to be federally qualified as an HMO. Although federal qualification is voluntary, many plans seek this status because it makes them more credible in the eyes of employers.[4] One of the review criteria in the federal qualification process is availability and accessibility of health services. A plan applying for federal qualification must submit maps designating its service area and identifying provider locations (and the number and type of providers at each location) to ensure that primary care and specialty services are available and accessible. However, federal legislation does not specify particular staffing ratios. Also, oversight of compliance with HMO Act requirements has been relatively weak in recent years.

HMOs are regulated by the states and must apply to the states for licensure.[5] Laws regulating HMOs vary by state, although 27 states have adopted the Model HMO Act, or substantial portions of it, developed by the National Association of Insurance Commissioners (NAIC). The NAIC Model HMO Act does not prescribe specific staffing ratios, although a few states specify minimum staffing ratios for closed panel plans in their regulations. For example, Pennsylvania requires 1 physician per 1,600 members (Kongstvedt 1993).

The growing concern by providers over the implications of being excluded from managed care networks has prompted a number of states to enact "any willing provider" laws. Such laws prevent plans from excluding from their networks providers that are willing to accept the plan's contractual requirements. Twenty-one states have enacted "any willing provider" laws for HMOs, although the laws in six states apply only to "any willing pharmacists" (Iglehart 1994a). In addition, nine states allow HMO enrollees to self-refer to non-network providers for specified services (GHAA 1993c). Eight states have "any willing provider" laws for PPOs and numerous other states are considering such statutes (Biskupie 1993). However, the extent to which these laws are enforced varies from state to state. The Supreme Court has decided not to review a lower court ruling upholding Virginia's "any willing provider" law. Such laws make it difficult for plans to exclude providers from their network but may also have loopholes allowing exclusion under given circumstances.

Physician Payment and Financial Incentives

The three basic approaches to paying physicians in managed care plans are salary, capitation, and fee-for-service (FFS). In addition, many plans include risk-sharing, bonus arrangements, or both in their compensation packages to encourage cost-conscious behavior by physicians. In reviewing what is known about these payment mechanisms, the distinction between two-tiered and three-tiered plans is critical. Specifically, in three-tiered plans, the incentives for physicians are determined not so much by the financial arrangements between the plan and the middle tier (e.g., a medical group), but rather by the arrangements between the middle tier and the physicians (Hillman, Welch, and Pauly 1992).

Payment Approaches

Much of the literature on physician payment approaches used by managed care plans has focused on how HMOs pay PCPs. In recent years, a number of cross-plan studies of payment mechanisms and financial incentives used by HMOs have appeared in the literature (Hillman 1987; Hillman, Welch, and Pauly 1992; Pauly, Hillman, and Kerstein 1990; GHAA 1992, 1993b; U.S. Department of Health and Human Services 1990). The literature also indicates considerable analysis and discussion of individual plan-specific payment approaches and strategies (see, for example, Goldfield et al. 1992, Cave 1993, Cave and Tucker 1990, Diller 1992, Gnessin 1990, Kouba 1991, Herrle 1992, Lipsitz et al. 1993). The most careful and comprehensive study of PCP payment approaches was conducted by Hillman, Welch, and Pauly (1992), who used data from a national survey of 260 HMOs in 1988. For two-tiered HMOs, the survey collected data on how the HMO paid its PCPs. For three-tiered HMOs, the survey collected data on how the HMO paid the middle tier and how the middle tier paid its PCPs. When the authors examined how individual PCPs were ultimately paid across all HMOs, they found that PCPs received payment through salaries in 23 percent of the plans, through capitation in 35 percent, and through FFS in 36 percent of plans.[6] The method of payment was not known in 6 percent of the plans, reflecting the fact that some managers at three-tiered HMOs did not know how PCPs were paid by the middle tier.

Hillman, Welch, and Pauly (1992) did not present findings for HMOs classified according to a standard typology (e.g., staff, group, network, and IPA), so comparison with other studies is not straightforward. They did present findings separately for two-tiered and three-tiered HMOs, however. The authors noted that previous studies, which failed to adequately distinguish three-tiered from two-tiered HMOs, have probably overestimated the extent to which HMOs pay physicians by capitation, because they failed to recognize that capitation payments made by the HMO to a middle tier are often converted to salary or FFS payments to PCPs. This makes it difficult to identify any trends in how individual PCPs are paid by HMOs.

The latest GHAA *HMO Industry Profile* to include data on financial arrangements with physicians indicates that in 1992, 14 percent of HMOs paid individual PCPs primarily by salary, 44 percent by capitation, and 42 percent by FFS (GHAA 1993b). Salary is by far the most common payment method among staff model plans, whereas group model plans nearly equally use salary, capitation, and FFS. In IPA model plans, FFS is the most common payment method (53 percent of plans), followed by capitation (47 percent) and salary (1 percent). In network model plans, capitation is the most common method (67 percent), followed by FFS (18 percent) and salary (15 percent). Among plans that pay PCPs by FFS, 77 percent use a fee schedule; 19 percent pay discounted usual, customary, and reasonable (UCR) charges; and 4 percent pay UCR charges. However, 62 percent of enrollees in traditional HMOs now are in plans that are known to pay their PCPs on salary or capitation (InterStudy 1994).

There is less evidence in the literature on how HMOs pay specialists. Hillman (1987) reports that 13 percent of the HMOs he surveyed paid specialists completely or partly by capitation. Payment to specialists was not the primary focus of the study, however, so no evidence was given either on the prevalence of salary and FFS payments to specialists or on the types of specialists that received capitation payments. Goldfield et al. (1992) assert that an increasing number of HMOs are capitating specialists, but no evidence was given on the number and types of HMOs that capitate specialists or on the types of specialists that receive capitation. The trade literature contains anecdotal evidence that increasing numbers of specialty groups such as radiologists are being capitated by HMOs. This is consistent with recent HMO survey data showing that 30 percent of all HMOs and 24 percent of IPAs mixed models capitate specialists (InterStudy 1994).

PPOs have traditionally paid physicians on a FFS basis. In a survey of 116 PPOs that submitted letters of interest for a Medicare PPO demonstration, 60 percent indicated that they base their payments to physicians on a fee schedule, 29 percent pay discounted UCR charges, 7 percent pay UCR charges, and 4 percent use mixed systems with one payment method for their PCPs and another for specialists (Langwell, Carlton, and Swearingen 1989). These findings are consistent with earlier published findings (de Lissovoy et al. 1987) and a more recent survey of PPOs (Marion Merrill Dow 1993). de Lissovoy et al. noted that some PPOs in their survey used a gatekeeper model in which the gatekeeper received a capitation payment or retainer for case management. Some analysts would regard such an arrangement as a point-of-service (POS) plan rather than a true PPO, although as noted above standard definitions have not been accepted on this distinction (Miller and Luft 1991).

There is little evidence in the literature on how payments are modified for physicians in POS products. Kongstvedt (1993) has described the challenges faced by POS plans that attempt to capitate a gatekeeper. Some plans reportedly adjust the capitation rate downward to account for expected out-of-network use by enrollees. Others reportedly make retroactive adjustments to capitation payments to account for actual out-of-network use. Both methods are unpopular with providers and difficult to administer, so many managed care firms that offer both an HMO and a POS plan reportedly capitate gatekeepers for HMO enrollees but pay FFS for POS enrollees. The extent to which these various payment methods are used in POS plans is not known. However, Kongstvedt argues that the increased popularity of POS plans has increased the need for managed care plans to use FFS.

If approximately 35 to 40 percent of HMOs pay their PCPs by FFS, and PPOs and POS plans are growing more popular, FFS payment plays an important role in managed care. The literature contains much evidence on the disadvantages of FFS payment in terms of the incentives for increased service use. To counteract these incentives, managed care plans can use a variety of techniques (discussion follows) including provider risk-sharing arrangements, utilization management procedures, and physician profiling to identify, educate, and possibly remove high-cost providers. Managed care plans can also attempt to influence physician behavior through the design and administration of FFS payment systems. For example, some plans could implement fee schedules based on the resource-based relative value scale (RBRVS) used in the new Medicare fee schedule. Blue Cross and Blue Shield of California recently decided to implement a resource-based fee schedule for 44,000 physicians belonging to its PPO network ("California Blue Shield Adopts" 1994). RBRVS does not eliminate the incentives inherent in FFS payment to provide more services, but it reduces the financial incentives for providing complex procedures relative to patient evaluation and management-oriented primary care services.

We know very little about whether and how managed care plans are using RBRVS. The latter point is particularly critical, as RBRVS can be used for many purposes short of pure payment (e.g., charge screening and input to setting salaries by specialty). Only 12 percent of HMOs report using some form of relative value scale for specialists and 11 percent for PCPs (InterStudy 1994). In any case, it is unlikely that many plans are adopting Medicare's system without any modification (e.g., higher conversion factors, blended rates, revised pediatric or obstetric weights). In December 1992, PPRC surveyed 20 Blue Cross and Blue Shield plans and 16 large commercial insurers and commercial managed care organizations to investigate how they have used, or plan to use, the Medicare RBRVS (Physician Payment Review Commission [PPRC] 1993).[7] This survey found that some PPOs and IPA model HMOs have used the Medicare RBRVS either to modify their existing fee schedules or to develop new fee schedules to replace a UCR system. Because the sample of payers with managed care plans was relatively small, PPRC was not able to infer anything about the percentage of managed care plans that have used the Medicare RBRVS. In its 1994 report, PPRC (1994) reviews more recent evidence indicating growing use of RBRVS by both private payors (especially BCBS) and Medicaid. However, although some studies touch on managed care arrangements, none focuses specifically on identifying the use of RBRVS by managed care plans.

Some managed care plans have reportedly negotiated specialized contracts with providers for certain high-cost services such as cardiac bypass surgery, organ transplants, oncology care, spinal and head injury care, and neurosurgery (Kretz 1991). This approach is similar to the Health Care Financing Administration's demonstration of "centers for excellence" for cardiac bypass surgery. Typically, a small number of providers are selected for such contracts according to their specialized expertise. Payment for such services is often reportedly based on a bundled rate that includes payment for physician services, inpatient hospital care, and ancillary services. Information on such payment approaches comes from the trade literature and is anecdotal in nature. Data are not available on the number and types of managed care plans that have negotiated such arrangements or the types of services that have been covered under these arrangements.

Another poorly researched question involves understanding how, if at all, managed care plans vary payment across payers. Medicaid studies document the apparently unique use of case management fees in primary care case management models of managed care delivery (Hurley, Freund, and Paul 1993). We know very little about how capitation and risk-based payments may be adjusted for differences in patient mix that distinguish Medicare, Medicaid, and commercial patients from one another, or about how payment rates may vary, if at all, for these different market sectors.

Risk Sharing and Bonus Arrangements

Many managed care plans use various risk-sharing mechanisms, bonus mechanisms, or both to influence physician behavior. Most of the literature on these financial incentives has focused on HMOs. Much of it discusses the merits or analyzes the effects of these incentives on cost and quality (see, for example, Bronow 1993, Berenson 1987, Church 1989, Hillman 1991, and Anders 1993), but only a few studies address the actual prevalence of different approaches. The most common is for the HMO to withhold a portion of the payment to the PCP until the end of the year. At year-end, actual costs for specialty referrals and inpatient care are compared with the amounts the plan allocated from premium revenue to pay for such services. If there is a deficit in the specialty and inpatient funds, the plan retains the withheld funds to cover the deficit. If there is a surplus, the plan may return some or all of the withheld funds. The amount of the withheld funds returned often depends on the economic performance of the individual physician, that is, the size of the surplus in the withholding fund for his or her own patients. However, it may also often depend on the performance of the risk pool with which that physician is associated.

In a survey of approximately 300 HMOs, Hillman (1987) found that approximately two-thirds of the contractual arrangements between HMOs and PCPs included a withholding provision. Only 21 percent of the plans that paid PCPs on a salary basis used withholding, while 82 percent of the plans that paid FFS and 67 percent of those that paid capitation used withholding, whereas 82 percent of the plans that paid FFS and 67 percent of those that paid capitation used withholding. Regardless of the basic method of payment, most HMOs in the study withheld between 11 and 20 percent of the payment amount. Kongstvedt (1993) reports that many HMOs include a provision in their contracts with PCPs authorizing them to increase the withholding percentage during the course of the year if the year-to-date deficits in the referral and inpatient funds exceed the amount of the funds withheld. In addition, some plans put physicians at risk for more than the amount withheld—for example, by increasing the withholding percentage or reducing the capitation rate for the physician the following year.

Plans that use withholding arrangements organize their physicians into risk pools. At one extreme, a risk pool can consist of individual PCPs; that is, the amount (if any) of the withheld funds received by a given PCP at year-end depends on the amount of any surplus or deficit in the referral and hospital funds for his or her own patients. At the other extreme, the risk pool may include all physicians in the HMO. Many HMOs define risk pools as subsets of the plan physicians, such as medical group practices or PCPs within a defined geographic area. Of the HMOs studied by Hillman, Welch, and Pauly (1992), 15 percent defined their risk pools as individual PCPs, 34 percent defined them as subsets of plan PCPs (such as medical groups), and 40 percent defined them as all PCPs in the plan.[3]

Even when risk pools include subsets of plan physicians or all plan physicians, risk is often shared with all physicians in the risk pool, but reward is tracked individually. That is, the amount of any surplus returned to an individual physician often depends on his or her own performance. Plans typically apply some type of stop-loss to protect PCPs in the case of expensive cases. For example, after referral or inpatient costs for a particular patient exceed a specified threshold, they are no longer counted against the physician's balance in his or her withholding fund—or in some plans, a percentage of such costs, say 20 percent, above the threshold is counted (Kongstvedt 1993).

Staff model HMOs rely more on bonuses than on withholding arrangements (Kongstvedt 1993). Bonuses are typically based on either total plan performance or how actual medical costs compare with projected costs. They are often also linked with formal performance evaluations, which may depend on factors such as productivity, medical knowledge, and management of patient care.

Concerned that rewards based only on cost and utilization may "send the wrong message," some plans have developed incentive systems that also account for such factors as quality of care or patient satisfaction as well as use and cost. Schlackman (1993) has described an innovative payment system developed by U.S. Healthcare to adjust the capitation payments paid to its PCPs. The base capitation rate received by a primary care office, which depends on the age and sex of the office members, is adjusted by a "quality factor" derived from three components: (1) quality review, (2) comprehensive care, and (3) use. The quality review component is based on member surveys, medical record reviews, the transfer rate of patients out of the PCP's office, and managed care philosophy. The comprehensive care component allows primary care offices to receive increases in the base capitation amount through such activities as serving large numbers of plan members or extending office hours. The adjustment to the capitation rate is derived from a formula in which the quality review and comprehensive care components receive a combined weight of 82 percent, whereas the use component receives a weight of 18 percent. Offices are re-evaluated at six-month intervals and receive continual feedback.

At least two other HMOs have reportedly implemented systems in which quality of care and patient satisfaction are used to determine PCP financial rewards, and such systems are being tested by other plans (Morain 1992). The approaches used by the other plans have not been described in detail in the literature. GHAA's surveys indicate that 22 percent of plans make some use of quality and 16 percent make some use of patient satisfaction information in paying providers (GHAA 1992). However, it is unclear what methods plans are using to do so and unlikely that large numbers of plans currently are doing so extensively or with well defined data. Anecdotal evidence suggests that managed care managers differ in their opinions about how valuable or feasible these approaches are, but these issues are not well researched. Hillman (1991) has conducted some research exploring physician manager's general attitudes about the value and impact of various financial incentives in HMOs.

The preceding research provides some insight into how risk is ultimately distributed between plans and physicians, particularly primary care physicians, taking into account both payment and incentive arrangements. Less is known about how the administrative costs or markup of these arrangements influences the amount of premium available for care delivery. Similarly, there is relatively limited information on how risk and incentive payments influence the variation in physician income. Such variation may be either theoretical (the maximum amount of spread possible in income) or empirical (the amount of spread that occurs in reality). In effect, incentive arrangements that place a great deal of risk on individual physicians are probably equivalent to a very tight individual capitation payment with no additional incentive payment. The federal government has recently enacted rules that limit financial risk to individual physicians for Medicare and Medicaid payments to 30 percent of payment for services ("HMO MD Incentive Rules Proposed" 1993).

Monitoring Physicians and Influencing Practice

Managed care plans rely on nonfinancial mechanisms as well as financial incentives to affect physician practice. It is important to understand the types of nonfinancial mechanisms plans used to monitor physicians and influence practice, the objectives plans seek to achieve with these mechanisms, and how, if at all, they relate to the plans' financial incentives. In this section, we discuss what is known and not known about five types of nonfinancial mechanisms: profiling systems, gatekeeper arrangements, utilization management techniques, focused studies and clinical indicators, and practice guidelines.

Profiling Systems

Surveys of HMOs and PPOs have found that significant numbers of plans maintain some type of physician profile system. For example, of 41 HMOs included in a case study of plans with Medicare risk contracts, 59 percent reported maintaining profiling data (Nelson et al. 1990). The majority of these plans had profiles for individual physicians, but some maintained them on an aggregate basis. The HMOs differed in how they used the profiles. Some used them to monitor the performance of individual physicians (i.e., to identify outliers). Others reported using aggregate profiles for overall monitoring of plan performance and physician education. Some HMOs also reported using profiles to monitor the behavior of capitated physicians to ensure that they were not skimping on care. InterStudy (1994) indicates that 90 percent of HMOs provide primary care physicians with some form of information on service use and 71 percent on rates of preventive measures but only 25 percent with rates of disease incidence and 22 percent patient health status. However, 81 percent reported tracking patient outcomes for specific conditions, including 58 percent using rates of complications or readmissions, 44 percent cost effectiveness measures, and 27 percent functional status measures.

Profiling is also done by many PPOs. Langwell, Carlton, and Swearingen (1989) report that 23 percent of the 102 PPOs that completed a survey expressing interest in a Medicare PPO demonstration reported that they maintained physician profiles. Hoy, Curtis, and Rice (1991) report that nearly all PPOs sponsored by commercial insurers maintain physician profiles, although they did not describe them.

The PPRC sponsored a conference on profiling to address concerns that "the ease with which profiling can be done may be outpacing the ability to use profiling effectively and responsibly" (PPRC 1992). The papers presented at the conference discussed key issues related to profiling, including what is being profiled (e.g., outcomes or process), the data needs for profiling, and the possible uses of profiling by plans and health care providers (such as feedback mechanisms, payment adjustment, and physician selection).

Although we have little evidence on the range of profiling systems used by managed care plans throughout the United States, there are several articles in the trade and research literature describing individual systems (Braham and Ruchlin 1987, Betty et al. 1990, Gottlieb, Margolis, and Schoenbaum 1990, Heinen et al. 1993, McGuirk-Porell et al 1991, Berwick and Coltin 1986, Winickoff et al. 1984). Findlay (1993) recently documented some other individual efforts, noting that a number of plans intend to substitute profiling systems for what they allege are more expensive and time-consuming utilization review systems. In this context, profiling can screen physicians as well as claims or bills. According to Findlay, most of the efforts are relatively new, and few plans have fully operating systems.

Most examples of the profiling systems referred to above are used by HMOs—some systems profile physicians throughout the HMO, and others are used by specific group practices within an HMO. The systems usually collect utilization statistics on individual physicians and compare them to peer group statistics (such as mean admission rates for a particular specialty group within the HMO) rather than to normative standards. One system, developed at the Harvard Community Health Plan, used practice guidelines developed by the physician staff as a benchmark comparison for its physician profiles (Gottlieb, Margolis, and Schoenbaum 1990). The profile comparisons primarily serve as feedback mechanisms for the physicians. Few of the articles describe plan actions to handle "outlier" physicians. How plans attempt to modify undesirable physician behavior identified through the profiling or whether plans actually remove physicians from networks based on profiles remain unanswered. There is also little discussion of adjustments for case-mix differences when comparing profiling measures across physicians or how data problems (e.g., faulty diagnosis codes or care excluded because it is not billed separately) constrain the results or detract from the perceived value of these approaches. (The one exception is an article on a profiling software package developed by the Medical Group Management Association that measures physician productivity and adjusts for relative intensity of services provided through the use of resource-based relative value units, Lazarus et al. 1989.) Also lacking attention in the literature are problems of profiling caused, for instance, by POS products or by the small number of patients any physician may serve, both in general and for that HMO.

Gatekeeper Arrangements

The literature indicates that the vast majority of HMOs in some way use primary care physicians as gatekeepers or case managers. According to a 1987 survey of HMOs by GHAA, over 90 percent use primary care gatekeepers (GHAA 1988). Nelson et al. (1990), in a case study of 41 HMOs operating under Medicare risk contracts, found that over 80 percent use primary care gatekeepers, although most plans prefer the term "case manager" to "gatekeeper." Franks, Clancy, and Nutting (1992) point out that the term gatekeeper has acquired a negative connotation, implying that the physician is the agent of the HMO, restricting patients' access to high-cost medical care, rather than the agent of the patient. They emphasize the role of the gatekeeper in coordinating patient care and protecting patients from the adverse effects of unnecessary care. Published data on the prevalence of gatekeeping do not tend to distinguish between the differences in gatekeeper models, which vary in the degree to which they are used to score (reward, or both) individual performance, serve as prior approval mechanisms, or organize and coordinate care.

Although most HMOs report that they use primary care gatekeepers, there is less information in the literature about the structure of gatekeeper systems and the responsibilities of gatekeepers. Physicians as gatekeepers may be family practice physicians, general practitioners, internists, pediatricians, and in some HMOs, obstetrician/gynecologists (OB/GYNs). It is not known how many HMOs permit women to select an OB/GYN as a gatekeeper. Plans in which women choose a physician other than an OB/GYN as a gatekeeper raise the question of whether women can self-refer to an OB/GYN or alternative providers, such as nurse midwives. More generally, can mental health or substance abuse be accessed on self-referral? Are subspecialists used as gatekeepers for particular categories of chronically ill patients, and if so, how? Similarly, little effort has been devoted to understanding the differences between arrangements involving assignment to individual physicians and those based on a larger number of providers in the group setting, where the paper record may substitute for a direct patient/physician bond.

The literature does not provide detailed information on the responsibilities HMOs assign the gatekeeper. Nelson et al. (1990), in a study of 41 HMOs with Medicare risk contracts, found that although over 80 percent of plans use primary care gatekeepers, only 42 percent require enrollees to obtain prior approval from the gatekeeper for specialty care. A survey of managers of 91 HMOs conducted by AMCRA found that about half of the plans that used gatekeepers allow members to self-refer to specialists (Traska 1988). Neither of these studies report whether there are certain types of specialists for which self-referral is permitted by HMOs. And in plans that require the patient to go through the gatekeeper, still more questions remain: How strict is the enforcement? Must patients visit the gatekeeper, or is a telephone call sufficient?

Relatively little is known about the use of gatekeeping in PPOs and point-of-service products. Although it appears that some PPOs are developing gatekeeper models, the extent of this effort is not known. Recent data show that 44 percent of PPOs offer an EPO product and that of these, 68 percent require that patients enroll (Marion Merrill Dow 1993).

Utilization Management Techniques

HMOs and PPOs have historically used a variety of utilization management procedures to control costs. In case studies of 41 HMOs with Medicare risk contracts (Nelson et al. 1990), plans report using the following utilization management procedures:

- 88 percent require prior authorization for nonemergency hospital admissions from either a gatekeeper, the HMO utilization review staff, or the medical director

- 95 percent conduct routine concurrent reviews of all hospital stays
- 90 percent use some form of discharge planning, the nature of which varied across plans from simply assigning an expected length of stay at admission to intensive planning for post-discharge service use to facilitate early discharge
- 56 percent conduct retrospective reviews of inpatient stays, although most do so infrequently (e.g., reviews of a random sample of stays or of stays for which a question arose about the claim)
- 42 percent require prior authorization from a primary care physician for referral physicians (i.e., specialists)—some all the time and others just for out-of-network care
- 49 percent conduct ambulatory utilization review, such as prior authorization for certain resource-intensive services (e.g., ambulatory surgeries and MRI) and ongoing review of continual treatment (e.g., psychiatric care)

Hoy, Curtis, and Rice (1991) report that practically all PPOs sponsored by commercial insurance companies use precertification, concurrent review, and discharge planning to control inpatient costs, and that 58 percent of the PPOs require second opinions for surgeries. However, the insurers report that the requirement for a second opinion was waived in cases where clinical guidelines indicated surgery was necessary. Langwell, Carlton, and Swearingen (1989) report that of 102 PPOs responding to a survey of their interest in a Medicare PPO demonstration, 78 percent require prior authorization for hospital admissions, 51 percent use concurrent inpatient review, 55 percent use retrospective inpatient review, 31 percent use discharge planning, 44 percent require second opinions for surgeries, and 29 percent require prior authorization for resource intensive ambulatory surgeries and treatments.

However, there is less information about differences in the structure of these programs across managed care plans. For example, we do not know the extent to which utilization review is based on formal criteria and whether there are exceptions for more difficult cases, which effectively leave criteria ambiguous or not explicit. It is not clear what happens when care deviates from the criteria.

Also not clear is how plans view the relative trade-offs between utilization management, physician profiling, physician financial incentives, and organizational culture. For example, plans that place physicians at financial risk for inpatient care and specialty referrals may choose to rely less on case-by-case utilization management procedures. Some plans may substitute careful provider selection, socialization on appropriate use, and peer review for more externally based reviews. Similarly, plans that maintain profiles of individual physician practice patterns may choose to spend fewer resources on utilization management. There is no evidence in the literature to support these hypotheses. Finally, there is a question that concerns three-tiered HMOs: We are not certain about the extent to which they delegate utilization review activities to the middle tier and with what, if any, constraints they may do so.

Focused Studies and Clinical Indicators

Continuous quality improvement (CQI) is a current popular concept in managed care (e.g., Schlackman 1991, Burns et al. 1992, and Burda 1991). Anecdotally, we understand that many plans claim to be striving to create population-based and other measures of quality to monitor and improve performance. However, there is little information on how many plans conduct such studies, what topics they include, what they use them for, and how they are developed or obtained. We understand that HMOs are gearing up both for NCQA accreditation and to prepare HEDIS information on quality and other indicators for purchasers, but it is not clear how many can report such indicators. Nor is it certain when they will be able to do so (11 percent say they report these data now [InterStudy 1994]). In addition, the administrative requirements on physician offices to support such systems are not clear. Such requirements might include administrative data or access to clinical records for chart review.

Practice Guidelines

There is considerable interest nationwide in practice guidelines because, even though they may have been oversold (United States Congress 1994), they focus on issues of both quality and cost-effectiveness. It is not known how many plans currently use formal, written practice guidelines, the specific health conditions or screening procedures for which they are used, or the sources of the guidelines. Plans using practice guidelines could potentially derive them from various federal agencies (most recently the Agency for Health Care Policy Research), from national professional associations (such as the National Cancer Society), or from the plan's parent company. It is also not known how plans monitor compliance with their guidelines, including, for example, the extent to which they rely on chart reviews or administrative/claims data to monitor compliance.

Conclusion

This literature synthesis shows how little we know about important features of the arrangements managed care plans make with their physicians. Most of the existing knowledge is dated, derived from a limited subset of managed care plans, inattentive to important structural differences between plans, and responsive only to relatively narrow issues such as compensation arrangements. And because many plans' features are not rigorously defined (e.g., credentialing, profiling, gatekeeping), the findings from methodologically sound studies are often not comparable to one another.

Addressing the enormous gaps in our current body of knowledge should be an urgent priority for the research community and for agencies and foundations that support research into medical care organization. The reason for this urgency can be found in the pervasive and fundamental impacts that managed care plans are having on the delivery of care and the practice of medicine. This transformation of our nation's health care system is proceeding at an accelerating pace and we have painfully little sound evidence to either describe or to understand it, let alone to shape it.

The new world of managed care has profound implications for physician supply, organizational arrangement, specialty mix, practitioner working conditions, compensation arrangements, performance appraisal, and physician satisfaction. In every one of these areas, there is minimal credible research that adequately addresses the implications. Writing in the 1930s, the prescient Committee on the Costs of Medical Care observed that our medical technology was advancing as if it were aboard an airplane while our knowledge of the organization of medical care was proceeding on a stagecoach (Starr 1982). This observation rings perilously true today, more than a half-century later.

Acknowledgments

Jack Hoadley, Principal Policy Analyst with the Physician Payment Review Commission, conceived of the need for the project upon which this article is based. We are also appreciative of the insights provided by both Jack and others in the research, managed care and purchaser communities on the critical issues and questions they perceive on this topic.

Notes

1. EPO products vary. Some simulate HMOs, with patients paying 100 percent for out-of-network care. Others have intermediate cost sharing (e.g., 50 percent) with a high out-of-pocket maximum for opting out of network.
2. For discussion of screening for improper billing practices, see Morreim (1991).
3. GHAA has collected information on the average share of a physician's practice representing members of the HMO, but no comparable data exist for other managed care forms. The HMO data show that, as expected, there is a much greater level of commitment within group and staff models (61 to 63 percent of these plans involve physicians with at least 80 percent of their patients from the HMO, compared with

6 to 8 percent for network and IPA model plans). Nonetheless, the data also show that there is considerable variation both within plans of the same model and within the same plan (Gold 1991).

4. In recent years, the concern that federal qualifications could constrain an HMO's ability to respond to market forces has led some plans not to seek qualification or to develop nonqualified products.
5. For a detailed review of the impact of state laws on managed care plans, see Cooper and Green (1991).
6. Some plans using capitation for individual physicians exclude selected services and pay for them on a FFS basis to encourage physicians to provide them or to encourage primary care physicians rather than specialists to provide them.
7. This survey examined the use of Medicare's RBRVS by private payers in general, some of which offered managed care plans. Thus, the focus was not specifically on managed care plans.
8. The information on risk pools was missing from the other 11 percent.

References

Aetna goes doc hunting to staff its new primary care offices. 1993. *Managed Care Week* November 1, p. 3.

Anders, G. 1993. More managed care systems use incentive pay to reward "best" doctors. *Wall Street Journal* January 25, p. B4.

Ballard, M., and M. Terze. 1993. Automated credentialing: A practical approach to quality measurement. *AAPPO Journal* 36: 10–13.

Berenson, R. 1987. Hidden compromises in paying physicians. *Business and Health* July: 18–22.

———. 1991. A physician's view of managed care. *Health Affairs* 10 (4): 106–19.

Berkowitz, E., and W. Wolff. 1988. *Group Health Association: A portrait of a health maintenance organization.* Philadelphia, PA: Temple University Press.

Berwick, D., and K. Coltin. 1986. Feedback reduces test use in a health maintenance organization. *Journal of the American Medical Association* 255: 1450–54.

Betty, W., H. Hendricks, H. Rucchlin, and R. Braham. 1990. Physician practice profiling: A valuable information system for HMOs. *Medical Group Management Journal* November/December: 68–75.

Biskupic, J. 1993. Justices uphold ruling on hospital-insurer contracts. *Washington Post* November 30, p. A16.

Braham, R. L., and H. S. Ruchlin. 1987. Physician practice profiles: A case study of the use of audit and feedback in an ambulatory care group practice. *Health Care Management Review* 12: 11–16.

Brasher, P., and C. Sweeris. 1991. Resolving the National Practitioner Data Bank Dilemma. *AAPPO Journal* September: 27–33.

Bronow, R. 1993. HMO physician shared risk pools are dangerous to patients' health. *HealthSpan*, 10 (1): 9–12.

Burda, D. 1991. The two quality faces of HCHP. *Modern Health Care* 21 (11): 28–31.

Burns, L., and D. P. Thorpe. 1993. Trends and models in physician-hospital organization. *Health Care Management Review* 18 (4): 7–20.

Burns, L., M. Denton, S. Goldfein, L. Warrick, B. Morenz, and B. Sales. 1992. The use of continuous quality improvement methods in the development and dissemination of medical practice guidelines. *Quality Review Bulletin* December: 434–39.

California Blue Shield adopts RBRVS-based fees for PPO docs. 1994. *Managed Care Week* January 17, p. 3.

Cave, D. 1993. Incentives and cost-containment in primary care physician reimbursement. *Benefits Quarterly* 9 (3): 70–77.

Cave, D., and L. Tucker. 1990. Can physician capitation survive in the 1990s—HMOs will need to offset systematic risk. Paper presented at the Group Health Association of America conference, Los Angeles, California, June.

Church, D. 1989. An alternative to primary care capitation in an IPA model HMO. *Medical Interface* 2 (11): 37–39, 41–42.

Cooper, P., and K. Green. 1991. The impact of state laws on managed care. *Health Affairs* Winter: 161–69.

Day, K. 1993. A rush to "buy" doctors. *Washington Post* November 5, p. A1.

de Lissovoy, G., T. Rice, J. Gabel, and H. Gelzer. 1987. Preferred provider organizations one year later. *Inquiry* 24 (Summer): 127–35.

DeLoitte and Touche. 1992. *U.S. hospitals and the future of health care.* Boston, MA: DeLoitte and Touche.

Diller, W. 1992. Physician fee schedules help employers control cost increases. *Business and Health* 10 (8): 22–26.

Ellenberger, A. 1993. Managed care and physician contracting skills: Questions to ask. *American College of Surgeons Bulletin* 7 (5): 30–33.

Felt, S., H. Frazer, and M. Gold. 1994. *HMO primary care staffing patterns and processes: A cross-site analysis of 23 HMOs.* Washington, DC: Mathematica Policy Research.

Findlay, S. 1993. Profiling systems aim to eliminate second guessing of doctors. *Business and Health* April: 58–64.

Fisher, N., S. Howard, and D. Pasternak. 1993. Critical factors in recruiting health maintenance organization physicians. *Health Care Management Review* 18 (1): 51–61.

Franks, P., C. Clancy, and P. Nutting. 1992. Gatekeeping revisited—Protecting patients from overtreatment. *New England Journal of Medicine* 327 (6): 424–29.

Freudenheim, M. 1993. Physicians are selling practices to companies as changes loom. *New York Times* September 1, p. A1.

Friedson, E. 1975. *Doctoring together: A study of professional control.* New York: Elsevier Scientific.

Group Health Association of America. 1988. Unique approaches to case management. *GHAA News* 29 (2): 7–11.

———. 1992. *Industry profile.* Washington, DC: Group Health Association of America.

———. 1993a. *The recruitment experience of health maintenance organizations for primary care physicians.* Washington, DC: Group Health Association of America.

———. 1993b. *Industry profile.* Washington, DC: Group Health Association of America.

———. 1993c. *Open-panel provisions applicable to HMOs: Laws and 1993 proposals.* Washington, DC: Group Health Association of America.

Gold, M. 1991. HMOs and managed care. *Health Affairs* 10 (4): 189–206.

Goldfield, N., H. Berman, A. Collins, R. Cooper, D. Fragalin, P. Kongstvedt, N. Payson,

P. Siegel, A. Southam, and E. Weis. 1992. Methods of compensating physicians contracting with managed care organizations. *Journal of Ambulatory Care Management* 15 (4): 81–92.

Gottlieb, L., C. Margolis, and S. Schoenbaum. 1990. Clinical practice guidelines within an HMO: Development and implementation of quality improvement model. *Quality Review Bulletin* 16: 80–86.

Gnessin, A. 1990. Discrete capitation elements and provider stop-loss. Paper presented at the Group Health Association of America conference, Los Angeles, California, June.

Heinen, L., E. Peterson, K. Pion, and S. Leatherman. 1993. Quality evaluation in a managed care system: Comparative data to assess health plan performance. *Managed Care Quarterly* 1 (1): 62–76.

Herrle, G. 1992. Physician compensation in the era of managed care. *Medical Group Management Journal* November/December: 8–9.

Hillman, A. 1987. Financial incentives for physicians in HMOs. *New England Journal of Medicine* 317 (27): 1743–48.

———. 1991. Managing the physician: Rules vs. incentives. *Health Affairs* Winter: 138–46.

Hillman, A., W. P. Welch, and M. Pauly. 1992. Contractual arrangements between HMOs and primary care physicians: Three-tiered HMOs and risk pools. *Medical Care* 30 (2): 136–48.

HMO MD incentive rules proposed with risk thresholds. *Managed Care Week* January 4, p. 1.

Hoy, E., R. Curtis, and T. Rice. 1991. Change and growth in managed care. *Health Affairs* 10 (4): 18–36.

Hurley, R., D. Freund, and J. Paul. 1993. *Managed care in Medicaid: Lessons for policy and program design.* Ann Arbor, MI: Health Administration Press.

Iglehart, J. K. 1994a. The struggle between managed care and fee-for service practice. *New England Journal of Medicine* 331 (1): 63–67.

———. 1994b. Physicians and the growth of managed care. *New England Journal of Medicine* 331 (17): 1167–71.

Jacobs, M., and P. Mott. 1987. Physician characteristics and training emphasis considered desirable by leaders of HMOs. *Journal of Medical Education* 62 (September): 725–31.

Kongstvedt, P. 1993. Primary care in closed panels. In *The managed care handbook*, edited by Peter Kongstvedt. Gaithersburg, MD: Aspen.

Kopit, W., and M. Lutes. 1993. Legal issues and antitrust considerations in the establishment of credentialing and other selection criteria. In *The managed care handbook*, edited by Peter Kongstvedt. Gaithersburg, MD: Aspen.

Korenchuk, K. 1991. Negotiating and analyzing managed care contracts. *Medical Group Management Journal* 38 (1): 17–18, 20–23.

Kouba, D. 1991. Primary care providers: Managing today's prepaid risk. *Medical Group Management Journal* January/February: 37–40.

Kretz, S. 1991. Quality focused contracting for specialized managed care services. *AAPPO Journal* June/July: 15–21.

Langwell, K., N. Carlton, and G. Swearingen. 1989. *Industry profile: An in-depth look at Medicare PPO applicants.* Princeton, NJ: Mathematica Policy Research.

Lazarus, S., M. Krill, D. Gans, and A. Bergstrom. 1989. Physician productivity measurement and comparison. *Journal of Ambulatory Care Management* 12 (1): 38–51.

Lipsitz, D. 1993. A physician incentive compensation program in a staff model HMO. *HMO Practice* 7 (2): 82–87.

Lutes, M., and D. Hastings. 1993. Regulatory and legal influences on managed care. In *Making managed healthcare work*, edited by Peter Boland. Gaithersburg, MD: Aspen.

Marion Merrell Dow. 1993. *Managed Care Digest* 8 (PPO ed.). Kansas City, MO: Marion Merrell Dow.

McGuirk-Porell, M., G. Goldberg, D. Goldin, G. Lenhart, N. Ober, and R. Bizier. 1991. A performance-based quality evaluation system for preferred provider organizations. *Quality Review Bulletin* November: 365–73.

Miller, R., and H. Luft. 1991. Perspective: Diversity and transition in health insurance plans. *Health Affairs* 10 (4): 37–47.

Montague, J. 1993. Straight talk: Doctor-driven systems tell how they've gained physician allies. *Hospitals and Health Networks* July 5, pp. 22–27.

Morain, C. 1992. HMOs try to measure (and reward) "doctor quality." *Medical Economics* April 6, pp. 206–15.

More employees demand HMOs get NCQA accreditation. 1993. *Managed Care Week* July 26, p. 3.

Morreim, E. H. 1991. Gaming the system: Dodging the rules, ruling the dodgers. *Archives of Internal Medicine* 151 (March): 443–47.

Murray, D. 1992. Managed care: The payoffs keep getting bigger. *Medical Economics* December 7, pp. 124–34.

Nelson, S., K. Langwell, R. Brown, B. Brown, N. Carlton, and G. Swearingen. 1990. *Organizational and operational characteristics of TEFRA HMOs/CMPs.* Princeton, NJ: Mathematica Policy Research.

Ogden, D. 1993. Physician/hospital organizations in managed care contracting. *Medical Group Management Journal* May/June: 12–17.

O'Kane, M. 1993. Outside accreditation of managed care plans. In *The managed care handbook,* edited by Peter Kongstvedt. Gaithersburg, MD: Aspen.

Pauly, M., A. Hillman, and J. Kerstein. 1990. Managing physician incentives in managed care: The role of for-profit ownership. *Medical Care* 28 (11): 1013–24.

Physician Payment Review Commission. 1992. *Conference on profiling.* Washington, DC: Physician Payment Review Commission.

———. 1993. *Use of the Medicare fee schedule by other payers. Annual Report to Congress.* Washington, DC: Physician Payment Review Commission.

———. 1994. *Annual report to Congress.* Washington, DC: Physician Payment Review Commission.

Schlackman, N. 1991. The quality care cycle. *Quality Review Bulletin* 17 (11): 360–64.

———. 1993. Evolution of the quality based compensation model: The third generation. *American College of Medical Quality* 8 (2): 103–10.

Shouldice, R. 1987. Negotiating with alternative delivery systems. *Medical Group Management Journal* 34 (1): 9–11.

Shortell, S. M., R. R. Gillies, and D. A. Anderson. 1994. The new world of managed care: Creating organized delivery systems. *Health Affairs* Winter: 46–64.

Smillie, J. G. 1991. *Can physicians manage the quality and costs of health care: The story of the Permanente Medical Group.* New York: McGraw-Hill.

Somers, A. R., ed. 1971. *The Kaiser-Permanente Medical Care Program: A symposium.* New York: Commonwealth Fund.

Starr, P. 1982. *The social transformation of American medicine.* New York: Basic Books.

Sullivan, C., M. Miller, R. Feldman, and B. Dowd. 1992. Employer sponsored health insurance in 1991. *Health Affairs* Winter: 172–86.

The InterStudy. 1994. *Competitive Edge* 3 (2): 34–38.

Traska, M. 1988. AMCRA: HMOs confused about gatekeeper's role. *Hospitals* 62 (15): 40.

United States Congress, Office of Technology Assessment. 1994. *Identifying health technologies that work: Searching for evidence.* Washington, DC: Office of Technology Assessment.

U.S. Department of Health and Human Services. 1990. *Study of incentive arrangements offered by HMOs and CMPs to physicians.* Washington, DC: Department of Health and Human Services.

Weiner, J. 1993. Razing a tower of Babel: A taxonomy for managed care and health insurance plans. *Journal of Health Politics, Policy, and Law* 18 (1): 75–104.

Welch, W. P., A. Hillman, and M. V. Pauly. 1990. Toward new typologies for HMOs. *Milbank Quarterly* 68 (2): 221–43.

Winickoff, R. N., K. Coltin, M. Morgan, R. Buxbaum, and O. Barnett. 1984. Improving physician performance through peer comparison feedback. *Medical Care* 22: 527–34.

Winslow, R., and E. Felsenthal. 1993. Physicians fight back as insurers cut them from health networks. *Wall Street Journal* December 30, p. A1.

Zalta, E. 1993. Provider selection standards as a quality indicator. *Managed Care Quarterly* 1 (1): 53–61.

CHAPTER

5

A NATIONAL SURVEY OF THE ARRANGEMENTS MANAGED-CARE PLANS MAKE WITH PHYSICIANS

Marsha R. Gold, Robert Hurley, Timothy Lake, Todd Ensor, and Robert Berenson

UNDER MANAGED care, the financing and delivery of health care are organized by a single entity. Managed-care plans are classified as health maintenance organizations (HMOs), preferred-provider organizations (PPOs), or various mixes of the two.[1] There are two major forms of HMO: group-model or staff-model HMOs and network or independent-practice—association (IPA) HMOs. Both types are usually at risk for the costs of care and therefore often control costs by requiring patients to be referred to specialists by primary care doctors. The doctors in network or IPA HMOs are usually in independent practice. A PPO, in contrast, consists of a group of doctors who agree to provide services to the plan's patients for discounted fees. Although managed-care plans are growing rapidly in the United States, they are controversial among physicians, who are concerned about their intrusion into medical practice.[2–4] Despite important studies of managed care,[5–7] there is relatively little information on the arrangements managed-care plans make to recruit,

From *The New England Journal of Medicine* 333: 1678–1683.

pay, and monitor physicians.[8] Much more is known about group or staff HMOs than about newer types, such as network or IPA HMOs and other forms of managed care, which account for much of its recent growth.[6,7,9] In contrast to group or staff HMOs, which use physicians in fully integrated group practices, network or IPA HMOs use community-based physicians in private practice and thus may intrude more on physicians' practices. The early network or IPA HMOs were loosely structured. Fee discounts and utilization review were the main new features.[6] Although many people assume that this loose structure continues today,[10,11] the assumption remains controversial.

To learn more about the arrangements different plans make with physicians, the Physician Payment Review Commission sponsored a telephone survey of managed-care plans, conducted in 1994 by Mathematica Policy Research.[12,13] The survey covered the recruitment of physicians, compensation and financial incentives, and nonfinancial influences on care, including oversight of quality, profiling, practice guidelines, and utilization review.

Methods

Samples and Response Rates

We restricted the survey to HMOs and PPOs. We used a two-stage selection process in which 20 market areas were chosen, and then a sample of plans operating in these areas was selected.[14] Plans were defined as entities in particular market areas rather than parent corporations. In the first stage, the 54 largest metropolitan areas (where 86 percent of HMO enrollees reside) were stratified according to size (under 1 million people or 1 million or more) and managed-care penetration (under 30 percent, 30 to 49 percent, or 50 percent or more). Within these strata, individual market areas were selected at random. The probability that any given metropolitan area would be selected was proportional to the size of its managed-care enrollment.

In the second stage, we selected one sample each of group or staff HMOs, network or IPA HMOs, and PPOs. An HMO was classified as a group or staff plan or as a network or IPA plan, and HMOs with more than one type of model were classified according to which type predominated, as reported in the Group Health Association of America's *National Directory of HMOs*.[14]

Although HMOs and PPOs enroll about the same number of people nationwide, we limited the PPO sample to 30 percent of the total, because PPOs have less diverse and less developed managed-care features than HMOs. We established the size of the group or staff HMO sample and the network or IPA HMO sample on the basis of their shares of total nationwide HMO enrollment (39 and 61 percent, respectively). The probability that a given plan would be selected was generally proportional to the size of the plan within its market. However, we did seek a minimum of one plan of each type from each market. Selecting the PPOs was complicated by the absence of a good list of PPOs from which to sample and by the need to obtain preliminary information by telephone.

Although the original sample consisted of 146 plans, the effective sample was 138 plans, because 5 also offered HMO products and thus were already in our study through the HMO sample and 3 had merged. The overall response rate was 78 percent: 78 percent for the group or staff HMOs, 83 percent for the network or IPA HMOs, and 70 percent for the PPOs (which were surveyed last). National data show that the HMOs that responded were generally similar to those that did not, except that the response rates were lower (17 of the 31 HMOs, or 55 percent) for the plans owned by commercial insurers.

Questionnaire

All plans received the same questionnaire, which contained more than 300 items. It was developed on the basis of a literature review and advice from a panel of researchers and experts in the delivery of managed care.

The plans were surveyed between June and September 1994. Each received a letter on Physician Payment Review Commission letterhead along with a list of panel members and letters of endorsement from industry trade associations. The respondents were senior clinical managers designated by the chief executive officers of the plans. Because of the length of the questionnaire, we allowed up to three respondents, whose areas of knowledge corresponded to the three major areas surveyed.

Sources of Error and Bias

Our results are limited in that they are based on what the respondents said rather than on an audit of what they do, how well they do it, and how strongly the plans' arrangements influence the practice of physicians. Any bias in the results probably arises from overreporting of managed-care approaches, especially those regarded as desirable.

The findings are reported according to the type of plan. Because of the small sample, we mention only differences that are large and that show a consistent trend across similar variables. Statistically significant differences were determined with use of the chi-square test.[15] Smaller plans are underrepresented relative to their number but are not underrepresented relative to their share of national managed-care enrollment.

Results

Table 1 shows the characteristics of the 108 study plans. Together they enrolled 33.5 million people; 15.2 million of these were in HMOs, representing 35 percent of the national HMO enrollment of 41.3 million people when the sample was selected. The plans usually had at least 100,000 members, and often more than 250,000. Nearly all had been formed before 1990, and many before 1980. For-profit plans accounted for 59 percent of the sample and for about three quarters of the network or IPA HMOs and the PPOs.

Forming and Maintaining the Network

When asked which of three statements best characterized their policy on selecting physicians, most respondents chose "careful selection" (71 percent) rather than "prune later" (18 percent) or "as broad as feasible" (11 percent). Some plans (38 percent) were subtracting physicians ("tightening" the network), and others (43 percent) were adding physicians ("widening" the network). The group or staff HMOs were somewhat more likely to report widening their networks (51 percent) than the network or IPA HMOs (42 percent) or the PPOs (34 percent).

Table 2 summarizes the procedures used in recruiting physicians. When selecting physicians, the group or staff HMOs tended to have more demanding requirements than the other types of plan. Ninety percent of group or staff HMOs, but only 48 percent of the network or IPA HMOs and 41 percent of the PPOs, required board certification or eligibility. Both types of HMO were more likely than the PPOs to require that new physicians either have privileges at network hospitals or be able to obtain them. Both types of HMO were also more likely than the PPOs (48 percent vs. 7 percent) to require physicians to provide care for a predetermined number of patients or to practice only within the plan.

A minority of the plans (37 percent) used quantitative information about physicians' performance and practice style in selecting new physicians. However, 63 percent of all the plans and 73 percent of the network or IPA HMOs took into account qualitative information, such as professional reputation and patterns of care. When asked how much previous patterns of costs or utilization of resources influenced the selection of physicians, 61 percent of the respondents characterized the influence as small, 26 percent as moderate, and 13 percent as large.

Before signing a contract with a new physician, virtually all plans verified the physician's license and credentials, and almost all screened for reportable disciplinary actions, substance abuse, or similar problems. Sixty-six percent of the network or IPA HMOs visited the physician's

Table 1 Characteristics of 108 Managed-Care Plans

Characteristic	All Plans (n = 108) %	Group or Staff HMOs (n = 29) %	Network or IPA HMOs (n = 50) %	PPOs (n = 29) %
Enrollment*				
<50,000	17	34	12	7
50,000–99,999	15	14	14	17
100,000–249,999	24	31	20	24
≥250,000	44	21	53	52
First year of operation				
Before 1970	10	34	0	3
1970–1979	26	41	30	0
1980–1984	24	14	18	45
1985–1989	35	7	48	41
1990 or later	4	3	2	10
For profit	59	34	74	72
Ownership				
Commerical insurer	8	7	10	7
Blue Cross–Blue Shield	16	10	20	14
National HMO or managed-care company	24	34	28	7
Other†	52	48	42	72
Federally qualified HMO‡	64	83	57	—
Managed-care penetration in market§				
Low (<30%)	28	24	26	34
Medium (30–49%)	23	24	20	28
High (>49%)	49	52	54	38
Market size				
<1 million	19	17	16	28
≥1 million	81	83	84	72

*Plans were asked to provide enrollment figures according to the benefit plan offered. For PPO and other point-of-service benefit plans, plans could provide the number of persons covered or the number of subscribers. To convert the number of subscribers to the number of persons, we used the ratio of 2.2 persons per subscriber, which is published by the Group Health Association of America.
†Other includes other national companies, independent owners, joint ventures, physician owners, community or regional groups, hospitals, and other nonprofit groups.
‡Federal qualification is generally not applicable to PPOs, except for the few that offer HMO products.
§Market penetration is the percentage of the area's population enrolled in managed-care plans.

office, reviewed whether the facility met set standards, and screened care by reviewing medical records. Only 7 percent of the PPOs took all these steps, and 52 percent took none of them.

Ninety-three percent of the plans had a formal process for recredentialing physicians, although 62 percent began to do this only in 1991 or later. Rates of physician turnover were low and were consistent with

Table 2 Procedures Used by Managed-Care Plans to Recruit Physicians

Procedure	All Plans ($n = 108$) %	Group or Staff HMOs ($n = 29$) %	Network or IPA HMOs ($n = 50$) %	PPOs ($n = 29$) %
Selecting physicians				
Require board certification or board eligibility[*]	57	90	48[†]	41[†]
Require privileges at network hospital or ability to obtain them	82	86	88	69[‡]
Require agreement to take predetermined number of patients or not to practice outside plan[§]	37	48	48	7[†¶]
State that the effect of previous costs or utilization patterns on the decision was large	13	4	18[‖]	14
Contracting with physicians				
Verify license and credentials[**]	100	100	100	100
Consult National Practitioner Data Bank, sources on substance abuse, or both	92	86	94	93
Visit physician's office, review facility, and screen care through medical records[††]				
Do all three	43	38	66[‖]	7[†¶]
Do none of these	27	34	8[†]	52[¶]
Review quantitative data from indemnity claims, hospital-discharge data, or both	37	24	38	48[‖]
Meeting four criteria for orienting new physicians[‡‡]	30	69	22[†]	3[†‡]

[*]Other plans may allow exceptions.
[†]$P < 0.01$ for the comparison with group or staff HMOs.
[‡]$P < 0.10$ for the comparison with network or IPA HMOs.
[§]Only 100 plans responded (27 group or staff HMOs, 45 network or IPA HMOs, and 28 PPOs).
[¶]$P < 0.01$ for the comparison with network or IPA HMOs.
[‖]$P < 0.10$ for the comparison with group or staff HMOs.
[**]Only 102 plans responded (25 group or staff HMOs, 48 network or IPA HMOs, and 29 PPOs).
[††]Because they are much more likely to hire than to contract with physicians who practice in their facilities, group or staff HMOs may find these steps unnecessary or address the underlying concerns in different ways (e.g., by contacting references).
[‡‡]The four criteria are as follows: plan has orientation meetings specifically for medical staff, 75 percent or more of physicians participate, top management is involved, and less than 75 percent of time is devoted to administation issues. Of all plans, 5 percent met none of the criteria, 17 percent one, 23 percent two, 26 percent three, and 30 percent four.

those in other recent studies.[16] Sixty-seven percent of the group or staff HMOs, 79 percent of the network or IPA HMOs, and 86 percent of the PPOs had an annual turnover rate (including both voluntary and involuntary departures) of 5 percent or less. The higher rate of turnover in the group or staff HMOs resulted from the turnover of newly hired physicians in their first two years of employment. The group or staff HMOs were more likely to have extensive orientation programs for new physicians than were the network or IPA HMOs or the PPOs.

Risk Sharing, Payment, and Financial Incentives

Risk sharing with physicians was usual in both types of HMO but rare in the PPOs (Table 3). Among the network or IPA HMOs, 84 percent had some sharing of risk with primary care physicians; 56 percent used capitation as a primary method of payment; and 28 percent used fee-for-service payments in some form along with withholding or bonuses. In contrast, only 20 percent of the network or IPA HMOs used capitation as a predominant method of payment for individual specialists; 54 percent had some form of risk sharing with specialists, 47 percent used capitated payment for certain specialties, and 33 percent used competitive bidding to obtain some specialty services. The specialties in which physicians were most commonly paid on a capitated basis were cardiology, mental health, radiology, orthopedics, and ophthalmology. The group or staff HMOs paid primary care physicians on a salary or capitated basis, but fewer than half did the same for specialists (data not shown). The PPOs primarily used fee-for-service payments.

Most of the HMOs adjusted payments to primary care physicians to create performance-based incentives. Fifty percent of the group or staff HMOs and 74 percent of the network or IPA HMOs adjusted payments according to utilization and cost patterns. More than half of the group or staff HMOs and the network or IPA HMOs adjusted payment on the basis of patients' complaints and measures of the quality of care. The group or staff HMOs were more likely than the network or IPA HMOs to reward productivity and tenure in the plan, whereas the network or IPA HMOs were more likely to adjust payments according to the results of consumer surveys.

Practice and Utilization Management

The plans used several different nonfinancial methods to influence medical practice (Table 4). Ninety-two percent of the network or IPA HMOs and 61 percent of the group or staff HMOs required patients to select a primary care physician, who was responsible for most referrals to specialists.

More than 95 percent of the HMOs and 62 percent of the PPOs had a written quality-assurance plan, a quality-assurance committee,

Table 3 Procedures Used by Managed-Care Plans to Pay Physicians

Procedure	All Plans (n = 108) %	Group or Staff HMOs (n = 29) %	Network or IPA HMOs (n = 50) %	PPOs (n = 29) %
Primary care physicians				
Predominant payment for sole or largest benefit plan involves:				
Some sharing of risk with providers[*]	60	68	84	10[†‡]
Capitation as predominant method	37	34	56[§]	7[†‡]
Salary with no withholding or bonus	8	28	2[‡]	0[‡]
Fee for service with no withholding or bonus	31	3	12	90[†‡]
Basis of payment adjustment[¶]				
Utilization or cost measures	57	50	74[§]	34[†]
Patient complaints or grievance	49	57	61	21[†‡]
Quality measures	46	54	64	7[†‡]
Consumer surveys	36	37	55	3[†‡]
Provider productivity	24	43	26	3[†‡]
Enrollee turnover rate	21	11	36[§]	3[†]
None of the above	28	29	14	55[†§]
Financial reward given for devoting a higher percentage of time to plan, increasing number of patients, longevity, exclusivity, or willingness to provide a wider range of services[‖]	52	69	64	14[†‡]
Specialty physicians				
Predominant payment for sole or largest benefit plan involves:				
Some sharing of risk with providers[*] [**]	43	59	54	3[†‡]
Capitation as predominant method	18	31	20	0[†‡]
Salary with no withholding or bonus	6	17	2[§]	0[§]
Fee for service with no withholding or bonus	52	24	42	97[†‡]
Capitation for individual specialties, pooled capitation across specialties, risk sharing based on withholding or bonuses, or competitive bidding				
Any of the above	69	97	86	10[†‡]
Capitation for individual specialties	42	69	47	7[†‡]
Competitive bidding	28	31	33	17

*Physicians are paid some form of capitation (with or without other withholding or bonuses), or withholding or bonuses are applied to salary or fee-for-service arrangements. Withholding is similar to a bonus, except that funds are initially withheld and then returned in part or in whole at the end of the payment period.

†$P < 0.01$ for the comparison with network or IPA HMOs.

‡$P < 0.01$ for the comparison with group or staff HMOs.

§$P < 0.10$ for the comparison with group or staff HMOs.

¶The number of plans responding to this item ranged from 104 to 106 (27 to 29 group or staff HMOs, 48 or 49 network or IPA HMOs, and 29 PPOs).

‖This question did not refer specifically to primary care physicians, but these approaches are most relevant to them.

**Only 107 plans responded (29 group or staff HMOs, 49 network or IPA HMOs, and 29 PPOs).

Table 4 Procedures Used by Managed-Care Plans to Monitor Practice and Utilization

Procedure	All Plans ($n = 108$) %	Group or Staff HMOs ($n = 29$) %	Network or IPA HMOs ($n = 50$) %	PPOs ($n = 29$) %
Clinical structure (traditional HMO benefit plans)				
Plan generally holds primary care physicians responsible for referral to most specialists	94	96	92	—*
Patients are required to select an individual primary care physician†	82	61	92‡	—*
Medical management				
Quality structure				
Plan has a quality-assurance document, quality-assurance committees, and active patient-grievance procedures	87	97	96	62‡§
Quality monitoring and focused studies				
Plan requires clinically focused or outcome studies for specific clinical conditions and targeted quality-improvement initiatives, and uses them to identify needed improvements and to gauge success¶				
All of the above	62	79	70	31‡§
Focused studies conducted regularly	83	100	96	45‡§
Profiling				
Plan uses profiling, provides physician feedback, and identifies areas for system-wide improvement‖				
All of the above	68	69	80	45§**
Any use of profiles	74	76	86	52§**
Practice guidelines				
Plan uses established, formal, written practice guidelines, does so fairly extensively (in more than a few areas), monitors compliance, and meets with physicians to review results††				
All of the above	26	31	34	7§**
Any use of guidelines	63	76	76	28‡§
Utilization review				
Preadmission review for all nonemergency admissions, concurrent and retrospective review, discharge planning (that does not rely on hospital staff), and ambulatory review for resource-intensive services‡‡				
At least four of five	62	72	70	37‡§
Any of the above	95	97	100	86§
Data				
Plan maintains patient-level claims or encounter data base for hospital stays	91	90	100**	76§

Continued

Table 5.4 Continued

Procedure	All Plans ($n = 108$) %	Group or Staff HMOs ($n = 29$) %	Network or IPA HMOs ($n = 50$) %	PPOs ($n = 29$) %
Plan has patient-level claims or encounter data base for in-plan physician and other services, requires dummy claims or encounter forms, and estimates that ≥90% of encounter forms are submitted				
Requires data base	88	93	94	72§**
Requires data base with dummy claims§§	74	82	69	—*
Requires data base with dummy claims§§ and ≥90% of encounter forms submitted	24	39	13**	—*

*Only applicable to six PPOs with traditional HMO benefits.
†Only 107 plans responded (28 group or staff HMOs, 50 network or IPA HMOs, and 29 PPOs).
‡$P < 0.01$ for the comparison with group or staff HMOs.
§$P < 0.01$ for the comparison with network or IPA HMOs.
¶Clinically focused studies were defined as studies of performance of patient outcomes in areas such as childhood immunization, pregnancy, diabetes, breast cancer or mammography, lead toxicity, and sickle cell disease. One of the items specified that these must be done on a regular basis.
||Profiling was defined as examining patterns of practice through various use or outcome rates aggregated over time for a defined population of patients and comparing them with other practice patterns.
**$P < 0.10$ for the comparison with group or staff HMOs.
††Practice guidelines were defined as an explicit statement of what is known and believed about the benefits, risks, and costs of particular courses of medical action to assist decisions about appropriate health care for specific clinical conditions.
‡‡Respondents were asked to characterize their process for preadmission review in various ways. Those not counted as "yes" include, for example, those in which no specific action is needed, although the pattern may be monitored, those in which an intermediate entity or patient is responsible for preadmission review, and those covering only some nonemergency admissions.
§§If applicable (excludes those using fee for service as the predominant way of paying primary care and specialty physicians in the sole or largest benefit plan).

and a patient-grievance system. Seventy-nine percent of the group or staff HMOs and 70 percent of the network or IPA HMOs required outcome studies for particular clinical conditions, had targeted quality-improvement initiatives, and used outcome studies to identify needs for improvement and to gauge success. Studies of the treatment of asthma and diabetes and the use of mammography were the most common. Sixty-nine percent of the group or staff HMOs and 80 percent of the network or IPA HMOs used physician profiles and applied them. Substantially fewer PPOs than HMOs used outcome studies (31 percent) or physician profiles (45 percent) in this way.

Practice guidelines were used less often than outcome studies or physician profiles. About three quarters of the HMOs and 28 percent of the PPOs used formal, written practice guidelines. These most commonly applied to childhood immunizations, the management of asthma, mammographic screening, and screening for colorectal cancer. Almost all plans had procedures for utilization review. In most plans, patient-level claims or encounter data on physicians' services and other ambulatory care services were collected even when providers were paid on a capitated or salaried basis. But physicians submitted more than 90 percent of encounter forms (dummy claims) in only a minority of plans. Such information is less likely to be available in the network or IPA HMOs than in the group or staff HMOs.

Similarities among HMO Plans

There were many similarities in structure between the group or staff HMOs and the network or IPA HMOs. Fifty-five percent of the plans identified as group or staff HMOs were actually mixed models, with traditional HMO coverage provided by a network or IPA. Only 59 percent of the group or staff HMOs used physicians in large multispecialty groups to provide care to more than two-thirds of their enrollees. Moreover, only 44 percent reported that their members made up 80 percent or more of the practice of a typical physician in their plan, whereas 45 percent of the network or IPA HMOs reported that their members accounted for at least 20 percent of a typical physician's practice.

Discussion

Our findings indicate that managed-care plans have complex systems for recruiting physicians, paying them, and monitoring their performance. Such systems are much more likely to be found in HMOs than in PPOs, perhaps because purchasers have recently encouraged the accreditation of such plans by the National Committee for Quality Assurance.[17]

Our study is descriptive, and the data come from unaudited reports from the plans themselves. Thus, it can offer little insight into how the arrangements between physicians and managed-care plans influence the accessibility, cost, or quality of care.

Our findings do suggest, however, that many of the differences between specific HMOs cannot be explained by their classification as group or staff HMOs or as network or IPA HMOs. The Congressional Budget Office's estimates assume that most cost savings attributable to HMOs result from group or staff plans, not from network or IPA plans, on the basis of the belief that most network or IPA HMOs do not create the conditions on which savings depend[10,11]: "These conditions include [the presence of] cost conscious providers, an effective network for information and control, [placing] providers at financial risk, and [generating] a substantial portion of each provider's patient load."[10] We found that many large network or IPA HMOs met at least some of these conditions and that the two types of HMO did not differ from one another as much as is often assumed. Diversity in managed care occurs within as well as across types of plans.

Common arrangements between managed-care plans and physicians appear to result in less independence and less control over income and practice for physicians. Nonetheless, the emphasis on outcome studies and enrollee-based clinical information may have beneficial effects for plan members, because this approach accounts for those who do not use services as well as those who do.

Acknowledgments

We are indebted to Jack Hoadley of the Physician Payment Review Commission for his guidance and support; to the following staff members at Mathematica Policy Research: Lyle Nelson for reviewing the research, Linda Mendenko for supervising the survey, Daisy Ewell and Susan Thomas for programming support, Barbara Foot and DeWayne Davis for coordinating production, Daryl Hall for editing the manuscript, and Kathleen Donaldson for assistance in the preparation of the manuscript; to the managed-care plans that participated in the study; to the Group Health Association of America, the American Managed Care and Review Association, and the American Association of Preferred Provider Organizations; to the expert panel of clinical leaders in managed care; and to Paul Ginsburg of the Center for Studying Health Systems Change for reviewing the manuscript.

References

1. Weiner, J. P., and de Lissovoy, G. Razing a tower of Babel: a taxonomy for managed care and health insurance plans. J Health Polit Policy Law 1993; 18: 75–103.
2. Gabel, J., Liston, D., Jensen, G., and Marsteller, J. The health insurance picture in 1993: some rare good news. Health Aff (Millwood) 1994; 13 (1): 327–36.
3. Berenson, R. A. A physician's view of managed care. Health Aff (Millwood) 1991; 10 (4): 106–19.
4. Hillman, A. L. Managing the physician: rules versus incentives. Health Aff (Millwood) 1991; 10 (4): 138–46.
5. *Idem*. Financial incentives for physicians in HMOs: is there a conflict of interest? N "Engl J Med 1987; 317: 1743–48.
6. Luft, H. S. Health maintenance organizations: dimensions of performance. New York: John Wiley, 1981.

7. Miller, R. H., and Luft, H. S. Managed care plan performance since 1980: a literature analysis. JAMA 1994; 271: 1512–19.
8. Gold, M., Nelson, L., Lake. T., et al. Behind the curve: a critical assessment of how little is known about the managed care arrangements with physicians. Med Care Res Rev 1995; S2: 307–41.
9. Freeborn, D. K., and Pope, C. R. Promise and performance in managed care: the prepaid group practice model. Baltimore: Johns Hopkins University Press, 1994.
10. The effects of managed care and managed competition. Washington, D.C.: Congressional Budget Office, 1995.
11. Effects of managed care: an update. Washington, D.C.: Congressional Budget Office, 1994.
12. Annual report to Congress. Washington, D.C.: Physician Payment Review Commission, 1995.
13. Gold, M., Hurley, R., Lake, T., et al. Arrangements between managed care plans and physicians. Selected external research series no. 3. Washington, D.C.: Physician Payment Review Commission, 1995.
14. National Directory of HMOs. Washington, D.C.: Group Health Association of America, 1994.
15. Blalock, H. M. Social Statistics. New York: McGraw-Hill, 1979.
16. Report card pilot project, technical report. Washington, D.C.: National Committee for Quality Assurance, 1995.
17. Standards for the accreditation of managed care organizations. 1993 ed. Washington, D.C.: National Committee for Quality Assurance, 1992.

CHAPTER

6

HOW HMOs STRUCTURE PRIMARY CARE DELIVERY

Suzanne Felt-Lisk

MANAGED CARE'S increased influence on health care delivery highlights the need to better understand how people in managed care obtain primary care and referrals. A recent literature search found that previously published research on the topic is generally dated, derived from a limited subset of plans, inattentive to important structural differences between plans, and responsive to a narrow set of related issues.[1] Here, results are presented from a detailed study of primary care staffing in 23 health maintenance organizations (HMOs). Differences among HMOs are explored: who they use as "gatekeepers," how they use nurse practitioners (NPs) and physician assistants (PAs), and their policies on how people obtain referrals to specialists. The study also explored plans' initiatives to expand or better define a scope of practice for primary care physicians. To conclude, the implications of the findings are discussed.

Study Design

The study design consists of on-site interviews with senior health plan officials in 23 HMOs nationwide in winter and spring of 1994. The study

Reprinted with permission from *Managed Care Quarterly* 4 (4): 96–105. © 1996 Aspen Publishers, Inc. It is reprinted here without change.

was conducted by Mathematica Policy Research, Inc. for the federal Health Resources and Services Administration.[2] This sample of HMOs was constructed using a two-stage process, in which markets of varying HMO penetration and provider supply level were selected, and then a variety of plans were selected within these markets. The final sample consists of nine group or staff model plans in eight large urban areas and one rural area, nine network or IPA model plans in the same eight large urban areas and in one small urban area, and five plans selected because they have relatively high Medicaid enrollment (25 percent or more of their total enrollment). Mixed-model plans were accommodated by selecting plans based on predominant model type and studying the staffing of each model type component.

The eight selected urban markets cover the range of the 54 largest metropolitan statistical areas in terms of their population, physician-to-population ratio, and HMO penetration rate. A greater proportion of large plans than exist nationwide was selected so as to include greater numbers of physicians and enrollees. Thus, the sample is more representative of HMOs that have enrollments greater than 50,000. It is also more representative of the distribution of enrollees in HMOs nationally.

At each HMO, the site visitors used semistructured interview protocols to interview the key personnel who make staffing decisions, usually the medical director, provider relations or network development director, and marketing representative, and often also the chief executive officer, a government programs staff person, and a regional representative if the plan was large and somewhat decentralized. Generally, one or two site visitors spent about a day on site.

The sample of HMOs was designed to represent the full range of HMOs in the nation and to facilitate an understanding of how differences in model type, high Medicaid enrollment, and market factors affect primary care staffing. However, about half the HMOs originally selected declined to participate, requiring substitution of another HMO with similar characteristics, and the sites were selected primarily through a judgmental rather than random process; thus, both the study design and the relatively small number of plans means that the results are more useful for providing insight about staffing processes than specific point estimates of prevalence.

Selection of a "Gatekeeper"

Basic to managed care is the idea that a patient accesses care through primary care providers chosen from a health plan's associated network of providers. However, the study found wide variation in the extent to which

Table 1 Types of Plans Requiring Selection of One Primary Care Provider

	Rules for Selecting a Primary Care Provider (n = 23) Percentage of HMOs			
	Encouraged but Not Required to Select an Individual	Required to Select an Individual	Neither Encouraged nor Required to Select an Individual	Plan Has No Preference/ Groups or IPAs Determine Rules
All plans (n = 23)	30	39	13	17
Predominant model type				
Group/staff (n = 11)	36	55	9	0
Network/IPA (n = 12)	25	25	17	33
Medicaid enrollment				
None (n = 12)	25	42	8	25
1–24 percent of total enrollment (n = 3)	0	100	0	0
25+ percent of total enrollment (n = 8)	50	13	25	13

enrollees were required, versus encouraged, to select a single primary care provider to act as a gatekeeper.

New health plan enrollees generally are asked to choose a specific medical group/IPA or health center in the plan's provider network; they are then encouraged or required to select one primary care provider. As Table 1 shows, just over half of the group/staff model plans and a quarter of the network/IPA model plans required enrollees to select a specific primary care provider (6 of 11 plans and 3 of 12 plans, respectively). Half of the network/IPA model plans delegate the selection rules to the contracted group or IPA—typically because of the plan's payment policy, which capitates the group or IPA only, not individual providers.

The plan's decision to require rather than encourage selection of a primary care provider may be related to its proportion of Medicaid enrollees, since plans with high Medicaid enrollment appear less likely to have this requirement. The reason for this is unknown, although the pattern is consistent with what plans cite as the challenges of treating Medicaid patients. For example, the basic challenge of promoting appropriate use of primary care providers rather than emergency departments might be more easily met than expectations for compliance with more strict requirements for contacting a particular provider.

Regardless of whether a plan requires enrollees to select a provider, the plan typically allows providers other than the one selected to also provide primary care to the patient. For example, group/staff model plans accommodate enrollee "crossover"; that is, enrollees sometimes seek care at two or more different health centers in the plan, and the plan accommodates this. Network/IPA plans that contract with large medical groups mentioned that some of the primary care providers in these groups see one anothers' patients freely (without restriction) within the same site.

Types of Providers Used as Gatekeepers

HMOs typically use a combination of family practitioners (FPs), general practitioners (GPs), pediatricians, and internists as gatekeepers. Obstetrician/gynecologists (OB/GYNs) and subspecialist physicians may deliver primary care but are not often used as gatekeepers. Similarly, plans generally do not offer NPs and PAs as gatekeepers.

Primary Care Gatekeepers for Adults

Generally, adult enrollees select a primary care provider from a list of FPs, GPs, and internists who focus most of their practice on primary care. (Plans told us some of these internists have specialist designations, but they have chosen to largely practice primary care and so the plan lists them with general internists as primary care providers.) Though these providers form the core of plans' primary care provider lists and are most often selected by enrollees for this role, most plans also allow some other providers to be selected. In a third of the network/IPA type plans, the contracted groups or IPAs have the flexibility to set their own rules on provider selection, with the result that some allow OB/GYNs and/or subspecialists to be selected as primary care physicians. In fact, a significant minority of plans (10 of 23) allow selection of OB/GYNs as gatekeepers, though the extent to which OB/GYNs actually play this role is reported to be minimal. Although not often selected as a primary care provider through which care is channeled, OB/GYNs appear to provide a substantial amount of primary care. Most plans reported that OB/GYNs provide well-woman and obstetric and gynecological care upon patient self-referral to complement care delivered by the regular primary care provider; about three fourths of plans allow at least some self-referral for OB/GYN care.

Other common policies on who acts as a gatekeeper are allowing specialists to serve as primary care providers on a case-by-case, approved basis, and allowing NPs and PAs to be selected if specifically requested by the patient although these providers are not on the publicized list of primary care providers. A few plans had a unique approach reflecting their particular philosophy or circumstances; for example, in remote rural areas served by one plan, PAs or OB/GYNs may be selected due to a lack of the types of providers the plan uses in other parts of its service area.

Plans do not frequently use subspecialists as primary care providers, though more than three fourths of the plans allow them to play this role on a rare or exceptions basis, and about a third freely allow enrollees to select these providers as gatekeepers. Many plans view subspecialists without additional primary care training as poor providers of primary care, reporting that they tend to do more specialty care than other primary care providers, to be unhappy and want to return to their specialty, and refer to others too much for conditions they, as primary care providers, should handle. The eight plans that allow subspecialists to be selected as a primary care provider on more than an exceptions basis generally reported they do so because (1) they believe this practice is cost-effective (e.g., the plan otherwise had excess specialist capacity), (2) there is a large number of subspecialists in the market area who would not be able to stay based only on the basis of demand for specialty care, or (3) they want to provide consumers with as much choice of providers as possible within their network. These plans generally reported that while subspecialists are permitted to act as primary care providers with few restrictions, they generally do not play this role often, either because they are not selected by patients or because they do not choose to act in this role.

Plans vary in the extent to which they rely on internists compared with FPs for primary care. (Plans almost never distinguished between FPs and GPs in their policies or statistics, so following their lead both groups are labeled FPs for simplicity.) In over 60 percent of the plans (14 of 23), internists greatly outnumber FPs, or vice versa—that is, the plan clearly prefers and has experience with one type of primary care provider or the other. The remaining nine plans (39 percent) have a relatively even mixture of internists and FPs. Table 2 shows plan differences in this mix by model type. The reasons for the fact that internists greatly outnumber FPs in some plans did not always surface in discussion, but seem likely to be related to the plan's origin, when it was closely associated with a multispecialty group, to restrictions in some areas on admitting privileges for FPs by the hospitals with which the plan contracts, and to plan-imposed restrictions on FP practice, such as not allowing FPs to see children under a certain age or not allowing them to deliver infants, which would make plans with these restrictions less desirable to FPs seeking a full range of patient types. Differences in the competitive environment of HMOs may be another reason for different use of internists versus

Table 2 Differences in Mix of Internists and Family Practitioners by Model Type

Primary Care Physician Mix*	Percentage of HMOs		
	Group/Staff ($n = 11$)	Network/IPA ($n = 12$)	All Types ($n = 23$)
Internists greatly outnumber family practitioners	46	17	30
Near even mix of internists and family practitioners	27	50	39
Family practitioners greatly outnumber internists	27	33	30

*Internists were considerd to greatly outnumber FPs if the number of internists providing primary care was at least 50 percent greater than the number of FPs, or the plan described itself as heavily reliant on internists relative to other primary care providers. (The two pieces of information never conflicted but we did not have both pieces for every plan.) The reverse was true for categorizing plans where FPs greatly outnumbered internists.

FPs, among network/IPA model plans. None of the network/IPA model plans in areas with high HMO penetration heavily used internists relative to FPs, although internists heavily outnumbered FPs in two of four plans in low penetration areas. If this pattern is real rather than coincidental, it could reflect greater pressure to reduce costs in areas with high levels of HMO competition.

Several plans now using some FPs expressed their intent to use more of them. For example, one found it more cost-effective when moving into a new area to hire one FP rather than both an internist and pediatrician. Several plans see them as more flexible than internists given the larger range of ages they treat. However, other plans are more ambivalent about FPs and thus are not planning to use them more relative to other primary care providers. One plan found that FPs are more acceptable in the lower income areas than in other areas in its market. Another noted that while adults in its market are indifferent to seeing an internist or FP, they prefer that their children see a pediatrician.

Primary Care Gatekeepers for Children

Children in the study plans have a pediatrician or an FP as their primary care physician gatekeeper. Plans in which internists heavily outnumber FPs tend to use more pediatricians for their enrolled children, since internists do not treat children. Few plans (only three) require children to see pediatricians rather than the FPs who are available. There were not many rules or specific policies on primary care for children. The exceptions were one plan that had a specific policy requiring contracted providers to arrange with other providers to ensure 24-hour coverage for their practice, and that those who agree to provide coverage must treat patients of the same ages as those treated by the provider being covered (many pediatricians restrict their practice to children under a certain age, e.g., 15 or 18; and many internists see patients only over a certain age, e.g., 15 or 18, but the age limits vary by practice). A second plan had specific guidelines for when children must be seen by a pediatrician rather than another type of provider (e.g., sick children under age 1). Plans generally do not specify an age at which a patient must switch from a pediatrician to an internist but allow this to vary by pediatrician and internist practice.

Using Nurse Practitioners and Physician Assistants

Only two plans (of the 23) allow routine selection of NPs or PAs as gatekeepers; two others allow enrollees to select an NP or PA as a primary care provider if they specifically ask to or if medical group/IPA rules allow. Importantly, however, NPs and PAs provide primary care as part of a patient care team in most of the HMOs we visited. NPs, in particular, make up a large part of group/staff model plans' primary care staff, as shown in Table 3. Nearly two thirds of group/staff model plans use NPs extensively, and one third use PAs to some extent (more than "rarely"). (Plans were classified by frequency of use of NPs and PAs to show the major patterns of use, but the classifications are rough rather than precise. For example, plans were considered "heavy" users of NPs or PAs if they had at least one NP or PA for every five primary care physicians, or, if this figure was not available, if they considered themselves or their physicians to be heavy users of these providers. In the case of a plan that used some NPs or PAs, did not qualify as a "heavy" user, and did not specifically describe use as "rare," we classified the plan as having "some use.") Only one group/staff model plan does not use NPs, all use PAs to some extent, and much but not all of this use was for primary care. The general pattern of use for NPs and PAs was similar, though PAs were used somewhat less than NPs.

Group/staff model plans in the sample in areas with high levels of HMO penetration use NPs more heavily than other plans; all four of the group/staff model plans in areas with high HMO penetration (25 percent or more of the insured population) heavily used NPs, versus only two of the four in lower penetration areas. If the difference is real and not only a result of the markets we selected or other contributing causes related to these markets (e.g., the location of markets with high penetration), potential reasons for it could include better consumer and physician acceptance of NPs in areas with a long history of managed care,

Table 3 Use of Nurse Practitioners by Model Type

	Group/Staff Model Plans (Percentage of HMOs)	Network/IPA Model Plans (Percentage of HMOs)
Heavy use	64	0
Some use	9	33
Rare use	18	59
No use	9	8

or increased pressure on plans to reduce service delivery costs in areas with heavy competition from other HMOs.

Plans reported that NPs and PAs most commonly work six areas:

1. general primary care (13 plans)
2. urgent care (7 plans)
3. specialized positions (6 plans)
4. pediatric care (6 plans)
5. OB/GYN care (5 plans)
6. telephone triage (3 plans)

Four plans expressed a desire to increase use of NPs or PAs, but were finding recruiting very difficult. For example, one plan reported having to raise NP and PA salaries twice by mid-1994 to keep up with the competition and retain its own providers. It has also begun to use market surveys on a continuing basis to gauge this trend and keep its salaries in line.

A large minority of plans (8 of 23) are very supportive of NPs and PAs, and the rest are less supportive, neutral, or negative. (The classification of plans into "very supportive" or "less supportive, neutral, or negative" was considered both in terms of their use of NPs and PAs, and in terms of any special actions or plans to enhance their role or increase their number.) Only one or two plans could be categorized as being generally negative toward these providers. As Table 4 shows, very supportive plans tend to be group/staff model plans and plans without Medicaid contracts. It is not surprising that group/staff model plans were found to be more supportive, given that their general structure (organized multispecialty group or medical center settings rather than individual offices) is more conducive to providing ample work for NPs or PAs. It is not clear how to interpret the finding that plans with Medicaid contracts tend to be less supportive of NPs and PAs. The box provides examples of how and why plans are more or less supportive of NPs and PAs. The most common reason for lower levels of support is that the plan views

Table 4 Types of Plans More and Less Supportive of Nurse Practitioners and Physician Assistants

	Very Supportive	Less Supportive, Neutral, or Negative*
All plans	35	65
Predominant model type		
Group/staff (n = 11)	64	36
Network/IPA (n = 12)	8	92
Medicaid enrollment		
None (n = 12)	50	50
1–24 percent of total enrollment (n = 3)	33	67
25+ percent of total enrollment (n = 8)	13	88

*Only one or two plans could be categorized as generally negative toward these providers.

decisions on NPs and PAs as being within the discretion of the medical group or physician.

Both plans that are generally supportive of NPs and PAs and those less supportive reported that a substantial proportion of their physicians have negative views on the usefulness or cost-effectiveness of these providers. Such views appear to be a major barrier to increasing the use of NPs and PAs.

Structuring Access to Referrals

The primary care provider selected by enrollees generally functions as a gatekeeper, authorizing referrals for all or most specialty care according to plan rules. In less restrictive plans, any primary care provider the patient sees may perform this function, or, rarely, patients are free to make their own referral choices. Even when gatekeeping policies are generally restrictive, plans normally specify certain services that patients may access without a referral. The most common clinical areas for which plans allow self-referrals are shown in Table 5.

Plan policies for gatekeeping and referral vary widely, and although there are not strong patterns by model type, there is some tendency for network/IPA plans to delegate gatekeeping policies to their contracted groups/IPAs. Thirty percent (7) of the 23 plans use a strict or fairly strict gatekeeper model. That is, these plans require enrollees to select a primary care provider, then limit self-referrals requiring most care to be referred by the primary care provider. Even among these plans, however, most permit self-referral for limited OB/GYN care (6 of 7 plans). At the other extreme, 30 percent have very open policies or practices. Enrollees

Nature of Support for NPs and PAs

Supportive Actions

- Two plans already heavily using NPs and PAs are considering expanding their use—one created a task force to review the advantages and disadvantages of more extensive use.
- One group/staff model plan was raising the status of NPs and removing their nursing duties in hopes of better retaining them.
- One plan had recognized some group physicians using NPs as nurses and influenced them to more appropriately use these providers.
- Heavy use of NPs by 7 plans and PAs by 2 plans.

Supportive Comments

- NPs and PAs are cost-effective providers.
- Consumers in the plan feel more comfortable talking to them than to physicians.
- Consumers like them (generally).
- NPs have a feel for preventive care and teaching due to their training.
- Physicians like them because it enables their practice to be more productive, thus benefiting them financially.

Other Comments

- Most network/IPA plans were neutral or offered verbal support only, because they viewed decisions on NPs and PAs as an IPA or medical group decision.
- Many of the network/IPA plans did not track NP or PA use by their contracted providers.
- Several plans reported physicians were mixed in their views on these providers:
  - — Some physicians favored using them.
  - — Others viewed them as not cost-effective, too inclined to refer patients back to them, too inclined to spend excessive time with patients, or requiring too much supervision.
- Some plans reported mixed views by consumers. One plan's consumer-based strategy was in part distinguishing itself from its competitor by not using NPs or PAs.
- One reported being cautious about contracting with groups that use PAs due to the medical director's past experience with finding they were used without appropriate supervision.
- One heavy-Medicaid plan reported that it does not view NPs and PAs as very useful for its enrollees because the Medicaid clients tend to be sicker than other populations.
- One plan cited lack of availability of hospital privileges as a factor for NPs and PAs.

Table 5 Common Clinical Areas Where HMOs Allowed Enrollees to Self-Refer

Clinical Area	Number of HMOs ($n = 23$)
Limited OB/GYN	15
Mental health	7
Optometry	7
Substance abuse	5
Dermatology	2
All or nearly all care	3
No self-referrals	1

in these plans are able to access a wide range of primary care and specialty providers without getting a referral from their gatekeeper (if they chose one). Two plans in this group allow any physician within a patient's chosen health center to treat the patient without a referral, although referrals are required for any other care. Seventeen percent (4 plans) lie between these extremes. For example, they require a primary care provider to be chosen but allow nearly unrestricted access to other providers. Or they encourage but do not require selection of a primary care provider. The requirements for referrals to specialists are more strict than those of the plans described in the preceding item.

The remaining 22 percent of plans (5), all of which are network/IPA plans, either allow their contracted groups or IPAs to make these policies (4 of the 5 plans), or the rules differ depending on whether the contracted entity is a group or an IPA. If the entity is an IPA, a primary care provider must be chosen on the theory that more loosely structured entities need this rule to manage care by their providers.

The higher level of competition that plans face in areas with high HMO penetration may tend to influence them toward more open gatekeeping policies, (e.g., because of consumer preferences for more open access) although the small numbers prevent conclusions on this point. Only 1 of 7 plans (14 percent) in areas with high HMO penetration maintained strict gatekeeping policies versus 4 of 8 plans in areas with low to moderate HMO penetration.

Referrals must usually be in writing, although some plans allow referrals by phone or are equipped for electronic referrals. Face-to-face contact between a patient and a physician is not always required for a referral, for example, if the physician knows the patient and has discussed his or her problem by phone. Most plans allow patients to self-refer to specialists for at least one or two types of care, most often for a limited amount of OB/GYN care (Table 5).

In general, plans appear to be moving toward tighter gatekeeping arrangements and self-referral policies. Even two of the three most open plans support tighter gatekeeping arrangements in theory; their policies are open only because of major transitions. The main reasons plans gave for tighter arrangements is the perception that they enhance access to and continuity of care, and permit the plan to hold a provider accountable for a patient's care. Concerns about access and accountability are perhaps best explained by one plan as follows. Before the plan required patients to select a primary care provider, they would sometimes diagnose themselves as needing a specialist and call the specialist's office for an appointment. The administrative assistant who received the patient's request would often have to inform the patient that the physician had no appointments for many weeks, and the patient would try another specialist, perhaps in a related field, to gain access to care, perhaps with a similar lack of success. The frustrated patient would complain to the plan, but the plan had no one to hold accountable for the care of the patient. In the current system, the primary care provider can (1) ensure the patient is referred to the correct specialist, (2) facilitate access to this provider, and (3) be held accountable by the plan if he or she does not perform the first two functions.

Plans that have recently tightened their gatekeeping arrangements or are considering doing so indicated that the process takes considerable time and effort. One plan just completed an 18-month process; another reported it would probably tighten its system in the near future, but the medical director knows from experience about the difficult and controversial nature of the process.

Plans are not uniformly moving toward tighter gatekeeping. Five plans reported having recently and selectively eliminated referral requirements, for example, for optometry, after finding that primary care providers do not do any related screening or care, and thus contact with the primary care provider seemed unnecessary. Further, several plans are content with an open policy of care at the chosen health center and require referrals for care from physicians outside the center. Two predominantly group/staff model plans feel this way, and one network/IPA model plan noted that it often finds the groups that are more experienced with managed care are open about on-site referrals (these tend to be large, organized multispecialty group or health center settings). Only one plan directly challenged the concept of gatekeeping as a useful tool for managing care or containing costs. This plan believes that patients can effectively refer themselves for many conditions, and that capitating specialists should be the main mechanism for encouraging appropriate allocation of both resources and care between primary and specialty care providers.

Scope of Practice

Overall, plans perceive that the scope of practice of primary care physicians has not changed much in recent years. Beyond this generalization, all agree that there is not one agreed-upon set of conditions or treatments that constitute the scope of practice of primary care. Thus, the level of care received from a primary care provider may vary depending on the provider's comfort level and experience with certain procedures or conditions more than on any consensus about the scope of practice for primary care providers.

Specific primary care responsibilities may be defined under primary care capitation arrangements; that is, to the extent that physicians are capitated for primary care, they will have responsibility for a defined set of services associated with the capitation amount. (Since examining individual physician payment arrangements was beyond the scope of the study, the evidence is suggestive rather than conclusive in terms of the link between the definition of primary care and payment strategy.) However, not all primary care providers are paid on a capitated basis; in some and perhaps many cases, the medical group or IPA is capitated but chooses to pay its physicians on a discounted fee-for-service basis.

While the content of care practiced by primary care physicians does not appear to have changed substantially, or while such changes are at most limited to a few areas, there is some evidence that changes may soon occur. The study identified three main factors affecting what services are provided by primary care providers rather than specialists: (1) plan financial or other incentives to increase the range of primary care practice (six plans); (2) malpractice liability risk, which has reduced the range of primary care practice in certain areas (two plans); and (3) plan efforts to standardize what is considered primary care; in theory the efforts could either increase or decrease the range of primary care practice (three plans). In practice, it seems likely that plans are interested in standardizing the definition in order to encourage a wider range of practice for those primary care providers who tend to do less than others in their plan.

The financial or other means to increase the range of primary care practice include expanding lists of procedures considered to be primary care. For example, one plan reported adding ECG, minor acne, and allergy injections to its list; another added immunizations, ECGs, pregnancy and other routine tests, colonoscopies, and endoscopies. One plan pays a higher capitation amount to the primary care provider if the patient sees him or her rather than an OB/GYN for a routine gynecological exam. Another provides a financial incentive to primary care providers for performing instead of referring flexible sigmoidoscopies. Other plans simply noted that their compensation models (e.g., capitation to a group that includes specialty services) encourage a broadening of primary care practice.

In addition to expanding the list of procedures, another effort to increase the range of primary care involves redirecting patients with defined borderline conditions back to primary care providers. The plan making this attempt has identified low back pain, minor lacerations, and mild inflammatory bowel disease, for example, as conditions that primary care providers, rather than surgeons, should be treating. The plan is assessing referral patterns for these conditions to develop practice guidelines.

On the other hand, plans in two markets reported that malpractice liability risk has reduced the scope of practice for primary care providers. Some of those who once provided obstetrical care or care for newborns have now reportedly discontinued these services because of the real or perceived high risk of malpractice suits.

The study found three examples of plan efforts to standardize the definition of primary care. The first plan is more specifically defining what primary care providers should do by using lists of procedures because of the current need for computer software packages that could identify payable bills versus procedures included in a primary care capitation amount. The second plan is circulating among providers medical management guidelines that define what primary care providers should be doing. Providers were to comment on the guidelines. The medical director's intent is to encourage physicians to buy into the list of guidelines. The effort stemmed from his observation of wide differences among individual primary care providers in the types of patients they feel comfortable treating. The third plan is analyzing the types of conditions that are being referred from primary care providers, then convening groups of specialists and primary care providers to attempt to reach a consensus on what can be done by primary care physicians. This plan reported that additional training for some primary care providers is the natural follow-up to such an effort, and that it is organizing and will support this training. The plan reported a positive outcome from the process it used to develop this list. It perceived that the primary care and specialist physicians left the meetings with stronger working relationships and a better understanding of each other's capabilities and responsibilities.

The second and third efforts were in progress at the time of the site visit, and therefore the nature of primary care has not yet substantially changed in these plans.

Implications

While HMOs generally pursue a more organized primary care delivery strategy than the fee-for-service sector, their strategies vary substantially across plans. Even the plans with tight gatekeeping systems allow patients access to some services without referral (OB/GYN self-referrals were allowed on a limited basis in 15 of the 23 plans) though beyond OB/GYN plans do not agree on which services patients should directly access. Also, not all plans required selection of a single primary care gatekeeper, though all at least encouraged it. Plans truly ranged from virtually unrestricted access to the plan's full network of providers at one extreme, to plans that strictly required nearly all care decisions be channeled through the chosen primary care provider.

Contracting provider groups have a large role in structuring primary care delivery in network/IPA model plans. This is an increasingly important observation since much of the growth of managed care is occurring in this type of plan.[3,4] Contrary to the popular notion that health plans determine most aspects of delivery, many of the network/IPA type plans we visited paid medical groups or IPAs on a capitated basis, then took a hands-off attitude toward delivery. It was often the medical group or IPA that was responsible for rules regarding choice of primary care provider, and use of NPs or PAs, for example.

Also, the care a patient receives from a primary care physician appears to vary depending on the provider's level of comfort and experience with certain procedures or conditions more than on any consensus about the scope of practice for primary care physicians. There are signs that the scope of practice of primary care physicians may expand for those physicians who now practice primary care within a narrower scope than their peers. For example, 6 of the 23 HMOs reported having financial incentives or educational initiatives to expand the content of primary care. However, they described these as small steps that were not likely to result in large changes in primary care practice in the near future.

Finally, plans' views on the use of subspecialists and OB/GYNs as gatekeepers raise a cautionary note. As policy makers and providers seek opportunities to balance the number of specialists relative to primary care providers, use of specialists in primary care roles may become more common. Yet the findings suggest that plans often view the primary care skills of such providers negatively. At a minimum, initiatives to retrain specialists to practice primary care will be critical to address the perceived problems of over-referral and specialty orientation. Further, some plans were skeptical that primary care was a fitting role for many subspecialists, since the skills used in primary care differ greatly from those attracting physicians to certain specialties (e.g., radiology).

In sum, the diversity among health plans in their primary care strategies is evident from the study. However, the relative desirability of the various strategies has to do with both value judgments (e.g., about what organization or person should be held accountable for an enrollee's care) and unanswered research questions about how different strategies and incentives toward expanded primary care practice affect health care costs, outcomes, and satisfaction with care.

Acknowledgments

The 23 health plans that volunteered senior management time to participate in the site visit interviews on a confidential basis are gratefully acknowledged. Marsha Gold, a Senior Fellow at Mathematica Policy Research, Inc., acted as a senior advisor to the study and provided useful comments on an earlier draft of the manuscript. Jessica Townsend, at the Office of Planning, Evaluation, and Legislation within the Health Resources and Services Administration, saw the need for this study, served as the project officer for the study, and also provided useful comments on a draft of this manuscript. Hilary Frazer, Karyen Chu, and Timothy Lake were other project team members who contributed to collecting the information for this analysis.

References

1. Gold, M., et al. "Behind the Curve: A Critical Assessment of How Little Is Known About Arrangements Between Managed Care Plans and Physicians." *Medical Care Research and Review* 52 (3) (September 1995): 307–41.

2. Felt, S., Frazer, H., and Gold, M. "HMO Primary Care Staffing Patterns and Processes: A Cross-Site Analysis of 23 HMOs." Washington, D.C.: Mathematica Policy Research, Inc., December 23, 1994R.

3. Group Health Association of America. *1995 National Directory of HMOs*. Washington, D.C., GHAA: June 1995.

4. Group Health Association of America. *1993 National Directory of HMOs*. Washington, D.C., GHAA: June 1993.

CHAPTER

7

DELIVERING WOMEN'S PREVENTIVE SERVICES UNDER MANAGED CARE: OPPORTUNITY AND PROMISE

Nancy Heiser and Robert St. Peter

MANAGED CARE plans have become increasingly responsible for providing preventive services to women, including breast and cervical cancer screenings. Even though these types of services detect cancer early and greatly improve cancer survival rates when followed by proper treatment, women have historically underused them. With its growing role in today's healthcare system, managed care offers a unique opportunity to improve the delivery of these services.

Managed care plans now provide healthcare to an unprecedented number of women, including many Medicaid and Medicare beneficiaries, who are at higher risk than others of not receiving preventive care. As such, studying how managed care plans deliver preventive care has grown in policy importance. In addition, the very structure of these plans may profoundly influence preventive care delivery. Because managed care plans integrate healthcare financing and delivery and provide care to a specific population, they may have greater incentives and capacity than

From *Improving the Delivery of Clinical Services to Women in Managed Care Organizations: A Case Study Analysis*, published by Mathematica Policy Research, Inc.

traditional fee-for-service plans to stress disease prevention and health promotion.

This publication summarizes the results of a study conducted by Mathematica Policy Research, Inc., to provide practical information to managed care plans about the types of prevention programs available to women and the potential contributions to their health. It also describes how plans design and implement preventive service programs in managed care settings. The study, conducted for the Commonwealth Fund, is based on analyses of disease prevention programs in six managed care plans and one medical group practice across the United States.

Findings in Brief

- The prevention programs we studied use their management systems and organized care delivery systems to improve the delivery of care.
- The plans use a population-based approach to develop prevention programs. Scientifically based screening guidelines are the programs' foundation.
- To increase the use of screenings, programs use a variety of strategies, such as patient and provider reminders, performance indicators and provider financial incentives, and standardized office procedures. The underlying data structure for these strategies may include tailored program databases or the plan's larger data management system.
- To develop and implement a successful data-driven prevention program, managed care plans must determine essential program features, engage patients and providers, establish good data collection strategies, and continually monitor and evaluate the program.
- Future research should examine the interventions that work in different managed care settings. Programs might benefit from public-private partnerships for promoting the use of preventive services and from purchasers' demands for better delivery of preventive care.

The Programs

We analyzed breast and cervical cancer screening programs because they have the potential to greatly improve the health of a large number of women. Furthermore, managed care plans have historically focused on establishing these services first when developing preventive service programs. As a result, breast and cervical cancer screening programs have the most to tell about plans' efforts and experiences in designing prevention programs.

The plans we studied use two strategies for improving the delivery of breast and cervical cancer screening:

- **Data-driven strategies** use administrative data, medical charts, patient surveys, ancillary data (for example, laboratory and pharmacy data), or a combination of these sources to support preventive service programs.
- **Office-based strategies** use office materials and standard procedures to help office staff monitor preventive services.

Both types of strategies offer great potential for improving screening services as managed care plans step up efforts to gather data as a way to manage their plans and refine their care delivery systems.

We identified screening programs for the case study by conducting a literature review and talking with knowledgeable individuals about prevention programs and managed care. We then selected seven programs that illustrated key points of interest and yielded a mix of managed care plans. We made no attempt to assess relative program effectiveness.

The programs operate in one of the following six health maintenance organizations (HMOs) or a medical group practice that works closely with an HMO but provides its own prevention programs:

- Comprehensive Health Services, Inc./The Wellness Plan
- Group Health Cooperative of Puget Sound
- Harvard Community Health Plan
- Kaiser Foundation Health Plan of Southern California
- Keystone Health Plan East
- U.S. Healthcare
- Park Nicollet Clinic (a medical group)

We collected information about breast and cervical cancer prevention programs in these seven organizations through written materials and telephone interviews with staff—usually the medical director and prevention program director. Next, we discuss how the programs are similar, as well as how they differ.

Program Focus

The programs focus either on one preventive service (we call these "stand-alone programs") or on a broad range of preventive services, including breast and cervical cancer screening ("comprehensive programs"). Comprehensive programs usually create a list of preventive services recommended for each patient and track a patient's status for each service. Providers review each patient's status prior to an office visit.

Scientifically based screening guidelines are a central feature of these programs. These guidelines, which are routinely reviewed and updated, are used to structure programs and develop measures of program success. The guidelines vary by plan, reflecting controversy over the appropriate use of services the guidelines recommend, variations in local provider practices, and differences in the characteristics of plans' enrollees.

The programs' target populations are driven by the screening guidelines. For example, if a plan recommends an annual mammogram for all women age 50 and over and one every other year for women ages 40 to 49, all women age 40 and over are the target population. Some programs also target subgroups of women at high risk for developing a particular disease, such as breast cancer. Information on risk factors, such as family history, is collected through patient surveys.

Support for the Intervention

The programs use different combinations of data to support their interventions. Plan enrollment files typically serve to identify many individuals in the target population. Some women, however, cannot be identified through existing data (for example, sexually active females under age 18, who the guidelines recommend receive Pap smears). To determine the service needs of the target population, the programs often use claims or encounter data and sometimes laboratory data. Some programs have designed databases to support their cancer screening intervention, while others use their plan's larger management or clinical information system or an automated patient medical record system.

Getting More Women Screened

The programs use one or more of the following procedures to increase the use of breast and/or cervical cancer screening:

- **Patient reminders.** These reminders, which encourage women to obtain preventive services, are the primary data-driven, patient-focused intervention used. They may target all women in a program or only those who are past due for a service. Reminders may take the form of letters, postcards, phone calls, or a combination of the three.
- **Provider reminders.** These reminders are designed either to (1) prompt a provider to review a patient's records before every visit to identify unmet preventive care needs, or (2) periodically remind a provider about preventive care needs through, for example, lists of patients needing a given service.
- **Performance feedback to providers.** This feedback may be in the form of performance indicators to encourage providers to improve

the delivery of preventive care. Programs often use the HEDIS (Health Plan Employer Data Information Set) mammography and Pap smear measures. Performance measures can be computed for a medical service area, a group of providers, or individual providers. Feedback includes performance information on other providers for comparison.

- **Financial incentives for providers.** Some programs link financial compensation to providers' performance. This approach involves assessing performance in the delivery of preventive care and using this information, usually in combination with other performance measures, to determine provider payments (such as adjustments in salary, annual bonuses, or capitation payments).
- **Office staff reminders and procedures.** Some programs use reminders, such as flowcharts and stickers placed in medical charts, or standardized office procedures to flag unmet needs for preventive care.

Looking to the Future

The breast and cervical cancer screening programs we studied illustrate how managed care plans and associated medical group practices integrate health promotion and disease prevention activities in healthcare delivery. Some managed care plans are taking an active role in promoting the use of preventive services and have long-standing, well-developed programs. Others have relatively new programs and are experimenting with ways to promote their services.

Prevention programs and supporting research efforts require substantial planning and resource commitments from sponsoring health plans. To improve the delivery of services, plans should use a population-based approach to identify the clinical conditions to be addressed. They also must select the target population, define the outcomes to be measured, and engage providers and patients in program design and implementation. After programs are up and running, plans need to monitor their success and use the information to change the behavior of patients, providers, or both.

Elements of Success

We identified the following areas as important in the success of data-driven preventive services programs. Although managed care plans have made progress within each area, they still face many challenges.

- **Determining program features.** As plans make decisions about developing prevention programs, they must consider several important design factors. Specifically, they must select the preventive services for which they will develop a program. They must also decide whether to implement stand-alone or comprehensive programs, and determine the extent to which resources will be used to target high-risk populations (such as low-income women). The programs we studied have formed committees and other mechanisms for selecting the preventive services to be included. They have also developed both stand-alone and comprehensive programs. Some have devoted resources to identifying high-risk populations, such as women at higher risk for developing breast or cervical cancer and women at risk for not receiving preventive services. The plans are struggling with many of their decisions, especially as they attempt to control costs while meeting external demands for positive performance indicators. Identifying and reaching high-risk populations is also difficult, since enrollment turnover in managed care plans is high.

- **Engaging patients and providers.** Most program administrators emphasize the need for support from providers and patients. Many plans try to involve them in the early stages of program development. It may be difficult to engage providers in loosely structured networks and determine how to influence their behavior —through financial and/or nonfinancial incentives—while minimizing their burden. Plans also face challenges in reaching more diverse patient groups and educating them about preventive services.
- **Collecting data.** The programs we studied illustrate how administrative and other forms of data can be used in innovative ways to support prevention programs. They have used data creatively to determine unmet preventive care needs, but the data quality and the ease with which data can be obtained vary considerably. Plans' biggest challenge is collecting accurate and timely data that can be used for a variety of purposes, such as monitoring performance and meeting external reporting requirements. Factors such as out-of-plan service use and discontinuous enrollment may complicate these efforts. Other challenges include using imperfect or incomplete data to identify and reach target populations, determine unmet preventive care needs, develop methods and algorithms for additional preventive services (such as counseling), and identify high-risk groups.
- **Monitoring and evaluating programs.** The monitoring process involves many challenges, including determining whom to include in the program population for evaluation purposes and how to identify them. Challenges also include determining what constitutes "success" and overcoming the data difficulties described above. Plans are facing increasing pressure to develop and monitor health outcome measures, a process that will require new data collection methods and efforts. The biggest hurdle involves

defining meaningful measures and integrating the data collection process for monitoring and evaluating with the prevention program and healthcare service delivery system.

The programs we studied can provide important information to others about resolving the challenges involved in improving the delivery of preventive care. Increasing external demands from purchasers and accreditation organizations may spur these programs to continue to develop and improve. Programs might benefit from forming partnerships with public health programs that are pursuing similar efforts to increase the use of preventive services.

Future research should attempt to shed light on the types of interventions that work in various managed care settings. It would also be useful to develop strategies for small network models entering the market as well as strategies for reaching the women most at risk for not receiving preventive services. Plans would also benefit from improved methods for collecting and managing data for prevention programs. Other research efforts might identify successful public-private partnerships for promoting the use of preventive services.

PART

3

MANAGED CARE AND PUBLIC PROGRAMS

Introduction: Why Do Policymakers Have a Special Interest in Managed Care for Public Programs?

The performance of publicly funded programs like Medicare and Medicaid has always been carefully scrutinized. These programs were established to improve access to care for groups of the U.S. population that might otherwise have limited access because of financial or other barriers. Medicare covers both the elderly and disabled people—groups that use a higher than average amount of services—and includes particularly vulnerable subgroups such as frail elders and individuals with disabilities (Moon 1996). Medicaid serves the poor and others with special needs, such as low-income pregnant women and young children; the sick whose limited incomes are eaten up by heavy health expenses; and groups such as the disabled, mentally retarded, and elderly people who need long-term care services (Rowland et al. 1992).

The performance of these programs has always been more closely monitored than that of the general healthcare system because of the groups served and the tax dollars consumed. As managed care has been introduced into Medicare and Medicaid, this scrutiny has continued and intensified. As a result, there is substantial interest in research that targets the role of managed care in these programs.

The first two of the seven articles in this section are based on recent studies to provide critical information to policymakers interested in the performance of Medicare managed care. Both articles examine risk-based Medicare HMOs, which have historically been the main managed care contracting vehicle in Medicare. While only a small share of Medicare beneficiaries were enrolled in Medicare HMOs in 1997, this share is rapidly rising.

The first article, "Do Health Maintenance Organizations Work for Medicare?", summarizes the findings from a four-year, multimillion-dollar evaluation of the program sponsored by the Health Care Financing Administration, the federal agency responsible for Medicare. The evaluation results are mixed: They are relatively encouraging about the ability of Medicare HMOs to reduce utilization without lowering quality of care. However, they also show that, because of adverse selection, costs to the government actually increased. These findings have fueled an ongoing debate over federal Medicare HMO payment policy.

The second article, "Access to Care in Medicare HMOs, 1996," is based on a national survey of Medicare managed care enrollees and disenrollees. Using a variety of measures and subgroup comparisons, the authors describe patterns of access to care and illustrate why both of these are important in monitoring access to care. The study was sponsored by the Physician Payment Review Commission, an agency established to provide objective analysis to Congress on Medicare physician payment and other program issues. The study provides baseline information for monitoring access in Medicare managed care as well as information that can be used to revise ongoing Medicare surveys to better support their use in monitoring performance.

Five articles in Part 3 are based on research about Medicaid managed care. Medicaid research is more challenging than in Medicare because of the variation in state Medicaid programs, the extreme diversity of the Medicaid population, and the dearth of uniform data on the program nationwide. The expansion of Medicaid managed care will exacerbate the problems, particularly because the 1997 Balanced Budget Act gives states greater flexibility to structure their programs, without special federal waivers.

The third of the seven articles in Part 3, "Changes in Health Plans Serving Medicaid, 1993–1996," provides a national context for understanding managed care plans in the Medicaid program. Using a database developed for this purpose, the authors describe recent trends in the characteristics of health plans participating in Medicaid managed care and the implications of these trends for oversight.

The next two articles describe the early experience of states that have been prominent in today's rapidly expanding Medicaid managed care market. "Medicaid Managed Care: Lessons from Five States" summarizes results from case studies documenting the design of and experience with Medicaid managed care in California, Minnesota, New York, Oregon, and Tennessee. The paper offers ten lessons for other states pursuing Medicaid managed care. "Reforming State Medicaid Programs: First-Year Implementation Experiences from Three States" presents the first reports from a multiyear, comprehensive, federally funded evaluation of states that have implemented Medicaid managed care as part of a broader Section 1115 waiver from the Health Care Financing Administration. The paper covers Hawaii, Rhode Island, and Tennessee and also describes lessons learned during implementation. Both these studies show that prior managed care experience and effective oversight structures are critical to a state's success in Medicaid managed care.

The last two articles focus on the design of these oversight structures. "Quality Assurance for Medicaid Managed Care" summarizes a three-year evaluation of the Quality Assurance Reform Initiative (QARI), a three-state demonstration that sought to define a framework for quality assurance functions in Medicaid managed care that involved health plans and their affiliated providers, states, and Medicaid beneficiaries. The demonstration showed that it is feasible to develop oversight structures like QARI, but doing so also takes a great deal of time and effort. "Medicaid Managed Care Encounter Data: What, Why, and Where Next?" focuses on how to create an information infrastructure to support performance monitoring in Medicaid managed care. This endeavor may arguably be one of the major administrative challenges of the future.

References

Moon, M. 1996. *Medicare Now and in the Future,* 2nd ed. Washington, DC: Urban Institute Press.

Rowland, D., J. Feder, B. Lyons, and A. Salganicoff. 1992. *Medicaid at the Crossroads.* Baltimore, MD: Kaiser Commission for the Future of Medicaid.

CHAPTER

8

DO HEALTH MAINTENANCE ORGANIZATIONS WORK FOR MEDICARE?

Randall S. Brown, Dolores Gurnick Clement,
Jerrold W. Hill, Sheldon M. Retchin,
and Jeanette W. Bergeron

Medicare Risk Program: Purpose and Evolution

As one of many efforts to control Medicare costs, HCFA has tried to use HMOs to generate the cost savings for Medicare that HMOs are widely believed to produce for employers providing health coverage to non-elderly people. HMOs, which act as insurers but have control over the set of providers from which members can choose and how much they are paid, have an incentive to provide care in the most cost-effective manner possible. This cost-effectiveness is achieved by reducing unnecessary services and providing health care in the least expensive but appropriate setting. The market power of HMOs can also help them negotiate favorable prices for provider services.

The Medicare risk program, which became operational in April 1985 under the Tax Equity and Fiscal Responsibility Act (TEFRA) of 1982 (Public Law 97-248), allows HMOs to assume responsibility for providing all Medicare-covered services to beneficiaries in return for a capitated payment. The capitation payment to an HMO for an enrolled

From *Health Care Financing Review* 15 (1): 7–23. It is reprinted here without change.

beneficiary living in a given county is equal to 95 percent of HCFA's actuarial estimate of the average amount that HCFA would spend in FFS reimbursements for a Medicare beneficiary who resides in that county. This county rate, the adjusted average per capita cost (AAPCC), is equal to the projected average Medicare reimbursement per beneficiary in the United States for the year multiplied by the historic average ratio of Medicare reimbursements per beneficiary for the county to Medicare reimbursements per beneficiary for the United States. The payment rate also varies with the individual's age, gender, reason for entitlement (age or disability), institutional status (residing in a nursing home or not), and Medicaid eligibility, to account for the possibility that those who enroll in HMOs may not be representative of the Medicare population in that county.

In return for the AAPCC premium, HMOs must provide or arrange all Medicare-covered services for enrolled beneficiaries. HMOs also cover the Medicare deductibles and coinsurance for which a beneficiary is responsible, but can charge a premium for this coverage, as well as for any other benefits covered by the risk plan but not by Medicare (for example, eye exams and lenses, hearing tests and aids, prescription drugs, and preventive care).

HCFA's primary goal in establishing the risk program was to reduce Medicare costs. HCFA also sought to achieve two other objectives: (1) to provide more efficient health care than that rendered by the FFS sector, while maintaining or improving the quality of care; and (2) to give Medicare beneficiaries access to the same range of choices of health care delivery systems available to younger individuals. HCFA also hoped that costs in the FFS sector would decline as more Medicare beneficiaries enrolled in HMOs. The expectation was that the risk program would be attractive to HMOs, causing rapid expansion in the number of participating risk plans and beneficiaries.

To determine whether the risk program accomplished these objectives, HCFA funded a 4-year evaluation conducted by Mathematica Policy Research, Inc. and the Medical College of Virginia. The overall results of this evaluation, which we summarize in this article, are reviewed in greater detail in Brown et al. (1993). The samples and analyses were designed to yield results that were representative of the entire Medicare risk program (Figure 1). HMO impacts were estimated by comparing the experience of Medicare HMO members to that of non-HMO Medicare beneficiaries residing in the same locations, controlling statistically for differences in the composition of the two groups. The methodology

Figure 1 Areas Served, by Medicare Risk Plans and Levels of Enrollment: January 1992

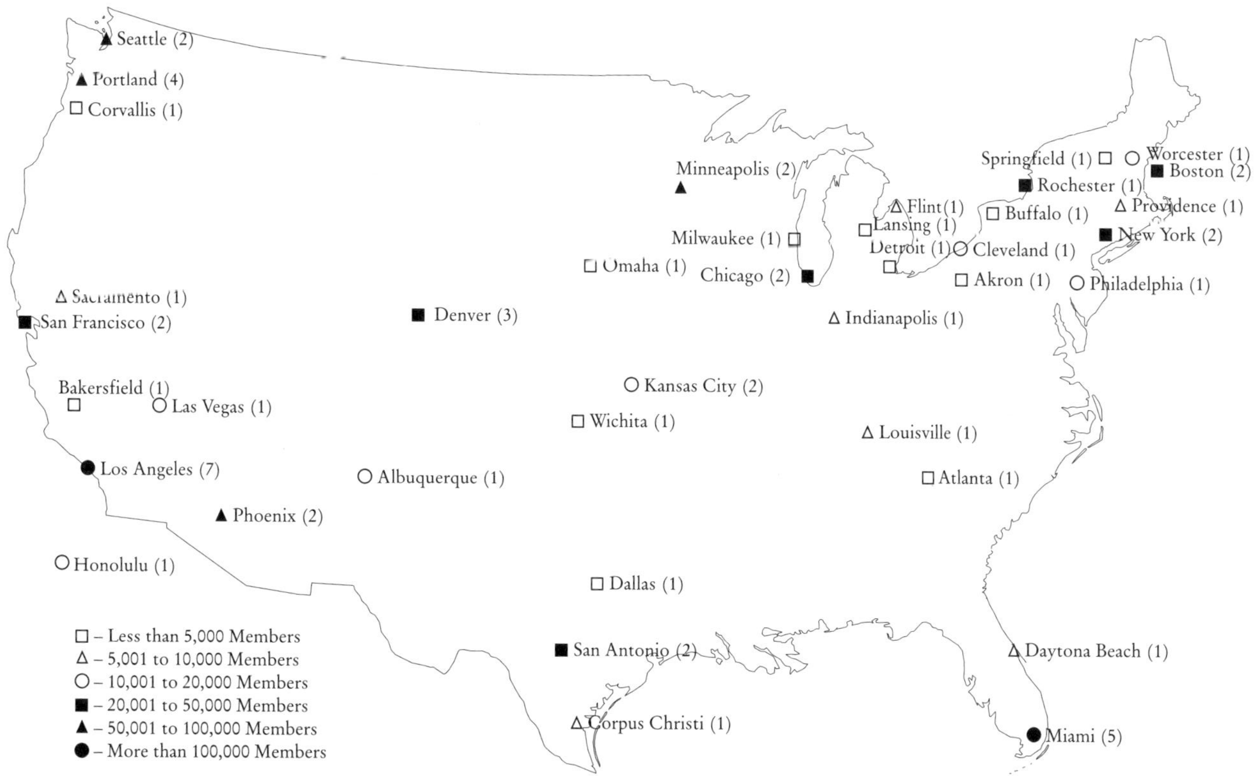

Source: Brown, R. S., and Bergeron, J. W., Mathematica Policy Research, Clement, D. G., and Retchin, S. M., Virginia Commonwealth University, and Hill, J. W., SANUS Corporation Health Systems, 1993.

Notes: In a few instances, a risk plan will have enrollees in more than one market area (for example, Miama and Tampa; Los Angeles and San Diego). In these cases, the enrollment for the entire plan is attributed to the market area of largest enrollment, unless the plan has separate contracts for the areas. The number of plans in the market area are shown in parentheses.

and research details are explained more fully in the 18 separate technical reports completed under the evaluation.

Do Medicare HMOs Save Money?

By design, the risk program should lower costs to HCFA by 5 percent, relative to what HCFA would have paid in FFS reimbursements, because the HMOs are paid only 95 percent of the AAPCC. However, if those who enroll in risk plans are not a representative mix of Medicare beneficiaries (after risk adjustment factors are considered), HCFA payments based on the AAPCC may not be a particularly accurate estimate of what FFS reimbursements would have been for this group. This potential problem exists even if the AAPCC methodology forecasts average costs for those in the FFS sector perfectly. In particular, if enrollees are healthier on average than other beneficiaries (that is, if the HMOs experience "favorable selection"), the program will save less than the intended 5 percent and may actually increase costs to HCFA. If HMOs experience "adverse selection," HCFA will save more than 5 percent, but risk plans may lose money and drop out of the program. The evaluation measured the extent of favorable or adverse selection and estimated the effects of the risk program on costs to HCFA.

Risk Plans Attract Healthier Beneficiaries

Risk plan enrollees had substantially lower Medicare reimbursements during the 2 years prior to enrollment than did non-enrollees during a comparable period, even after controlling for differences between the two groups in the demographic risk factors incorporated in the AAPCC payment mechanism (Hill and Brown, 1990). Prior reimbursements for a sample of nearly 100,000 new enrollees in 1987 and 1988 were about 20 percent lower overall than the risk-adjusted reimbursements for non-enrollees from the same market areas. About two-thirds of the 98 risk plans examined experienced clearly favorable selection according to this measure, and the other one-third experienced slightly favorable or neutral selection. None of the plans experienced adverse selection. Similar results were obtained from comparing the proportions of the two groups of beneficiaries with a prior hospital stay for a condition associated with high costs in subsequent years.

Enrollees also had fewer functional disabilities and other indicators of chronic health problems than non-enrollees, were less likely to rate their health as poor, and expressed less inclination to use health care services when they were not feeling well (Hill and Brown, 1992). Even after controlling for enrollee and non-enrollee differences in health status that could be a result of differences between the groups in factors accounted for by the AAPCC payment mechanism (enrollees were less likely to be on Medicaid, in institutions, 80 years of age or over, or Medicare-entitled because of disability rather than age), enrollees were 15 to 30 percent less likely than non-enrollees to exhibit various health problems. For example, 27 percent of enrollees had a history of cancer, heart disease, or stroke, compared with 32 percent of non-enrollees (a 16-percent lower rate of incidence), even after adjusting for the demographic risk factors. These findings were obtained from a 1990 survey of more than 6,400 randomly selected enrollees from 75 risk plans and a comparable number of non-enrollees from the same market areas. The sample was drawn from the full set of enrollees, unlike the prior-use analysis samples, thereby providing a more representative picture of the risk program as it matured.

The differences between enrollees and non-enrollees appear to be due primarily to the self-selection of enrollees, because HMOs must enroll any interested Medicare beneficiary. Beneficiaries with chronic health problems are less likely than those in good health to change doctors or give up their freedom to use the primary care physicians, specialists, and hospitals of their choice.

Costs to Medicare Increased

We estimate that HCFA expenditures for the risk program were approximately 5.7 percent more than they would have been for FFS care, primarily as a result of favorable selection into Medicare risk plans. Although HCFA paid the HMOs 95 percent of the AAPCC estimate of what FFS costs would have been, our estimates of these FFS costs for the survey sample of enrollees were only 90 percent of the AAPCC projection. To project what FFS reimbursements would have been for the enrollees, we inserted data on various characteristics for enrollees in the survey sample (demographic risk factors, health status, access to care, attitudes, and socioeconomic traits) into a Medicare reimbursements equation that was estimated for the non-enrollees in the survey sample. We used a similar approach based solely on the AAPCC demographic risk factors to project the AAPCC payment that would prevail if it predicted average FFS costs perfectly for the non-enrollees in each market area. The estimated effect—the difference between projected AAPCC payments and the projected FFS costs for enrollees—is statistically significant at the 0.01 level. The 95 percent confidence interval for the estimated increase in cost to HCFA resulting from the risk program is 2.4 to 9.1 percent. Our estimates indicate that Medicare Part A costs (for hospital, skilled nursing facility [SNF], and home health care) increased by 8.5 percent; Part B costs (for physician services, laboratory tests, and X-rays) increased by only 2.7 percent.

The difference between projected AAPCC payments and projected FFS costs for enrollees was due almost entirely to health status differences between enrollees and non-enrollees that were not fully captured by the demographic risk factors—that is, age, gender, residence in a nursing home, Medicaid eligibility, reason for entitlement, and county of residence. Differences in self-ratings of health, the ability to perform activities of daily living (ADLs) and instrumental activities of daily living (IADLs) without assistance, and a history of serious illness (cancer, heart disease, or stroke) accounted for 83 percent of the difference between the projected AAPCC rate and the projected FFS costs of enrollees. The history of serious illness indicator alone accounted for 38 of the 83 percent. Differences in attitudes toward health and health care accounted for 14 percent of the difference, and socioeconomic factors and access to care accounted for the remaining 3 percent.

Cost increases to HCFA were greatest for enrollees in the areas with the highest AAPCCs, HMOs that did not charge a premium, and staff model plans. Costs to HCFA for enrollees in plans that did not charge a premium were more than 8 percent higher than FFS costs would have been, whereas costs increased by only 2 percent for enrollees in plans that charged beneficiaries $50 or more per month. Thus, although costs to HCFA have increased, the program requirement that excess payments be used to lower premiums or increase benefits to beneficiaries is clearly working as intended. The higher estimated cost increases to HCFA in areas with high AAPCC rates indicate that selection into risk plans is more favorable in these areas. Our estimates, because of their construction, are driven only by observable differences in the characteristics of enrollees and non-enrollees and do not reflect any additional effects on costs that would result from errors in the AAPCC in predicting average FFS costs for a given county or market area.

Do HMOs Reduce Service Utilization?

The premise of the Medicare risk program is that HMOs can prosper while providing Medicare coverage for less money than the FFS sector, primarily by reducing unnecessary service use and inefficiency in the delivery of health care. HMOs are believed to achieve most of their savings by reducing hospital use, presumably by substituting less expensive types of care, including ambulatory care, home health visits, and nursing home care, and by practicing preventive care.

We estimated the impact of the risk program on the utilization of hospital services, SNFs, home health care, and physician visits by comparing service use reported on the survey by enrollees and non-enrollees for the year prior to the interview, controlling for differences in health status measures, attitudes toward health care, and demographic variables.

HMOs Reduce Hospital Days

HMOs shortened the average hospital length of stay (LOS) by 1.5 days (16.8 percent) relative to FFS, but did not affect the number of hospital admissions (Table 1). The finding that HMOs reduce total hospital days by shortening stays rather than by reducing admissions is contrary to expectations generated by some previous studies (Manning et al., 1984; Luft, 1981), and is especially surprising given that Medicare's prospective payment system (PPS) provides a similar incentive for hospitals to reduce LOSs among FFS patients. (Under PPS, which was implemented in 1983, hospitals are paid a fixed, pre-determined amount on the basis of a patient's diagnosis.) However, our findings are supported by recent literature (Stern et al., 1989) and by our independent analysis of the quality of inpatient care (described later), which showed that LOSs among two groups of HMO patients with particular conditions (colon cancer and stroke) were 18 to 23 percent shorter, on average, than LOSs among FFS patients with the same conditions in the same metropolitan areas. Further support for these findings comes from an evaluation case study (Hurley and Bannick, 1992) indicating that many successful risk plans use case management (preadmission planning for each patient by a specially trained nurse, together with the patient's physician, to determine how long the patient should be in the hospital) to shorten hospital stays. Case managers also identify the type of post-discharge care likely to be required and arrange for the care well in advance to ensure that it is available when needed. The lack of an effect on admission rates suggests that few hospital stays for elderly people are discretionary now and that FFS providers are using new technologies to treat individuals as outpatients. Hospital admissions per 1,000 aged Medicare beneficiaries in the FFS sector declined by 25 percent from 1985 to 1989, indicating that Medicare HMOs may have much less opportunity now than they did in the past to save money by reducing hospital admissions.

HMOs Increase Some Services but Reduce Intensity

Medicare risk plans increased the likelihood that beneficiaries visited a physician at least once during the year from 84 to 89 percent but slightly reduced the likelihood of having one or more visits per month (on average) from 14 to 12.5 percent (Hill et al., 1992). HMOs also increased the likelihood that beneficiaries had a physical exam by 6 percent, consistent

Table 1 Medicare HMO Effects on Hospital Use

Hospital Use Measure	HMO	FFS	Impact
Sample Size	6,457	6,071	—
Probability of 1 or more hospitalizations in percent	15.0	15.9	−0.9
Hospital stays per 1,000 beneficiaries	218	212	6
Hospital days per 1,000 beneficiaries	1,530	1,839	−309*
Averge length of stay	7.25	8.69	−1.44*

Source: (Hill et al., 1992).
Notes: HMO is health maintenance organization. FFS is fee-for-service.
*Statistically significant at the .05 level (one-tailed test).

with HMOs' emphasis on and coverage of preventive care. However, these plans had no effect on the average number of visits per beneficiary in the month preceding the interview. This absence of an effect on number of visits reflects competing HMO incentives: to reduce the number of visits per patient to control costs, while encouraging patients to obtain routine preventive care to reduce the need for more expensive services later.

Similarly, risk plans increased by a large proportion (but a small absolute amount) the likelihood of a beneficiary's receiving care in an SNF, but they did not increase the total number of SNF days relative to those beneficiaries in FFS care. These estimates are consistent with the expectation that HMOs may shorten hospital stays by substituting SNF care for more expensive hospital days. We found that, for stroke patients, HMO members were discharged sooner and to less intensive types of care arrangements (SNFs instead of rehabilitation hospitals) than FFS patients. However, HMOs appeared to reduce the intensity of use, because there was no effect on the total number of SNF days despite the increase in SNF admissions.

HMOs had no effect on the proportion of individuals with some home health care utilization, but they reduced the number of home health visits by 50 percent. Again, HMOs do not limit initial access to services but do control costs by reducing the intensity of the service rendered. HMOs reduced visits by registered nurses for nursing care and physical therapy and visits by home health aides for assistance with personal care.

Effects Are Greatest for the Seriously Ill

HMOs increased the use of some services by beneficiaries whose health was poorest, but they reduced the intensity of services more for this group than for other beneficiaries. For example, although HMOs had no effect on hospital admissions overall, they increased the probability of admission for enrollees in poor health and those with functional impairments. On the other hand, the largest HMO reductions in hospital days and home health visits were associated with beneficiaries who were in poor health, had ADL or IADL impairments, or died within 9 months after the interview. Our results for quality of care (reviewed later) suggest that these reductions are more likely the result of eliminating unnecessary services or substituting other types of care than of restricting access to needed care.

Effects Vary with Plan Characteristics

Staff model plans, plans that charged high premiums, and plans in low AAPCC areas were less successful than other risk plans at controlling utilization. Staff model plans, which pay physicians a salary and do not expose them to financial risk, were unable to reduce hospital days and home health visits, in contrast with the sizable reductions achieved by individual practice associations (IPAs) and group plans. Staff plans also increased the number of physician visits substantially, unlike the other model types. The much larger reductions in hospital days per 1,000 enrollees by HMOs in high AAPCC areas suggest that FFS hospital use in these areas may be especially inefficient. Finally, the HMOs that charged 1990 monthly premiums of $50 or more were unable to reduce hospital use or home health use and showed an increase in physician visits relative to the FFS sector. This finding suggests that their utilization management practices or incentives did not yield more efficient medical practices than FFS and therefore did not enable these HMOs to provide coverage at rates substantially below medigap rates. However, it is possible that competition from HMOs in some of these areas has forced the FFS sector to be as efficient as the HMOs.

HMOs Use Fewer Medical Resources

The combined HMO effects on hospital, physician, home health, and SNF use suggest that HMOs may have spent about 10.5 percent less for all Medicare-covered services combined than the amount HCFA would have spent in reimbursements to FFS providers. This estimate is a weighted average of the proportionate HMO effects on the four types of services examined (with weights equal to the share of that service in total projected Medicare FFS reimbursements for enrollees). It has no bearing on whether the risk program affects the costs to HCFA, because payments to HMOs are predetermined by the AAPCC and are unaffected by the HMOs' actual resource use. However, the estimate does imply that the potential for cost savings to HCFA may exist. The reduction in medical resources consumed is reasonably large (resulting almost entirely from the 17 percent reduction in hospital days) and may be sufficient to allow HMOs to cover their administrative costs, even if their AAPCC payments were reduced. This estimate is quite rough, however, because the marginal service use eliminated by HMOs may not be as expensive as service use that could not be eliminated (for example, the last days of a hospital stay may be less resource-intensive), thus lowering the amount of potential savings. On the other hand, because HMO members undergo fewer tests and are more likely than FFS patients to be treated by primary care physicians rather than by specialists, the difference between AAPCC payments and the amount paid by an HMO for medical services may exceed the 10.5 percent estimate. Furthermore, HMOs may negotiate more favorable rates for services than those paid by Medicare.

Do HMOs Affect Quality of Care?

The quality of care delivered by HMOs has the potential to be better or worse than that rendered by FFS providers. In responding to the financial incentives to provide care more efficiently, HMOs may restrict services too much, leading to lower-quality care. Efforts to economize can also lead to poorer care if the HMOs' physicians, other service providers, or facilities are inferior to those in the FFS sector. On the other hand, the features that distinguish HMOs from FFS providers—the coordination of care, the emphasis on preventive care, and lower out-of-pocket costs to members—can lead to higher-quality care for enrollees.

We assessed the impacts of risk plans on quality of care by: comparing the services received by HMO and FFS patients who were hospitalized for colon cancer or stroke and their outcomes; comparing the ambulatory care received by HMO and FFS patients for three chronic problems (joint pain, urinary incontinence, and recurring chest pain); and comparing the satisfaction of HMO enrollees and non-enrollees with various aspects of the care they received.[1]

Inpatient Outcomes Are Similar to FFS

The rates of death, hospital readmission, and post-admission complications among HMO and FFS patients were similar, indicating no differences in outcomes (Table 2). Furthermore, HMOs achieved these outcomes with significantly lower use of various procedures, tests, or services. HMOs reduced hospital LOS by 23 percent among colon cancer patients and by 18 percent among stroke patients, consistent with the 17 percent shorter LOS observed overall among the survey sample (which

Table 2 Medicare HMO Effects on Hospital Outcomes

	Stroke Patients			Colon Cancer Patients		
Outcomes	HMO	FFS	Impact	HMO	FFS	Impact
Sample size	402	408	—	412	401	—
Percent readmitted within:						
31 days after discharge	9.3	12.4	−3.1	7.6	7.9	−0.3
61 days after discharge	14.4	14.9	−0.5	11.6	12.2	−0.6
91 days after discharge	17.3	17.2	0.1	15.2	14.8	0.4
Percent of in-hospital deaths	12.2	14.7	−2.5	3.4	4.8	−1.4

Source: (Retchin et al., 1992).
Notes: HMO is health maintenance organization. FFS is fee-for-service.

did not control for diagnosis). HMO members also spent about one-third less time, on average, in intensive care units for both conditions. In addition, HMOs substantially reduced the use of various laboratory tests and procedures that appeared to be discretionary, such as multiple computerized axial tomography scans and electroencephalograms for stroke patients.

Although the similarity in outcomes suggests no major differences in quality of care, a few differences do indicate that HMOs may be providing less adequate care in some situations. The most striking evidence for this inference was the significantly shorter distance between the tumor and the margin of resection (the portion of the colon that was removed) for HMO patients. For these patients, the average distance was approximately equal to the minimum recommendation. However, various other indicators of quality of surgical care revealed no differences between the two systems of care—for example, the amount of colon removed, the amount of blood lost during surgery, and the average number of lymph nodes removed. HMO stroke patients received significantly less physical therapy while in the hospital and had greater motor and speech deficits at discharge, yet were not more likely to have post-discharge speech or physical therapy planned. This pattern suggests that HMOs may economize on rehabilitative care; on the other hand, HMO patients were discharged sooner and may well have recovered an equivalent level of functioning with the passage of an equivalent number of days after the date of admission. Finally, HMO patients were not more likely to have post-admission complications, and the responses of HMOs to complications were similar in most cases. However, HMOs were less likely than FFS providers (49 versus 64 percent) to give chest X-rays to colon cancer patients who experienced post-operative fevers. (A review of the literature indicates X-rays are called for in 80 to 100 percent of such patients.) HMOs also administered pre-operative antibiotics less frequently than did FFS providers. This precaution is recommended for all colon surgery patients by the American Society of Hospital Pharmacists as protection against wound infections. This difference between enrollees and non-enrollees did not produce a higher incidence of post-operative fevers among enrollees in our sample, however. Although there is no evidence that these differences in care led to poorer patient outcomes, they cause some concern because of their potential adverse effect on outcomes.

In addition to providing less resource-intensive care while a patient is in the hospital, HMOs also discharged both stroke and colon cancer patients to lower-cost settings than did FFS providers. For stroke patients, HMOs discharged a higher proportion to nursing homes and a lower proportion to rehabilitation hospitals, which tend to be substantially more expensive and provide more extensive rehabilitative services. For colon cancer patients, HMOs discharged patients to their homes more often and to nursing homes or rehabilitation hospitals less often. We have no followup data on the quality of life or recovery time for either group of patients, so it is not possible to determine whether these differences in post-hospital care are evidence of HMOs' greater cost-effectiveness or of poorer care. We know only that these differences did not affect hospital readmission rates for patients with either condition.

Access to Ambulatory Care Matches FFS

We observed no consistent pattern of differences between HMO and FFS patients in the likelihood of receiving medical attention for three common, chronic problems of elderly people (Table 3). HMOs consistently use resources less intensively, however. HMO members and FFS beneficiaries were equally likely to have experienced each of the three health problems—joint pain, urinary incontinence, and chest pain. There were differences between the two groups in the proportion seeking and receiving medical attention, ranging from HMO members being significantly more likely than nonenrollees to visit a physician for their joint pain, equally likely to see a physician for incontinence, and significantly less likely to see a physician for chest pains. Further investigation of HMO patients with chest pain who did not see a doctor revealed that none of these individuals had sought care. This absence of evidence of differences in access to care contrasts markedly with the sizable differences in the type and quantity of resources used in their treatment. For each of these conditions, HMO members were less likely than FFS patients

Table 3 Medicare HMO Effects on Ambulatory Outcomes

	Joint Pain			Urinary Incontinence			Chest Pain		
Symptom Response	HMO	FFS	Impact	HMO	FFS	Impact	HMO	FFS	Impact
Sample size	2,243	2,009	—	946	764	—	556	524	—
Percent no longer experiencing problem	22.7	22.1	0.6	46.6	51.2	−4.6	43.7	45.1	−1.4
Percent whose symptoms improved (for those still experiencing symptoms)	29.3	36.5	−7.2*	35.6	29.2	6.4	39.3	44.4	−5.1

Source: (Clement et al., 1992).
Notes: HMO is health maintenance organization. FFS is fee-for-service.
*Statistically significant at the .05 level (two-tailed test).

to see a specialist, less likely to have a followup visit scheduled, and less likely to have their progress monitored. HMOs also administered X-rays less often (but only for patients with urinary incontinence). However, HMOs prescribed medication more often for patients with joint pain. No differences were observed in prescribed treatments or use of specific diagnostic tests.

As with inpatient care, ambulatory outcomes were quite similar for HMO and FFS patients, despite the lower use of resources by HMOs. The estimated effect of HMOs on the likelihood that a patient was symptom-free at the time of the interview was not statistically significant for any of the three conditions. Of those who were still experiencing joint pain, HMO patients were less likely than FFS patients to indicate that their symptoms had improved; no such difference was observed among patients still experiencing urinary incontinence or chest pain. Taken together, these outcome measures suggest that the ambulatory care received by HMO patients is of comparable quality to that received by FFS patients. The lower level of services rendered appears to be due to the elimination of discretionary services.

Enrollees' Satisfaction with HMOs Is Mixed

More than 90 percent of both HMO enrollees and FFS beneficiaries rated various dimensions of their care as good or excellent. On virtually every dimension examined except cost, however, enrollees were significantly less likely than non-enrollees to rate their care as excellent. Enrollees were less likely to rate their level of satisfaction as excellent for measures of the care process (for example, explanations given by their physicians or attention they received as a patient), the structure of care (ease of obtaining care, waiting times, and ease of seeing the physician of their choice), and the perceived quality and outcomes of care (thoroughness of examinations and overall results of care received). On the other hand, enrollees were much more likely to rate their satisfaction with out-of-pocket costs as excellent and identified significantly fewer instances of needing various types of health care for which they did not have coverage.

Another rough indicator of satisfaction—the proportion of enrollees who left the risk program within the first year of enrollment—suggests that a sizable proportion of new enrollees are not satisfied. Of the beneficiaries who joined a risk plan voluntarily, 20 percent dropped out within 12 months after joining, although the rates varied widely across risk plans.

Most enrollees, however, seemed to feel that HMOs' lower costs and wider set of benefits more than compensated for their lower level of satisfaction with care received. About 93 percent of HMO enrollees indicated that they would recommend their HMO to a friend or relative.

Implications for Medicare Risk Contracting

The Medicare risk program has increased beneficiaries' range of choices in health care delivery systems, and risk plans do appear to be able to reduce utilization rates without affecting the quality of care. However, the primary goal of the risk program—to reduce costs to HCFA—has not been realized. Our estimate of a 5.7-percent increase in costs implies that the $578 million paid out to HMOs in capitation payments for the month of June 1992 was about $31 million more than HCFA would have spent in FFS reimbursements for the 1.4 million enrollees. Although HMOs channeled much of this increase in costs into lower out-of-pocket expenses and additional benefits for enrolled beneficiaries, the intent of the program was to lower costs to HCFA, rather than to subsidize the health care of beneficiaries in selected areas. However, our estimates suggest that the potential exists for such cost savings, as a result of sizable reductions in utilization of hospitals and home health services.

The difficulty in achieving these cost savings is that adjusting the payment mechanism to account for the favorable selection experienced by risk plans will lower the average AAPCC payment to most HMOs, which is likely to reduce profits and discourage HMOs from participating. One-half of the participating risk plans are already losing money (Shin and Brown, 1993), nearly one-half of the plans that were active at some time from 1987 to 1990 had discontinued their risk contracts by 1991 (McGee and Brown, 1992), and very few new risk contracts have been signed. Furthermore, reductions in AAPCC payments may cause

HMOs to increase their premiums, which is likely to slow growth in the rate of enrollment in existing risk plans. Changing the AAPCC in order to save money for HCFA may compromise the objective of offering a managed care option to more beneficiaries.

Finding a solution that will enable HCFA to hold the current costs of the risk program to FFS levels while not driving HMOs and beneficiaries out of the program is important, because managed care has many inherent advantages that should lead to greater efficiency in the long run. The incentives in the risk program are structured to minimize costs rather than to maximize revenues, as in the FFS sector. Risk plans also do not have an incentive or opportunity to shift costs to other types of providers, as often occurs in response to a HCFA initiative to control Medicare costs for a particular service. Finally, HMOs are organized to facilitate the coordination of care (which should eliminate provision of overlapping services to beneficiaries), and their emphasis on preventive care could lead to better long-term outcomes and perhaps lower costs. However, these potential efficiencies will not affect costs to HCFA unless the AAPCC payment mechanism is changed to reflect favorable selection.

HCFA could take several actions to help make the potential cost savings of the risk program a reality without driving HMOs away. One change, modifying the AAPCC, must occur to eliminate the cost increases to HCFA. Several other actions would help HMOs accomplish three key cost-cutting objectives: (1) enrolling a sufficient number of beneficiaries to spread the financial risk and fixed costs adequately; (2) bringing administrative costs for Medicare plans under control; and (3) holding service utilization rates down (especially for hospital care). The burden is not solely HCFA's; HMOs must also make some changes to increase their likelihood of succeeding in the Medicare market.

Revise Payment Methodology

Our results suggest that adding one additional factor to the AAPCC payment rate formula—a history of cancer, heart disease, or stroke—could eliminate the increase in costs to HCFA. Our simulations show that if this change were implemented and the plans were still paid only 95 percent of the revised AAPCC, HCFA would actually save 1.1 percent relative to FFS costs, rather than losing money. This approach is similar to the diagnostic cost group (DCG) method developed by Ash et al. (1986) but is simpler, includes a larger proportion of beneficiaries in the high-cost group (about one-third of Medicare beneficiaries have had cancer, heart disease, or a stroke), and is not limited to the experience of the previous year. Data from HMOs on a refined version of this type of indicator would be much easier to verify than some of the risk factors proposed by others, such as measures of functioning. In addition, these data would only need to be updated when a beneficiary experiences such a health problem for the first time. This change would reduce AAPCC payments the most for plans that create the greatest cost increases to HCFA—that is, those experiencing the most favorable selection. Our estimates suggest that the change would not yield the full 5 percent savings originally intended but would at least eliminate cost increases to HCFA.

Modifying the AAPCC formula by adding an adjuster for health status is likely to force HMOs with particularly favorable selection to charge beneficiaries a higher premium. Because a number of these plans charge no premium, and others charge a rate well below the market price for the benefits they offer, premiums could increase significantly without driving enrollees out of these plans. Enrollees would still receive a favorable price, but the price would no longer be subsidized by the Medicare program.

Several other changes to the AAPCC could benefit HMOs without increasing costs to HCFA—in particular, standardizing the rate paid within a given metropolitan area, reducing the year-to-year volatility in payment rates, and tying changes in payment rates to current market factors rather than to outdated trends. These changes, which we and others have proposed before, would make payments to risk plans more consistent with their costs for particular members or in a particular year, enable them to plan more effectively, and smooth out the erratic annual changes in their revenue flow. These changes should be cost neutral and relatively easy to implement.

Finally, although the relative accuracy of AAPCC rates for different counties was beyond the scope of our analysis, there is widespread belief in the industry that the rates are much more generous in some market areas than others. These differences account in part for the fact that risk plans in some areas are able to offer, at no charge to beneficiaries, extensive services beyond what Medicare covers, while risk plans in other areas struggle to survive. Until these disparities are eliminated, there will continue to be great differences across areas in the number, size, and financial success of Medicare risk plans.

Increase Plan Enrollments

Increasing the average enrollment in risk plans and enrolling a greater proportion of individuals who require the most health care are perhaps the best ways to offset the adverse effects that a more accurate payment formula might have on HMO revenues. Having more Medicare members (the median enrollment in 1990 was only 4,733 members) would help HMOs reduce their costs per member month by spreading the large fixed portion of administrative costs over more members and diluting its influence. (Boles [1992] estimates that few HMOs whose administrative costs exceed 10 percent of revenues make a profit overall.) Enrollment growth would also reduce the risk that a few seriously ill members would create overall losses for a risk plan. (A risk plan with 5,000 members that would normally break even has a 12-percent chance of losing 5 percent or more in a given year, simply because of variability in health care costs for beneficiaries.) Encouraging the enrollment of sicker beneficiaries to create a more neutral mix of enrollees would keep AAPCC payments from shrinking as the change was implemented. This change could be especially beneficial in light of the evaluation finding that HMOs achieved their greatest resource savings for the beneficiaries who normally have the greatest health care use. Implicit HMO profit margins on these individuals should be higher than average.

Two changes could make enrollment more attractive to beneficiaries, including those in poor health: (1) increasing the number of area physicians affiliated with a Medicare risk plan; and (2) increasing the number of employers that provide health care coverage to their retirees through a Medicare risk plan. The proposed reduction in AAPCC payment rates would probably engender higher risk plan premiums for beneficiaries, which will dampen their interest in the program. Increasing the likelihood that beneficiaries could join a Medicare risk plan without changing their physicians would offset this adverse effect substantially and could create a more neutral mix of enrollees. Various ways to encourage the participation of physicians in HMOs could be devised, including offering some form of incentive to either physicians or HMOs. However, adding physicians who are not necessarily agreeable to managed care concepts will be unattractive to HMOs. Alternatively, HMOs could be offered financial incentives for net increases in enrollments of a given size or percentage. Employers could be given financial incentives to offer risk plan membership as a health care option for their retirees. All of these incentives that involve payments to physicians, HMOs, or beneficiaries would have to be temporary, in order to avoid further net increases in long-term costs. The objective of incentives is to help risk plans reach a size at which they can at least break even.

One frequently proposed option for increasing enrollment growth that should not be adopted is reducing the Part B premium of beneficiaries who enroll in an HMO, because it would be very expensive and probably ineffective. It would be difficult and probably illegal to restrict such benefits to new enrollees; hence, unnecessary Part B premium rebates would be made to 1.4 million current enrollees. Furthermore, because only about 20 percent of Medicare beneficiaries enroll in Medicare risk plans in areas where the plans do not charge any premium (a savings of $50 to $100 per month relative to medigap coverage), offering beneficiaries a rebate of $5 to $10 per month on their Part B premium is unlikely to attract many new members.

Minimize Administrative Burdens

HCFA could also look for ways to minimize the administrative burden that risk program rules and requirements impose on participating plans. For example, HMOs have long complained that the mandated peer review organization (PRO) process for ensuring quality of care is burdensome and redundant, given their own quality assurance procedures. A number of changes have been made to reduce the PRO and other administrative burdens in recent years, but there may still be areas where administrative demands of the program could be reduced without compromising HCFA's ability to comply with its oversight responsibilities.

Reduce Certain Legislative Constraints

HCFA could encourage States to eliminate regulations that require HMOs to pay fixed rates per hospital admission on the basis of diagnosis; these rates vitiate hospitals' incentive to reduce hospital LOS and force them to pay higher effective prices than they might be able to negotiate for hospital care. HCFA could also advocate eliminating regulations that reduce HMOs' ability to impose reasonable levels of financial risk on physicians. Similarly, States could be encouraged to allow the market to determine the appropriate price for medigap policies. These changes would introduce more competitive pressure into the market, increasing the likelihood that the twofold goal of cost reductions for HCFA and growth in the risk program can be attained.

HMOs Must Adapt to Medicare

Although HCFA can take some actions to facilitate HMOs' ability to operate successful risk plans, much of the burden must fall on the HMOs themselves. Many risk plans are simply too small to achieve the stable utilization patterns and low administrative cost per member month needed to plan effectively and operate efficiently. These plans will need to be more aggressive about growth if they expect to prosper under a payment system that eliminates the benefits of favorable selection. Larger plans may also have high administrative costs that are incompatible with acceptable financial performance—these plans must look for ways to reduce these costs.

HMOs can also be more innovative about finding ways to control utilization, especially hospital care. We found that successful risk plans now tend to be proactive rather than reactive in seeking ways to lower utilization, try to foster a spirit of cooperation between the plan and the physicians in managing member services, and emphasize educating physicians rather than attempting to control their behavior (Hurley and Bannick, 1992). These HMOs tend to rely heavily on case management of hospital stays to keep them as short as possible, planning strategies for individual patients' treatment and recovery and arranging for needed post-discharge services well in advance. They also are continually seeking ways to improve their performance. Risk plans that find it difficult to control utilization for their Medicare beneficiaries may want to explore these approaches and look for other innovative ways, such as risk sharing, monitoring, practice guidelines, and other mechanisms, to manage the care of their elderly members.

Conclusions

These suggestions for change clearly require a much more thorough examination of the possible consequences and operational concerns. The recommendations are put forth simply to illustrate the potential to improve the risk program, from the perspective of both HMOs and taxpayers. At present, HMOs in the risk program provide care that is approximately equal in quality to that rendered in the FFS sector, with more extensive benefit coverage and at a much lower price to beneficiaries than alternative supplemental coverage. HMOs successfully reduce utilization by sizable margins by practicing cost-effective care. They are also capable of generating savings that can be shared among beneficiaries, HCFA, and HMOs. Furthermore, although a number of HMOs have left the risk program and others complain of financial difficulties, the non-renewal rate has declined and a high proportion of plans that have left the program would be interested in reentering if the payment mechanism were reformed. With a carefully planned package of changes by HCFA and continued efforts on the part of HMOs, HMOs' ability to deliver Medicare services more efficiently could bring savings to HCFA, beneficiaries, and HMOs.

Note

1. We assessed the effects on quality of care separately for stroke and colon cancer patients by comparing, for each group, the treatments received by a sample of about

400 HMO patients (from 19 HMOs) with those received by an equal number of comparable FFS patients at hospitals serving the same counties; the data for this analysis were abstracted from the records of 154 hospitals. (See Retchin et al. [1992] for a detailed discussion of methodology and results.) Data for analyzing the effects on access to care and satisfaction with care came from the same survey of beneficiaries that we used to estimate effects on cost and utilization. Statistical models were used to control for differences between enrollees and non-enrollees that could create differences in access or satisfaction not resulting from the influence of an HMO. (See Clement et al. [1992] for a detailed discussion of the study procedures and findings.)

References

Ash, A., Porell, F., Gruenberg, L. et al.: Adjusting Medicare Capitation Payments Using Prior Hospitalization Data. *Health Care Financing Review* 10 (4): 17–30, August 1989.

Brown, R. S., Bergeron, J. W., Clement, D. G. et al.: *The Medicare Risk Program for HMOs—Final Summary Report on Findings from the Evaluation.* Contract Number 500-88-0006. Princeton. Mathematica Policy Research, Inc., February 1993.

Boles, E.: Insolvency in Managed Care Organizations: Financial Indicators. *Topics in Health Care Financing* 19 (2): 40–57, Winter 1992.

Clement, D. G., Retchin, S. M., Stegall, M. H., and Brown, R. S.: *Evaluation of Access and Satisfaction with Care in the TEFRA Program.* Richmond. Williamson Institute for Health Studies, October 1992.

Hill, J. W., and Brown, R. S.: *Biased Selection in the TEFRA HMO/CMP Program.* Princeton. Mathematica Policy Research, Inc., September 1990.

Hill, J. W., and Brown, R. S.: *Health Status, Financial Barriers, and the Decision to Enroll in Medicare Risk Plans.* Princeton. Mathematica Policy Research, Inc., June 1992.

Hill, J. W., Brown, R. S., Chu, D., and Bergeron, J. W.: *The Impact of the Medicare Risk Program on the Use of Services and Cost to Medicare.* Princeton. Mathematica Policy Research, Inc., December 1992.

Hurley, R. E., and Bannick, R. R.: *Utilization Management Practices in HMOs with Medicare Risk Contracts.* Richmond. Williamson Institute for Health Studies, October 1992.

Luft, H. S.: *Health Maintenance Organizations: Dimensions of Performance.* New York. John Wiley and Sons, 1981.

Manning, W. G., Liebowitz, A., Goldberg, G. et al.: A Controlled Trial of the Effect of a Prepaid Group Practice on Use of Services. *New England Journal of Medicine* 310 (23): 1505–11, June 1984.

McGee, J., and Brown, R. S.: *What Makes HMOs Drop Their Medicare Risk Contracts?* Princeton. Mathematica Policy Research, Inc., May 1992.

Retchin, S. M., Brown, R. S., Cohen, R. et al.: *The Quality of Care in TEFRA HMOs/CMPs.* Richmond. Medical College of Virginia, December 1992.

Shin, R. T., and Brown, R. S.: *HMOs' Profits on Their Medicare Risk Plans.* Princeton. Mathematica Policy Research, Inc., February 1993.

Stern, R. S., Juhn, P. I., Gertler, P. J., and Epstein, A. M.: A Comparison of Length of Stay and Costs for Health Maintenance Organizations and Fee-for-Service Patients. *Archives of Internal Medicine* 149: 1185–88, May 1989.

CHAPTER

9

ACCESS TO CARE IN MEDICARE HMOs, 1996

Lyle Nelson, Randall Brown, Marsha Gold,
Anne Ciemnecki, and Elizabeth Docteur

ENROLLMENT IN Medicare managed care increased about 50 percent between the end of 1994 and the beginning of 1997.[1] Although fewer than 11 percent of Medicare beneficiaries are now enrolled in health maintenance organizations (HMOs) in the Medicare risk program, the proportion is growing and may accelerate further as Congress debates Medicare financing reform. A key point of contention is whether Medicare managed care will restrict access to needed care by trying to control costs and improve access by better coordinating care for Medicare beneficiaries.[2] In the most comprehensive national study of the Medicare HMO program to date, Randall Brown and colleagues concluded that Medicare HMOs used resources more efficiently, with fairly minor differences in access, quality, and beneficiary satisfaction compared with fee-for-service Medicare.[3] Yet this study and others identify areas in which Medicare HMOs perform more poorly, particularly for some vulnerable subgroups such as the chronically ill.[4]

A better understanding of access to care in Medicare HMOs clearly is of interest, particularly because existing studies are now more than five years old and the Medicare HMO program has changed considerably since then.

This study provides a nationally representative access profile from the perspective of Medicare beneficiaries. It is based on a 1996 national survey of 3,080 Medicare managed care enrollees and disenrollees and provides information on access to care for the Medicare population in general and for vulnerable subgroups. Finally, it highlights lessons for strengthening the monitoring of these issues.

Methods

Sample Design

We conducted a telephone survey of a stratified random sample of 3,080 Medicare beneficiaries who were enrolled in a Medicare managed care risk plan for at least two months during the year ending February 1996.[5] We selected the sample from the Group Health Plan (GHP) file maintained by the Health Care Financing Administration (HCFA). We restricted the sample to beneficiaries who were enrolled for at least two months because we wanted to study access to care among beneficiaries who were likely to have had some experience in their plan.[6]

The sample design was structured with sufficient sample sizes to provide relatively reliable estimates for vulnerable subpopulations and disenrollees. We stratified the sample by enrollment status, age, race, and plan size. We defined four strata based on enrollment status: continuous enrollees (those enrolled throughout the year), new enrollees (those who joined a risk plan within the past year), switchers (those who disenrolled from one risk plan and joined another), and disenrollees (those who returned to fee-for-service Medicare). We refer to the first three of these strata as current enrollees, since they were all enrolled in a risk plan as of 1 March 1996. We oversampled disenrollees and switchers to obtain adequate sample sizes for analysis.

Using data from the GHP file, we oversampled subgroups of particular policy interest: African Americans, the nonelderly disabled, and the oldest old (age eighty-five and older). We undersampled beneficiaries in the five largest Medicare risk plans—four in southern California and one in Miami—which together contain nearly one-third of all Medicare risk enrollees. This allowed us to obtain more precise estimates for newer plans and markets that will be more dominant in the program's future.

Survey Instrument

The telephone survey asked detailed questions on access to care, service use, satisfaction with care, health status and conditions, and demographics. Although we built on questions from existing surveys, we also developed new items to tap important concepts of access that are ignored or poorly reflected in those surveys. We developed a conceptual framework for examining access in a managed care environment.[7]

The survey was conducted during a twelve-week period that began on 13 May 1996. Proxy respondents accounted for 12 percent of all interviews and 20 percent of those for the oldest old. The overall response rate was 64 percent, similar to that for other recent telephone surveys of Medicare beneficiaries. Respondents and nonrespondents had similar characteristics, but the response rate was lower for African Americans (60 percent), persons covered by Medicaid (53 percent), and the nonelderly disabled and oldest old (61 percent for each).

Analytic Methods

The analysis is based on data weighted to compensate for oversampling of selected strata and to provide nationally representative estimates of those enrolled in Medicare HMOs during the reference period. We used the SUDAAN software package to account for the stratified sample design and weighting in computing standard errors. The subgroup analyses included comparisons across groups that were defined by enrollment status and comparisons of vulnerable subgroups with others.

To the extent feasible, we compared access estimates from this study with estimates for the national Medicare fee-for-service population based on the 1994 Medicare Current Beneficiary Survey (MCBS). Fee-for-service observations were weighted to match the Medicare HMO population on age, race, and health status and were restricted to those in metropolitan areas, since 98 percent of Medicare risk enrollees live in such areas. Comparisons were limited by differences in design and content between the two surveys.

Profile of Medicare HMO Enrollees

Medicare beneficiaries enrolled in the study population were most often continuous enrollees (63 percent), followed by new enrollees (29 percent), switchers (4.7 percent), and disenrollees to fee-for-service Medicare (2.8 percent).[8] Of those who left their plan during the year for reasons other than death or plan termination, nearly two-thirds enrolled in another plan. In the total population, 76 percent paid no premium, and 83 percent had prescription drug coverage. Just under half cited costs and benefits as their most important reason for enrolling.

More than half of all enrollees were in HMOs in California and Florida. Nearly one-third were enrolled in one of the five plans (out of 178 participating in the risk program) that had more than 100,000 Medicare enrollees. One-quarter had been enrolled for more than four years. The average duration of enrollment was lower for disenrollees (twenty-four months) than it was in general (thirty-six months). Although 31 percent of continuous enrollees were in plans outside of California, Florida, and Arizona, 57 percent of new enrollees were in plans outside of these states.

Of the weighted sample, 5.5 percent were disabled; 45 percent of current disabled enrollees were new enrollees. The oldest old accounted for 7.7 percent of the sample; 8 percent of the sample were African American, and 8 percent were Hispanic. Four percent were jointly eligible for Medicaid (dually eligible). Twenty percent had incomes under $10,000 per year, and 40 percent had incomes over $20,000 per year. Fewer than 1 percent were institutionalized.

Access to Care

Overview of Selected Access Measures

The great majority of Medicare beneficiaries who are enrolled in risk plans report having no problems with access to care and are satisfied with their plans (Exhibit 1). Only 8 percent said that they had problems making appointments. Six percent reported that their primary care physician had not referred them to a specialist when they thought a referral was needed; more than half of these beneficiaries reported that the lack of a referral had no consequences. One percent said that their plan physician did not admit them to a hospital when they thought it was needed; 44 percent of these beneficiaries said that the lack of an admission had no consequences. Among those who had been hospitalized, 6 percent felt that their plan physician had discharged them from the hospital too soon; 70 percent of these beneficiaries reported some type of adverse consequence, such as a worsening of their condition or a delay in their recovery (42 percent), or the need to arrange for home care or nursing home care (19 percent).

Beneficiaries were more likely to report problems with access to home health care. Of the 8 percent who received home health care through their plan during the past year, 17 percent felt that they needed more care than the plan provided. However, fewer than half a percent felt that they needed home health care from their plan but did not receive it. Seventy percent of beneficiaries who felt that they needed more home health care than their plan provided reported some type of adverse consequence.

Most Medicare beneficiaries who are enrolled in HMOs are satisfied with the overall health care covered by their plan and with the specific dimensions of care we examined (Exhibit 1). Only 4 percent said that they intended to disenroll from their plan or wanted to disenroll but felt that they could not do so for financial reasons.

Exhibit 1 Selected Access and Satisfaction Measures for Medicare HMO Enrollees, 1996

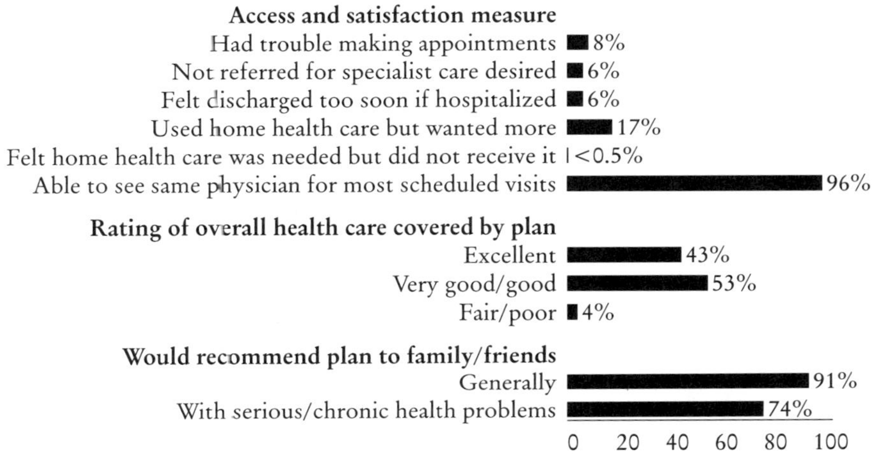

Source: Mathematica Policy Research/Physician Payment Review Commission survey of Medicare HMO enrollees, 1996.
Notes: Sample size = 3,080. HMO is health maintenance organization.

Access and Integration of New Enrollees

Nearly all of the new enrollees (including plan switchers) reported that they were provided with enough information on how to obtain care. Of the 25 percent who had questions or wanted more information, 69 percent obtained the information without any problem, 11 percent said that they did not try to obtain it, and 20 percent experienced problems or were unsuccessful. Ninety-six percent had a primary care physician in the plan, and more than 80 percent selected their physician rather than being assigned a physician by the plan. Forty-two percent of recent enrollees kept the same primary care physician as they had before joining their plan—a nearly two-fold increase from 1990.[9] Only 44 percent with a new primary care physician were encouraged to come in for an exam or assessment after enrolling.

Use of Preventive Services

Compared with beneficiaries in fee-for-service Medicare, those enrolled in risk plans were more likely to have received a flu shot during the past winter (66 percent versus 58 percent) and (among women) more likely to have received a mammogram in the past year (62 percent versus

39 percent).[10] The HMO/fee-for-service differential for flu shots and mammograms was greatest among beneficiary subgroups that were least likely to receive them in the fee-for-service sector. Thus, for flu shots, the differential was greatest for the nonelderly disabled (51 percent versus 36 percent), African Americans (53 percent versus 37 percent), and persons with low incomes (62 percent versus 47 percent).

Access for Vulnerable Subgroups

Vulnerable subgroups—the nonelderly disabled, the oldest old, persons with functional impairments, and persons in fair or poor health or with worsening health—were much more likely than the general population to report access problems (Exhibit 2). Differences are particularly striking for home health care, an area in which some vulnerable subgroups are three or more times more likely to report problems. In addition, beneficiaries in vulnerable subgroups are more likely to disenroll from HMOs and enroll in fee-for-service Medicare. Relative to an aggregate disenrollment rate of less than 3 percent, disenrollment rates were higher for the nonelderly disabled (4.7 percent), the oldest old (4.2 percent), African Americans (4.6 percent), persons in fair or poor health (4.7 percent), and persons with functional impairments (5.5 percent). These disparities may be accounted for in part by differences in the length of enrollment across subgroups, because disenrollment is higher early in enrollment, and new enrollees account for a particularly large share of some subgroups, such as the disabled.

To control for differences between vulnerable subgroups and others in relative need for care, we computed the percentage of beneficiaries who reported access problems among those we defined as having a need for particular services. Enrollees were considered to be in need of a service if they either received the service or did not receive the service but felt that they needed it. Controlling for differences in need in this way greatly reduces (and in some cases eliminates) the difference between vulnerable subgroups and others in the proportion who reported access problems. However, in the case of home health care, the service for which we found the greatest unmet need, the nonelderly disabled were still twice as likely as beneficiaries ages sixty-five to eighty-four to report access problems (Exhibit 3). In general, the higher probability of reported problems obtaining specialty referrals and inpatient care among vulnerable subgroups appears to be only partially related to a greater need for care among such groups.

Despite their greater likelihood of encountering access problems, the vulnerable subgroups were just as likely as others to say that they would

Exhibit 2 Selected Access and Satisfaction Measure for Subgroups of Medicare HMO Enrollees, 1996

	Enrollee Subgroups						
Access and Satisfaction Measure	All Beneficiaries (n = 3,080)	Nonelderly Disabled (n = 419)	Oldest Old (85+) (n = 390)	African Americans (n = 456)	In Fair or Poor Health (n = 603)	In Worse Health than One Year Ago (n = 466)	Has Functional Impairments (n = 450)
Not referred for specialist care enrollee thought was needed	6.2%	9.5%[a]	5.8%	4.4%	8.8%	11.4%[b]	4.7%
Felt discharged too soon if hospitalized	6.2	10.0	9.8	8.3	7.0	8.3	13.2[a]
Did not receive home health care enrollee thought was needed[c]	1.6	4.1[b]	5.4[b]	2.7	5.6[b]	6.4[b]	7.6[b]
Rate overall health care covered by plan as excellent	43.2	41.1	36.7[a]	26.5[b]	32.3[b]	38.0	38.9
Would recommend plan to family/friends with serious or chronic health problems	74.4	75.4	70.4	73.8	69.9	74.5	74.0

Source: Mathematica Policy Research/Physician Payment Review Commission survey of Medicare HMO enrollees, 1996.

Note: The counterparts for the vulnerable subgroups are as follows: beneficiaries ages sixty-five to eighty-four (for the nonelderly disabled and the oldest old); whites; enrollees in excellent health; enrollees whose health is the same as a year ago; and enrollees without functional impairments.

[a]Difference between vulnerable subgroup and counterpart is significant at the .05 level.

[b]Difference between vulnerable subgroup and counterpart is significant at the .01 level.

[c]Defined as the percentage of enrollees who either (1) received home health care from their plan but felt that they needed more, or (2) did not receive any home health care from their plan but felt that they needed such care.

Exhibit 3 Relative Likelihood of Reporting Problems with Access to Home Care, Adjusted and Unadjusted Estimates for Vulnerable Subgroups of Medicare HMO Enrollees, 1996

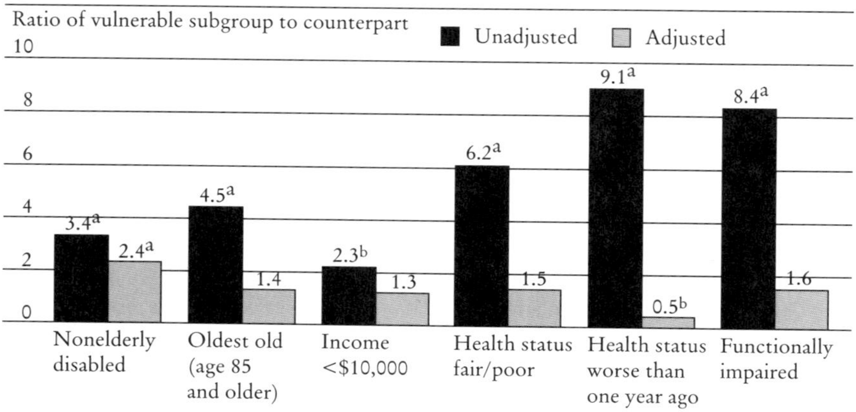

Source: Mathematica Policy Research (MPR)/Physician Payment Review Commission (PPRC) survey, 1996.
Notes: Ratio of vulnerable subgroup to counterpart in likelihood of reporting access problems. Counterparts for vulnerable subgroups are beneficiaries ages sixty-five to eighty-four (for the nonelderly disabled and the oldest old); those with incomes more than $20,000; those whose health status is excellent; those whose health is the same as a year ago; and those who are not functionally impaired. Adjusted measures include only enrollees who used or perceived a need for home health care in the past year.
[a]Difference between vulnerable subgroup and counterpart is significant at the .01 level.
[b]Difference between vulnerable subgroup and counterpart is significant at the .05 level.

recommend their plan to a family member or friend with a serious or chronic health problem (70–75 percent) (Exhibit 2).

African American beneficiaries were no more likely than white beneficiaries to report access problems. This finding is noteworthy, given the evidence that African Americans are more likely than whites to experience access problems in fee-for-service Medicare.[11] However, African American beneficiaries were much less likely than white beneficiaries to be satisfied with the overall health care covered by their plans (27 percent rated their care as excellent, compared with 45 percent of whites) and were less satisfied than whites were with each dimension of care we examined. However, African Americans were as likely as other beneficiaries to recommend their plan. African Americans in the fee-for-service sector also were less satisfied than whites were with their care.[12]

Access for Disenrollees

Fewer than 3 percent of persons enrolled in Medicare risk plans during the one-year sampling period disenrolled and returned to fee-for-service

Medicare. Disenrollees to fee-for-service were more likely than those in Medicare managed care to report access problems and less likely to be satisfied with their plans. They are a heterogeneous group, however, varying both in their experiences in their plans and their reasons for disenrolling. Fourteen percent of disenrollees reported that their primary care physician had not referred them to a specialist when they thought it was needed (versus 6 percent for current enrollees), and 57 percent said that they would recommend their plan to a family member or friend (versus 91 percent for current enrollees). About a quarter of disenrollees who returned to fee-for-service said that they disenrolled because they moved out of their plan's service area. The other main reasons for returning to fee-for-service were dissatisfaction with plan physicians (26 percent), financial issues (18 percent), and access problems (10 percent).

Comparisons with Medicare Fee-for-Service

Medicare beneficiaries enrolled in HMOs appear to be more likely than fee-for-service enrollees to report access problems, although the size of the difference probably is overstated because the measures for the two sectors differ. Twelve percent of the HMO sample reported one or more specific access problems in the past year, compared with 4 percent in the fee-for-service sector. The fee-for-service estimate is based on a single question in the MCBS about whether beneficiaries had any trouble obtaining health care they wanted or needed in the past year, whereas the HMO estimate is computed as a percentage of those who reported one or more access problems covered in a series of questions about particular problems.

Vulnerable subgroups typically have more access problems than other beneficiaries have in Medicare fee-for-service.[13] Our study shows that this also happens in Medicare HMOs (Exhibit 4). The reported incidence of access problems is higher in HMOs. However, our results indicate that, except for the oldest old, the differences between vulnerable subgroups and their less vulnerable counterparts in the likelihood of encountering access problems are smaller in managed care than in the fee-for-service sector.

Discussion

This study provides the most comprehensive and nationally representative profile of access to care in Medicare managed care available today. Its main strengths relative to previous studies rest in the broader range of access measures included and in the targeted analysis of beneficiary subgroups considered most vulnerable to access problems. Such analysis

Exhibit 4 Comparison of Reported Access Problems, by Vulnerable Subpopulations in Medicare HMOs and in the Fee-for-Service Sector, 1996

	All Beneficiaries	Nonelderly Disabled	Oldest Old (85+)	African American	Low Income[a]	Fair or Poor Health
Percent of fee-for-service beneficiaries who had trouble getting care in past year[b]	4.0%	14.1%	3.1%	8.2%	7.8%	9.3%
Percent of HMO enrollees who have ever experienced access problems in their plan[c]						
All enrollees	13.3	24.9	16.1	12.6	15.9	23.6
Enrolled for one year or less	12.0	21.3	23.1	13.6	16.5	26.1
Likelihood of access problems by vulnerable subgroups relative to their counterparts (ratio)[d]						
Fee-for-service beneficiaries	—	5.2	1.1	2.4	3.9	11.6
HMO enrollees						
All	—	2.0	1.3	0.9	1.3	2.2
Enrolled for one year or less	—	2.1	2.2	1.2	1.9	4.5

Sources: Mathematica Policy Research/Physician Payment Review Commission survey of Medicare HMO enrollees. Fee-for-service estimates from 1994 Medicare Current Beneficiary Survey.
[a]Low income is defined as annual household income of less than $10,000.
[b]For fee-for-service beneficiaries, the access measure shown is the percentage who reported having trouble getting health care they wanted or needed within the past year.
[c]For HMO enrollees, the access measure shown is the percentage who reported one or more of the following problems since enrolling in their plan: not being referred for desired specialist care, not being admitted to a hospital when desired, being discharged from a hospital before feeling ready, not receiving the home health care desired, experiencing delays obtaining care, and experiencing any other problems obtaining care.
[d]The counterparts to vulnerable subgroups are as follows: beneficiaries ages sixty-five to eighty-four (counterparts to the nonelderly disbled and the oldest old); whites (for African Americans); those with an annual household income of more than $20,000 (for those with low income); and those in excellent health (for those in fair or poor health).

is not now feasible with data from the MCBS because the HMO sample is too small (although it is being expanded).[14] There also are inconsistencies and limitations in how the MCBS measures access to care for HMO and fee-for-service enrollees.[15]

The results of our study provide a mixed but generally encouraging picture. The great majority of Medicare managed care enrollees do not report access problems, are relatively satisfied with the care they receive, and would recommend their plan. This holds true for vulnerable subgroups as well as for the population in general. However, these findings are based on data from persons who voluntarily joined an HMO, attracted by the lower out-of-pocket costs and greater benefits.

There are some areas, however, in which HMOs can and should provide better access than they do now. Access to home health services is particularly problematic, which is consistent with other studies that find fewer visits and poorer outcomes for home health recipients in HMOs.[16] As in fee-for-service plans, access for vulnerable subpopulations is worse than that for other enrollees. Although definitive comparisons of access in HMOs vis-à-vis fee-for-service plans are not possible, some findings, such as those for the oldest old and persons in fair or poor health, are of particular concern. The fact that one in four beneficiaries would not recommend their plan to someone with a serious or chronic health problem is also a potential concern. Our findings suggest that HMOs need to address the needs of frail and more vulnerable Medicare beneficiaries more effectively.

Finally, the results of this study illustrate the utility of timely, high-quality data in considering public policy concerns, particularly when they involve controversial issues such as Medicare managed care. Having nationally representative data, from surveys or other sources, allows concerns to be systematically tested against experience. Such data provide a rich base for debating legitimate differences in policy perspectives and help to avoid "policy by anecdote." Yet few reliable sources of information exist to inform a policy debate that is highly charged with emotion. This study illustrates why representative and timely data that support standardized and appropriate comparisons of Medicare beneficiaries in HMOs and fee-for-service plans are essential to effective monitoring, oversight, and policymaking.

Acknowledgments

This study was conducted under a contract from the Physician Payment Review Commission (PPRC) to Mathematica Policy Research (MPR). The views expressed are those of the authors, and no endorsement by the PPRC is intended or should be inferred. Several staff were critical to this study. At MPR, Anna Aizer served as project analyst and manager, Karen CyBulski managed the development and conduct of the survey, Sara Yang provided the main programming support, and Sharon Clark was lead secretary. At the PPRC, Sally Trude contributed to the development of comparison estimates from the Medicare Current Beneficiary Survey, and David Colby provided guidance on project design. Elsewhere, Lucy Rose Fisher, Marshall McBean, Sheldon Retchin, and Shoshanna Sofaer consulted on the design of the survey instrument.

Notes

1. Health Care Financing Administration, *Medicare Prepaid Health Plans Monthly Report* (Baltimore: HCFA, December 1994 and January 1997).
2. M. Moon and K. Davis, "Preserving and Strengthening Medicare," *Health Affairs* (Winter 1995): 31–46.
3. R. S. Brown et al., "Do Health Maintenance Organizations Work for Medicare?" *Health Care Financing Review* 15, no. 1 (1993): 7–24.
4. J. Ware et al., "Differences in Four-Year Health Outcomes for Elderly and Poor, Chronically Ill Patients Treated in HMO and Fee-for-Service Systems: Results from the Medical Outcomes Study," *Journal of the American Medical Association* 276, no. 13 (1996): 1039–47.
5. L. Nelson et al., "Access to Care in Medicare Managed Care: Results from a 1996 Survey of Enrollees and Disenrollees," Selected External Research Series no. 7 (Washington: Physician Payment Review Commission, November 1996).
6. If we had included beneficiaries enrolled for only one month in our sample, the rate of disenrollment to fee-for-service would increase from 2.8 percent to 3.3 percent. We excluded beneficiaries who were in a plan for only one month (14 percent of disenrollees during the year), since many of these persons may not have realized that they had enrolled or may have changed their mind about enrolling before having any real experience obtaining care within the plan (frequently because they had not realized that they were required to obtain care only from HMO-affiliated physicians).
7. E. R. Docteur, D. C. Colby, and M. Gold, "Shifting the Paradigm: Monitoring Access in Medicare Managed Care," *Health Care Financing Review* 17, no. 4 (1996): 5–21.
8. Our disenrollment figures are lower than those recently reported in U.S. General Accounting Office, *Medicare: HCFA Should Release Data to Aid Consumers, Prompt Better HMO Performance*, GAO/HEHS-97–23 (Washington: GAO, October 1996). The GAO presented only plan-specific estimates of disenrollment (which vary greatly) and included only plans in California and Florida. The GAO estimates did not distinguish between switching risk plans and disenrolling to fee-for-service, and they included beneficiaries whose disenrollment date was identical to their enrollment date (those who canceled their HMO membership before their effective enrollment date) and those who were enrolled for only one month. Such persons were excluded from our study for the reasons described above.
9. R. S. Brown et al., "The Medicare Risk Program for HMOs—Final Summary Report on Findings from the Evaluation," HCFA Contract no. 500–88-0066 (Baltimore: HCFA, February 1993).
10. These estimates were adjusted to account for differences between HMO enrollees and fee-for-service beneficiaries in age, race, and health status. However, the difference in mammography rates may be attributable in part to differences between the two groups in the age distribution of women in the sixty-five to eighty-four age range, since some guidelines do not recommend annual mammograms for women over age seventy-five.
11. Physician Payment Review Commission, *Monitoring Access of Medicare Beneficiaries*, No. 95-1 (Washington: PPRC, May 1996).
12. Nelson et al., "Access to Care in Medicare Managed Care."

13. PPRC, *Monitoring Access of Medicare Beneficiaries.*
14. Docteur et al., "Shifting the Paradigm."
15. Ibid.
16. P. W. Shaughnessey, R. E. Schlenker, and D. F. Hittle, "Home Health Care Outcomes under Capitated and Fee-for-Service Payment," *Health Care Financing Review* 16, no. 1 (1994): 187–222.

CHAPTER

10

CHANGES IN HEALTH PLANS SERVING MEDICAID, 1993–1996

Suzanne Felt-Lisk and Sara Yang

THE RECENT growth in Medicaid managed care has dramatically changed the way Medicaid beneficiaries in many states obtain health care. In 1996, 7.7 million Medicaid beneficiaries (23 percent of all Medicaid beneficiaries) received care under fully capitated Medicaid managed care programs in thirty-five states, compared with 2.6 million beneficiaries in 1993. This change suggests a need to track the types of health plans in which beneficiaries are enrolling, to better understand the changing health care market, and to identify any policy implications. The changes of interest include changes in participation by commercial-based plans, the rate at which new health plans are forming to serve Medicaid, the extent to which patterns and changes vary by region or state, and the role of health plans that are Medicaid-only or Medicaid-dominated relative to other plans. In this paper we address these issues using a new data set that we developed specifically for this purpose.

Tracking full-risk health plans serving Medicaid is important for policymakers because these are the plans that face the strong financial incentives to reduce service use that are inherent in fully capitated payment. Lack of adequate oversight for such plans can result in problems

From *Health Affairs* 16 (5): 125–133.

such as possible instances of underservice or inadequate documentation.[1] Further, shifts over time in participation by these plans create a changing landscape for consumers who are navigating a Medicaid program that presents them with more choices than in the past.

Overall, we found that the number and proportion of plans serving Medicaid beneficiaries grew dramatically between 1993 and 1996, although the size and other characteristics of the plans remained relatively stable. Commercial plans' participation increased substantially over the period, yet more than half of the new plans entering the Medicaid market were newly formed plans, and most of these were Medicaid-only plans. There are now at least 144 Medicaid-only plans, and by June 1996, 3.6 million Medicaid beneficiaries were enrolled in plans in which Medicaid enrollees comprised at least 75 percent of the total enrollment. We therefore suggest that more attention should be paid to including these plans in future analyses of market trends and to ensuring that they maintain a baseline level of quality of care while taking into account their special strengths and limited resources.

Objectives and Methods

The trends identified here for 1993–1996 cover a critical period in the expansion of Medicaid managed care and use an expanded data set of health plans relative to prior studies. This analysis builds on previous research on types of health plans serving Medicaid by updating it to include 1995 and 1996 and by including all full-risk health plans serving Medicaid as identified through Health Care Financing Administration (HCFA) enrollment data.[2] Thus, for the first time in this type of analysis, we include the many plans that bear full financial risk for serving Medicaid beneficiaries but that are not listed in the industry directories and are likely not state-licensed as health maintenance organizations (HMOs). In contrast to some previous analyses, we also present results two ways: unweighted by enrollment, to profile the plans in the industry; and weighted, to profile the plans in which Medicaid beneficiaries are concentrated.

We focused on several major characteristics: (1) size of plan as measured by total enrollment, (2) number of Medicaid enrollees and percentage of plans' total enrollment that is Medicaid, (3) plans' affiliation with a major system, (4) the state in which the plan is located, and (5) whether the plan served the disabled Medicaid population in 1995. We focused on these areas both because they are of interest and because the data were available for plans listed in industry directories as well as for plans identified only through HCFA data.[3]

We defined the managed care plans of interest as those that were fully capitated for general medical services. This group includes many HMO-like organizations that are not licensed as HMOs but that carry similar responsibilities. That is, they are responsible for making available the same wide spectrum of medical services that HMOs provide; they are offered to beneficiaries when they select a health plan, just as HMOs are offered; and they must comply with HCFA requirements for quality assurance addressing enrollees' grievances.

Using Medicaid definitions, our group of interest thus includes HMOs, prepaid health plans that are fully capitated, and seven organizations classified by HCFA as health-insuring organizations, which also receive full capitation for general medical care for Medicaid beneficiaries.[4] We chose not to include other managed care arrangements such as partially capitated plans and primary care case management (PCCM) programs because they are generally structured very differently from full-risk plans and are not responsible for providing such a broad range of services under the strong financial incentives that full capitation brings. Although some of those we excluded may operate like HMOs, we had no way to distinguish these from the majority of PCCM programs and partially capitated plans that are very different.

Data Sources

To create the database for analysis, we merged data on HMOs nationwide that were available from industry sources with data from HCFA Medicaid managed care enrollment reports for 30 June 1993, 1994, 1995, and 1996. The industry sources were the *Group Health Association of America (GHAA) Directory of HMOs* for the years 1993, 1994, and 1995 and InterStudy directory data for 1996. We used the latter as an alternative data source for 1996 because the American Association of Health Plans (AAHP) (formerly GHAA) data for 1996 were not yet available. We also used a list of national HMO companies and multiregional HMOs previously developed for the Center for Studying Health System Change to identify plans that had more than 100,000 enrollees and were part of a major health plan system.[5]

Limitations

Matching health plans across years and data sources was challenging and required hand-matching addresses to correct instances in which plans with slight name variations appeared as separate plans and telephoning state Medicaid officials to clarify ambiguous information. We devoted considerable effort to eliminating plans on the HCFA listings that only provided specialized services (most often behavioral health and dental managed care plans) and to obtaining total enrollment data or verifying Medicaid-only status for plans not listed in the industry directories. Although we believe we have developed a useful and highly accurate database, a few errors undoubtedly remain.

In addition, it was not possible to use fully consistent matching dates of enrollment for total enrollment and Medicaid enrollment. Total enrollment data from GHAA are only available for 31 December of each year, and Medicaid data are only available for 30 June of each year. Thus, we matched total enrollment for 31 December 1992 with Medicaid enrollment for 30 June 1993 and labeled it "1993" and so on for each year.[6]

Full-Risk Plans in 1996

In 1996, 355 managed care plans served 7.7 million Medicaid beneficiaries in fully capitated programs in thirty-five states.

How Much Medicaid?

Nearly half (48 percent) of those Medicaid beneficiaries—3.6 million people—were in Medicaid-dominated plans (that is, plans in which Medicaid enrollees comprise 75 percent or more of the total enrollment), while 28 percent were in low-Medicaid plans and 24 percent were in mixed Medicaid/commercial plans. The 156 Medicaid-dominated plans operating in 1996 constituted 38 percent of all health plans serving Medicaid. Most were small—90 percent of Medicaid-dominated plans had fewer than 50,000 members. Probably because of this, Medicaid enrollees were three times more likely than commercial enrollees to be enrolled in small plans.

Among the Medicaid-dominated plans, 92 percent (144 plans) were basically Medicaid-only plans, with Medicaid comprising 90 to 100 percent of their total enrollment. At least sixteen of the Medicaid-only plans operating in 1996 were owned wholly or in part by federally funded community health centers.[7] Others may be other types of provider-based plans, newly formed independent plans, subsidiaries of commercial-based plans, or plans formed separately by companies focusing on Medicaid. There is no information about the nature of these plans, since most of them (105) are not listed in either the 1996 InterStudy directory or the 1995 GHAA directory.

Health plans serving Medicaid tended to be either Medicaid-dominated or low-Medicaid. Only 16 percent of the plans participating in Medicaid in 1996 had a relatively even emphasis on Medicaid and other enrollees, with Medicaid representing 25–74 percent of their total enrollment. This is not surprising since the Medicaid population is relatively concentrated in low-income areas. In total, more than three-fourths of Medicaid managed care enrollees are in plans at one extreme or the other in terms of Medicaid's role in the plan.

Large or Small Plans?

A majority of participating plans are small and serve a small number of Medicaid enrollees, but most enrollees are in large plans and those that serve a large number of Medicaid enrollees. Although 59 percent of participating health plans in 1996 had fewer than 50,000 enrollees, these small plans enrolled only 30 percent of the Medicaid beneficiaries in managed care (Exhibit 1). Similarly, nearly half (48 percent) of participating plans served fewer than 10,000 Medicaid enrollees in 1996, and they enrolled only 8 percent of Medicaid managed care enrollees. In contrast, more than half (52 percent) of enrollees were in the forty-three plans that served a large number of Medicaid enrollees (45,000 or more). And a majority of Medicaid enrollees (54 percent) were in large health plans (100,000 or more members). In fact, nearly a third of enrollees were in the very large plans (250,000 or more members). Enrollees in large plans were about evenly split between independent plans and plans affiliated with a major system.

Who Serves the Disabled?

Medicaid-dominated plans were more likely than other Medicaid-serving plans to serve the Medicaid disabled population (those receiving Supplemental Security Income [SSI] benefits) in 1995.[8] Fifty-eight percent of the Medicaid-dominated plans in states where at least one plan served disabled Medicaid beneficiaries, served these beneficiaries, compared with 45 percent of the other Medicaid-serving plans. These Medicaid-dominated plans accounted for 45 percent of the plans serving Medicaid/SSI.

Scope of Participation

Health plan participation in Medicaid is relatively widespread; only the South-Central and South Atlantic regions of the United States lag far behind. Thirty-six percent of commercial plans served Medicaid in 1996 (Exhibit 2).[9] Large plans tended to participate more often than smaller plans did (72 percent versus 23 percent). Independent plans tended to participate more often than did those affiliated with a major system (43 versus 29 percent). Only the South-Central and South Atlantic regions

Exhibit 1 Distribution of Medicaid and Participating Plans, by Plan Enrollment Characteristic, 1993 and 1996

	Distribution of Participating Plans		Distribution of Medicaid Managed Care Enrollees	
Plan Characteristics	1993	1996	1993	1996
Number of plans and enrollees	166	355	2,636,000	7,660,000
Total enrollment				
0–49,999	58%	59%	35%	30%
50,000–99,999	12	14	14	16
100,000–249,999	18	17	26	22
250,000 or more	11	11	25	32
Medicaid proportion of enrollment				
Less than 25 percent	48	40	25	28
25–49 percent	7	10	22	14
50–74 percent	6	6	7	11
75–89 percent	4	3	11	14
90 percent or more	34	41	36	34
Number of Medicaid enrollees				
Fewer than 10,000	61	48	13	8
10,000–19,999	19	18	17	11
20,000–44,999	12	22	24	29
45,000 or more	8	12	46	52

Source: Mathematica Policy Research analysis for the Center for Studying Health System Change, supported by The Robert Wood Johnson Foundation.

had less than a third of their health plans participating in Medicaid managed care. The South-Central region includes Tennessee, a state with high Medicaid managed care enrollment, but the rest of the states had low enrollment in 1996. Some of those states now are implementing Medicaid managed care, although not always on a full-risk basis.

In all, thirty-five U.S. states had at least one full-risk plan serving Medicaid. Sixteen states had 150,000 or more Medicaid enrollees in their capitated managed care programs in 1996. These sixteen high-enrollment states accounted for 87 percent of Medicaid enrollment in capitated plans nationally. The high-enrollment states are Arizona, California, Connecticut, Florida, Illinois, Michigan, Minnesota, Missouri, New Jersey, New York, Ohio, Oregon, Pennsylvania, Tennessee, Virginia, and Washington.

Changes in Number and Types of Plans

Although the number and proportion of plans serving Medicaid grew dramatically between 1993 and 1996, the size and other characteristics of

Exhibit 2 Participation Rates for Commercial Health Plans, 1993 and 1996

Plan Characteristics	Participation Rate	
	1993	1996
All plans	21%	36%
Total enrollment		
0–49,999	12	23
50,000–99,999	24	38
100,000–249,999	37	51
250,000 or more	58	72
Region[a]		
East North-Central	25	35
Mid-Atlantic	45	71
Mountain	14	35
New England	37	49
Pacific	27	65
South Atlantic	12	22
South-Central	0	8
West North-Central	14	34
System affiliation		
Affiliated with major system	15	29
Independent	26	43
State's Medicaid managed care enrollment		
150,000 or more	26	49
Less than 150,000	13	21

Source: Mathematica Policy Research analysis for the Center for Studying Health System Change, supported by The Robert Wood Johnson Foundation.
Note: This analysis excludes plans in which Medicaid makes up 75 percent or more of total enrollment. The participation rate is the percentage of plans of a given type that are serving Medicaid enrollees.
[a] The states in each region are as follows: East North-Central: OH, IN, IL, MI, WI. Mid-Atlantic: NJ, NY, PA. Mountain: AZ, CO, ID, MT, NM, NV, UT, WY. New England: CT, ME, MA, NH, RI, VT. Pacific: AK, CA, HI, WA, OR. South Atlantic: DE, District of Columbia, FL, GA, MD, NC, SC, VA, WV. South-Central: AL, AR, KY, LA, MS, OK, TN, TX. West North-Central: MN, IA, MO, ND, SD, NE, KS.

the plans remained relatively stable. The number of health plans serving Medicaid rose from 166 to 355 between 1993 and 1996, both because of growth in existing plans' participation in Medicaid and the formation of new plans designed to serve Medicaid (discussed below). Enrollment grew rapidly in every region of the country and in most states. Yet, despite these very large increases, there was relatively little shift in the types of plans serving Medicaid or in the types of plans in which beneficiaries tended to enroll. Enrollees in 1996 were about as likely as in 1993 to be in Medicaid-dominated plans (48 percent versus 47 percent), about as likely to be in plans affiliated with a large system (29 percent versus 28 percent), and about as likely to be in large plans as in small plans.[10]

Commercial Plans

Commercial-based plans' participation in Medicaid increased from 1993 to 1996. The percentage of all commercial-based plans that participated in Medicaid grew from 21 percent in 1993 to 36 percent in 1996, and the percentage of large commercial-based plans (100,000 or more total enrollees) participating grew from 43 percent to 59 percent during the period. Seventy-two percent of the largest plans (250,000 or more total enrollees) participated in Medicaid in 1996. Most of this increase in participation was in states with high Medicaid managed care enrollment by 1996. Outside these high-enrollment states, only about 21 percent of the commercial-based plans participated in Medicaid, compared with 49 percent of those plans in states with at least 150,000 Medicaid managed care enrollees in full-risk plans.[11]

Increasing Enrollments

Participating plans substantially increased their Medicaid enrollment, and this increase slightly outpaced increases in enrollment from other payer groups. The rapid growth in Medicaid enrollment in managed care plans was enough both to support additional health plans seeking to participate in Medicaid and to increase the volume of Medicaid enrollees of plans already in the market. During this period, a participating plan's average Medicaid enrollment grew by 36 percent, from 15,880 to 21,537. Increases in Medicaid enrollment slightly outpaced other enrollment growth—the average Medicaid portion of a participating plan's enrollment increased from 26 percent to 31 percent during the period. Of the 218 plans that were operating from 1993 through 1996 and that served Medicaid at some point during that time, 23 percent had large, consistent increases totaling 10,000 or more enrollees, and 49 percent had a consistent increase at some level. Nearly all of the rest had an inconsistent pattern of change or no change; only nine plans showed a consistent decline in Medicaid enrollment.

The number of Medicaid-dominated plans doubled during the period, as did the number of more evenly mixed plans (those in which Medicaid constituted 25 to 74 percent of total enrollment). Plans in which Medicaid accounted for a very small percentage (less than 10 percent) of total enrollment were the only type to grow more slowly, increasing from sixty-four plans in 1993 to ninety-four plans in 1996. This could reflect plans' becoming more decisive about their interest in serving Medicaid. That is, plans that did not market or emphasize their Medicaid service may have been pressured by Medicaid program changes and/or market forces to more aggressively market their services to Medicaid to stay in the Medicaid market.[12]

The Medicaid Market

Health plans entered the Medicaid market at a dramatically higher rate in 1995 and 1996 than in 1994. Some plans also left the Medicaid market. Overall, the number of plans in the Medicaid market nearly doubled over this period (Exhibit 3).

New Plans

More than half (63 percent) of plans entering the Medicaid market were newly formed plans, and nearly 81 percent of these were Medicaid-only plans. In all, 157 newly formed plans entered the Medicaid market, 127 of which were Medicaid-only plans (Medicaid comprised 90–100 percent of enrollees). We do not know if these plans intended to remain Medicaid-only or if some or all intended to enroll commercial members in the future.

Entry of the largest commercial-based plans into the Medicaid market dropped off between 1995 and 1996. Between 1994 and 1996, 120

Exhibit 3 Plans Entering and Exiting the Medicaid Market, 1993–1996

	Number Serving Medicaid in 1993	Entering Plans			Exiting Plans			Number Serving Medicaid in 1996	Net Change, 1993–1996
		1994	1995	1996	1994	1995	1996		
Operating status in 1993									
Operational	166	27	33	34	19	13	19	209	+43
Not operational	0	27	78	52	0	2	9	146	+146
Role of Medicaid[a]									
Medicaid-only	57	25	64	38	12	5	11	144	+87
Medicaid-dominated	7	2	1	1	0	2	0	12	+5
Commercial-based	102	27	46	47	7	8	17	199	+97
Total	166	54	111	86	19	15	28	355	+189

Source: Mathematica Policy Research analysis for the Center for Studying Health System Change, supported by The Robert Wood Johnson Foundation.

[a] Medicaid-only plans are those in which Medicaid comprises 90–100 percent of total enrollment. Medicaid-dominated plans are those in which Medicaid comprises 75–89 percent of total enrollment. Commercial-based plans are all other plans.

commercial-based plans, including forty-one large plans (100,000 or more enrollees), entered the market.[13] Thirteen of the largest plans (250,000 or more enrollees) entered the market in the two-year period 1994–1995, but only one did so in 1996 (not shown). This decline could reflect either a change in these health plans' views on the Medicaid market or differences in the configuration of plans in states where Medicaid managed care activity was gaining momentum.

Exiting Plans

Sixty-two plans left the Medicaid market between 1994 and 1996, with nearly half of those plans exiting during 1996. Although recent anecdotes suggest increased concern about whether commercial-based plans will pull out of the Medicaid market as states reduce their capitation rates, we did not find that pattern. Older, commercial-based plans did not represent an increasing proportion of plans leaving the market relative to other plans in 1996, but there was an increase in the number of commercial-based plans that left the market in 1996 compared with 1994 and 1995 (seventeen in 1996 compared with seven in 1994 and eight in 1995). Some of the plans that appeared to leave the Medicaid market because they were listed as serving Medicaid one year but not in subsequent years were actually still in the market under another name after being bought by or merging with another plan or having simply changed names. Plan failure or a sudden termination of Medicaid service likely has more dramatic implications for enrollees than other changes in organizational structure have.

We tried to obtain information on the reasons for plans' disappearance from the list of participating plans. We ascertained (largely from state Medicaid officials) that thirty-three of the plans that left the market had indeed been bought or merged or had changed names, that eight additional plans went out of business, and that four dropped off the list because they shifted from a fully capitated to a partially capitated program. We remain unsure about what happened to the seventeen other plans. Of the sixty-two plans that exited, it appears that thirty-two were commercial-based plans that stopped serving Medicaid during the period.

Implications for Policy

As Medicaid managed care has spread across the country since 1993, health plans of diverse sizes, missions, and system affiliations have viewed the Medicaid population as a potentially attractive market and either entered the market or increased their Medicaid enrollment. While the share of Medicaid enrollees served by commercial-based plans remained about the same during the study period, the proportion of participating commercial-based plans rose from 21 percent of participating plans in 1993 to 36 percent in 1996.

Although the overall trend was toward increased participation during the study period, sixty-two plans dropped off the list of Medicaid-serving plans for a variety of reasons, including business failure, merger with another organization, or a decision to drop their Medicaid service. Given today's dynamic Medicaid program environment, along with the potentially adverse effects on beneficiaries of plans dropping out of the market, policymakers should work with organizations that are tracking market trends to develop a routine, central means for determining why plans stop serving Medicaid enrollees.

Medicaid-dominated health plans, new and old, play an important role today in serving the Medicaid managed care population. Equally interesting, they have played this role at least since 1993, caring for 47 to 48 percent of Medicaid managed care beneficiaries throughout the period. Although the role of Medicaid-dominated plans relative to other plans has not changed much over the years, there are 127 new Medicaid-only health plans enrolling Medicaid beneficiaries and 1.6 million more beneficiaries enrolled in this type of plan than there were in 1993. This growth may interest policymakers for several reasons.

Oversight

First, more plans means a greater oversight burden for states and greater likelihood that problems may arise.

Monitoring Quality

Second, many of the Medicaid-dominated plans have been somewhat invisible to national-level researchers and policymakers; information about these plans is scarce and rarely integrated with information from licensed HMOs (or health plans known to AAHP and InterStudy), except perhaps by the state Medicaid programs. This makes it hard to understand national trends or to monitor changes and identify problems.[14] Because they do not have to meet the demands of large employers, Medicaid-dominated plans do not face the same pressures as commercial plans do to seek accreditation from the National Committee for Quality Assurance or to produce statistics on quality and utilization based on the Health Plan Employer Data and Information Set. Nor are they likely to have the resources to do so, at least in the near term. Besides tending to be smaller than other plans, as our data show, anecdotal evidence also suggests Medicaid-dominated plans tend to have fewer resources and reserves and to be based in underserved urban areas. Policymakers may need to be especially vigilant in monitoring these plans, since Medicaid provides the main means for ensuring that a quality improvement system is in place.[15]

The 75/25 Rule

Third, the Medicaid program has traditionally relied on a requirement commonly known as "the 75/25 rule" as a proxy for quality. The theory behind the rule is that if health plans can attract a substantial amount of business from paying customers who presumably have multiple options, they must have a reputation for providing good care and service with good physicians. Therefore, the rule states that for health plans that serve Medicaid, at least 25 percent of their enrollees must be non-Medicaid beneficiaries. Exceptions have always been granted for community health centers and plans or states that have been granted waivers. Even without a waiver, new plans have three years to meet the requirement.

With the major role that the Medicaid-dominated plans are playing and the high volume of beneficiaries they serve, policymakers may need to acknowledge the demise of the 75/25 rule, simply to reflect the reality of the day, and pursue other mechanisms to ensure acceptable quality of care. For example, states that have been granted federal waivers for their Medicaid managed care programs are committed to developing a quality improvement system for Medicaid managed care based on HCFA guidelines for the Quality Assurance Reform Initiative (QARI).[16] An evaluation of an earlier QARI demonstration found that the QARI guidelines were useful overall, but that they needed to be updated and revised.[17]

Role of Medicaid-Dominated Plans

Fourth, the presence of Medicaid-dominated plans and their likely continued role in the future argue for information on what they may contribute to the system, as well as what demands they place on it. A number of states have welcomed the formation of Medicaid-only plans to increase the managed care choices available to Medicaid beneficiaries, and some have actively supported development of such plans. These plans form their provider networks largely around physicians and health centers with practices focused on low-income populations, which may mean that the providers are more culturally sensitive than those in other plans. It may be that plans specializing in serving a particular Medicaid population deliver better care to that population cost-effectively. They also may use other nonmedical community resources more effectively than commercial plans do.

Thus, additional research is needed to document the relative strengths of Medicaid-dominated plans. In the meantime, the role of the state Medicaid and other health-related agencies is more critical than ever in ensuring acceptable quality of care in these plans and in supporting the quality improvement efforts of Medicaid-dominated plans while taking into account their limited resources.

Acknowledgments

This research was conducted in collaboration with the Center for Studying Health System Change, with funding from The Robert Wood Johnson Foundation. The authors gratefully acknowledge the helpful advice of Paul Ginsburg and Marsha Gold.

Notes

1. U. S. General Accounting Office, *States Turn to Managed Care to Improve Access and Control Costs*, GAO/HRD-93-46 (Washington: GAO, March 1993).
2. J. Gabel et al., "Growing Diversification in HMOs, 1988–1994," *Medical Care Research and Review* (March 1997): 101–17.
3. Other characteristics of interest for which we did not have data for many plans included for-profit/not-for-profit status, extent of service to urban versus rural enrollees, and characteristics of a plan's provider network.
4. Because CalOptima is the largest of the full-risk health-insuring organizations (HIOs) and thus potentially has a significant effect on our results, we obtained data from the organization on which plans it subcontracts with on a full-risk basis and their enrollment each year. It is likely that one or more of the other smaller HIOs also subcontracts with full-risk plans, in which case our figures may slightly underestimate the number of full-risk plans serving Medicaid.
5. J. Corrigan et al., "Trends toward a National Health Care Marketplace," *Inquiry* (Spring 1997): 11–28.
6. Because we used mostly InterStudy data rather than AAHP data for 1996, the total enrollment data for 1996 are for 1 January 1996, rather than 31 December 1995. This could affect the results since reenrollment occurs irregularly and in the commercial market is particularly extensive in January of each year. However, we did not view this as a major problem, given our focus on large differences in types of plans. In a few cases, where the AAHP and InterStudy data appeared to conflict because of reporting differences, we were able to substitute total enrollment for 31 December 1995 from prepublication data.
7. Bureau of Primary Health Care, Health Resources and Services Administration, U.S. Department of Health and Human Services, unpublished data, March 1997.
8. HCFA enrollment data only included an indicator for SSI service in 1995, not other years. Plans that are subcontractors to CalOptima in California are excluded from

this analysis because we do not have HCFA data indicating whether or not they serve the SSI population.

9. Medicaid-dominated plans were likely formed to serve Medicaid, so excluding them from this analysis gives the reader a better sense of the extent to which health plans with other options are participating in Medicaid.
10. The apparent trend toward enrollment in larger plans is a function of the national growth trend in plans rather than a change in where beneficiaries tend to enroll. (We examined this by reanalyzing the trend using plan sizes that were standardized for the national growth trend in total enrollment.)
11. The increase in participation was not attributable to a few major health plan systems' shifting all of their health plans into Medicaid managed care. The data show that plans that are affiliated with a particular system do not tend to move in or out of the Medicaid market all at one time.
12. Twenty-four of the eighty-nine new Medicaid-only plans that began operations in 1994 or 1995 grew to 20,000 or more members by 1996.
13. Those for whom Medicaid enrollment comprises less than 75 percent of their total enrollment.
14. There are several potential types of Medicaid-only plans, but these types are not identified in current data sources. At least twenty-four plans nationally are owned or operated at least in part by community health centers, and most of these are Medicaid-only plans. Bureau of Primary Health Care, unpublished data, March 1997. Other Medicaid-only plans may be run by commercial health plans. A commercial plan may, for example, establish a Medicaid-only plan in a state where it does not have a commercial health plan. Or it may license a Medicaid product separately from its commercial product. We recombined this latter type of plan, even when listed separately in an industry directory, so that it was counted as a commercial-based plan.
15. S. Felt-Lisk and R. St. Peter, *The Quality Assurance Reform Initiative (QARI) Demonstration for Medicaid Care: Final Evaluation Report* (Washington: The Henry J. Kaiser Family Foundation, November 1996). In the evaluation, which involved twenty-one health plans in three states, the plans with less-developed quality systems tended to be Medicaid-dominated plans.
16. Health Care Financing Administration, *A Health Care Quality Improvement System for Medicaid Managed Care: A Guide for States* (Washington: U.S. Department of Health and Human Services, July 1993).
17. Felt-Lisk and St. Peter, *The Quality Assurance Reform Initiative.*

CHAPTER

11

MEDICAID MANAGED CARE: LESSONS FROM FIVE STATES

Marsha Gold, Michael Sparer, and Karyen Chu

Introduction

Medicaid is in the midst of fundamental change. Medicaid officials in nearly every state are encouraging or requiring beneficiaries to enroll in managed care. This trend is largely a response to the continued rise of Medicaid expenses as well as an attempt to address the ongoing problems of access to care. These remain, even though this federal/state insurance program accounts for much of the nation's progress over the past thirty years in improving access to health care for low-income populations.

By 1994 forty-three states and the District of Columbia had a Medicaid managed care initiative.[1] Between 1990 and 1995 Medicaid managed care enrollment more than quadrupled. Thirty-two percent of all Medicaid beneficiaries are now in managed care.[2]

The shift to Medicaid managed care needs to be carefully monitored. For example, Medicaid managed care initiatives have had more problems than commercial managed care efforts have had, because of the unique

From *Health Affairs* 15 (3): 153–166.

nature of the Medicaid population (primarily low-income women and children, disabled persons, and the elderly) and sometimes inadequate state oversight.[3] There is a fear that these problems may escalate with increased state flexibility. In this context, policymakers need to understand quickly how best to shape Medicaid managed care initiatives so that access and care systems for low-income persons are improved and transition problems minimized. Because of the pace of change, timely insights are critical, even if they are less conclusive than they ultimately could be with a longer and more thorough evaluation.

In this paper we draw on the insight developed through site visits to five very different states in late 1994 to early 1995 to identify issues and early lessons from the states' experiences with implementing managed care. After a brief review of methods, we summarize the program features, the administrative and delivery issues raised, the effects on the health care system, our conclusions, and lessons.

Study Methods

We selected the five study states—California, Minnesota, New York, Oregon, and Tennessee—to provide diversity in size, strategies, and experience. The study was based on site visits by a team of two or three people that lasted from four to five days.[4] We interviewed state officials and others who are attempting to influence policy from the standpoint of consumers, providers, and insurers/health plans. Using interviews and, where available, documents, we prepared lengthy case studies for each state. These studies were circulated among diverse interviewees and revised using the comments we received. This paper compares the states and their experiences to identify common threads, cross-cutting issues, and general lessons. Our goal was to be well enough grounded in operational reality to catch the nuances but also general enough to see the "big picture." Some findings or conclusions may seem obvious but bear repeating, particularly given the pace of change.

Our study draws on recent work to build a framework for looking at managed care and its relationships with the broader health system.[5] Our focus on operations and effects in states leads us to expand on John Holahan's three-part framework to consider diverse aspects of eligibility and enrollment, managed care plan and provider participation, and state oversight.[6] Our focus is on access to care more than on financing, and we examine how the movement to managed care affects low-income persons and the safety net.

The strengths of the case-study method rest in its ability to provide timely, in-depth information from a variety of perspectives. The limitations are (1) the limited number of persons who can be interviewed; (2) the limited ability to go beyond identifying issues and problems to estimating their magnitude or empirical effects; and (3) the inherent subjectivity in interpreting complex and sometimes contradictory information. Programs are developed for operations, not for researchers. States vary in how they document policies, and many important facts and policies are not in writing. Thus, we rely heavily on interviews. We report facts that are supported by multiple sources and consistent with other information on hand. The systems we studied are evolving rapidly, so specific features may have changed since our visits.

Summary of State Initiatives

Exhibit 1 summarizes each state's Medicaid managed care initiatives, the states' history with managed care, and the implementation status of the initiatives. Briefly, the five initiatives are as follows.

- **California.** The state is developing a managed care strategy within its Medi-Cal program (California Medicaid). The goal is to have half of the projected Medi-Cal enrollment in managed care by late 1996. This is to be accomplished through a variety of managed care models that are now in different stages of development across the state.
- **Minnesota.** Minnesota has several initiatives that eventually will be integrated under a federal Section 1115 research and demonstration waiver. The state is expanding mandatory Medicaid managed care statewide. MinnesotaCare, the state's reform initiative, includes state-subsidized health insurance. Under the waiver, MinnesotaCare and Medicaid will be integrated under a managed care strategy, and MinnesotaCare will be supported in part with federal Medicaid funds.
- **New York.** Working through localities, New York is expanding managed care enrollment in Medicaid voluntarily, for the most part. Its goal is to achieve 50 percent penetration by the year 2000. In 1995 New York submitted an 1115 waiver application through which nearly all Medicaid beneficiaries would be enrolled in managed care on a mandatory basis, but it has not yet been approved.
- **Oregon.** As part of its broader health reform initiative involving both private and public initiatives, the Oregon Health Plan's Medicaid component expands coverage to all Oregonians below the poverty level. Savings are generated by managed care and by a benefit package that is defined by a "priority list" of covered condition and treatment pairs.

Exhibit 1 Characteristics of Managed Care Initiatives in Five States

	California	Minnesota	New York	Oregon	Tennessee
Size of State (1993)	31.4 million	4.5 million	18.1 million	3.0 million	5.1 million
Prior managed care experience					
Commerical	Extensive	Extensive	Limited	Extensive	Limited
Medicaid	Limited	Extensive	Limited	Extensive	Limited
Mandatory programs	A few counties	Yes	One small program	Yes	None
Eligibility expansions	No	Yes	No[a]	Yes	Yes
Benefits/cost sharing	Traditional Medicaid	MinnesotaCare, more limited benefits	Traditional Medicaid	Priority list	Extensive cost sharing
Capitation	Yes	Yes	Yes	Yes	Yes
Population focus	Families and children (SSI in a few counties)	Families and children with some others in demonstrations	Families and children	Those below poverty; disabled, aged, and blind being phased in	Comprehensive
Federal waivers	Freedom-of-choice waivers[b]	1115 submitted (now approved)[c]	1115 submitted[c]	1115 approved[c]	1115 approved[c]
Status at visit	Mandatory model in only some counties	Medicaid managed care expanding; MinnesotaCare not yet using managed care	Political transition; voluntary model except for one small demonstration project	One year's experience 1115	One year's experience 1115

Source: Authors' research.
Note: SSI is Supplemental Security Income.
[a]In its 1115 waiver application, New York proposes to add its Home Relief population to Medicaid, thereby generating federal matching funds for persons already covered by what previously was a program financed only with state funds.
[b]These are Section 1915(b) programmatic waivers that were established in 1981 to facilitate transition to managed care.
[c]Section 1115 waiver programs draw on the discretion of the secretary of health and human services to authorize statewide Medicaid managed care demonstrations that include eligibility, benefits, and service delivery charges.

- **Tennessee.** TennCare is an ambitious effort to rapidly revamp Tennessee's Medicaid program. In TennCare's first year enrollment increased from 770,000 to 1.1 million persons. Managed care enrollment is mandatory for virtually all TennCare insured persons. Subsidized, income-related coverage is available up to 400 percent of poverty, although new enrollment was limited after the first year. The system is financed through a complex structure that involves preexisting public and private health expenditures.

Given the scope of the issues covered, it is not possible to provide details on all of them. The individual case studies provide these details as well as additional documentation for our findings and conclusions.[7] Because none of the five states had much experience with managed care for disabled and other Supplemental Security Income (SSI) populations, who tend to be more vulnerable, this study provides little insight in this area.

Administrative Issues

Enrollment and Marketing

Shifting Medicaid beneficiaries from traditional Medicaid to managed care means that each beneficiary ultimately must be enrolled in an available plan. This process generally involves (1) informing beneficiaries of the change and the available choices; (2) explaining the procedures for making choices and helping beneficiaries understand the implications of those choices; (3) assigning those who do not make a choice to default options; and (4) notifying plans and beneficiaries of their choices in a timely manner so that enrollment cards and new-member materials can be distributed.

Administrative issues include determining who conducts the enrollment process (county, contractor, or health plan); whether enrollment is done in person or by mail; and how much, if any, direct marketing individual health plans may do. Additional tasks involve assuring that plans and accessible networks exist to serve the new enrollees.

Exhibit 2 summarizes key features of each state's approach to these issues. The processes functioned much more smoothly in two states (Minnesota and Oregon) than in others. Both states had much more experience to build on, and both also invested considerable time and resources in educating and communicating with beneficiaries. In Minnesota enrollees attend an educational session run by specially trained county staff when they come in for eligibility recertification. This eliminates extra steps for beneficiaries and almost does away with the need to assign beneficiaries to plans.[8] In Oregon a contractor handles information dissemination and holds numerous information sessions (in eight languages). Beneficiaries enroll in person or by mail, unless they also receive cash assistance, in which case they must enroll in person.

The overall experience of the five states is that plans' enrollment/selection processes are central to smooth implementation and that considerable attention must be paid to their design and funding. Problems arise even with good planning, especially when the volume of persons making the transition is high. For example, Oregon expected 5,000 calls in a month and received 4,000 in a day early in its program. Higher-than-expected telephone volume, illiteracy among beneficiaries, marketing

Exhibit 2 Enrollment and Marketing Features of Each State Medicaid Managed Care Initiative

	California[a]	Minnesota	New York	Oregon	Tennessee
Enrollment	Mail	In person	Mixed model (mail and in person)	Mixed model (mail and in person)	Mail
Central beneficiary education	Limited	Extensive	Limited	Extensive	Limited
Use of contractor support	Yes	No	No	Yes	No
Direct marketing					
Any	Yes	No	Yes[b]	No	No set policy
Door to door	Varies by county	No	Varies by Social Service District	No	No set policy
Voluntary selection rate in mandatory programs	86 percent	Virtually all	75–80 percent of subset at demonstration education sessions[c]	Over 90 percent	50–60 percent
Experience	Confusion	Smooth	Not applicable[d]	Smooth	Confusion

Source: Authors' research.
[a]Applies to Sacramento except where noted.
[b]Suspended in New York City as of summer 1995.
[c]Of the approximately 38,000 enrolled in Southwest Brooklyn, about 9–12 percent were assigned to a plan, about 37 percent were enrolled by county workers after one-on-one meetings, and the remaining 51–54 percent were enrolled directly by health plan marketers.
[d]New York State had only a limited mandatory program; hence, experience with this feature was limited. New York allegedly experienced considerable marketing problems under its voluntary program, especially in New York City.

abuses, low rates of plan selection, and inappropriate selections of plans because of poorly designed enrollment forms were among the problems states encountered.

TennCare's experience illustrates the serious problems that can arise when timing is tight and experience is limited. TennCare used a mail-in enrollment process exclusively. In the first year the state, the plans, and individual providers were overwhelmed by the volume of telephone calls and the confusion generated by the initial mailing. The state received 50,000 calls in one day and finally resorted to pulling state staff from non-health care agencies into temporary telephone duty. Because enrollment occurred before provider networks were fully in place, eligible persons could not effectively consult with their providers, as instructed, to select a plan. As many as half of the beneficiaries had to be assigned to a plan, and those who selected a plan did not always get their choice. Because of delays in notification, some patients apparently did not know which plan they were in for some time until after the system became effective, nor did they have new-member materials. Many persons appear to have continued their old care patterns despite the transition to managed care; fortunately, many providers responded with flexibility to this situation. For persons who were unsatisfied with the plan that was listed on their notification, the switch to another plan was difficult and often was not carried out in a timely manner. Meanwhile, at least one plan was totally overwhelmed by exceptionally rapid growth, partly driven by assignments made by the state. The plan's enrollment grew from 35,000 to 275,000 overnight.

Some states are more strict than others about health plan marketing. Both Oregon and Minnesota prohibit any direct marketing by health plans. New York recently suspended door-to-door marketing in New York City, and California, too, is adopting this policy. Some small Medicaid-only plans expressed concern that restricted marketing could put them at a disadvantage because they have less name recognition and cannot take advantage of commercial advertising authority to circumvent Medicaid restrictions. Direct marketing by plans has been associated with some of the historic abuses in Medicaid managed care.[9]

Eligibility

Several states use simplified enrollment processes for newly eligible persons, thereby encouraging enrollment. However, these efforts have had unintended effects. Oregon's attempt to simplify by considering only one month's income generated negative publicity about potential fraud or abuse. In addition, the eligibility criteria in Oregon are apparently generous enough so that many persons chose to join the Oregon Health Plan directly rather than traditional Medicaid and welfare (along with its associated stigma and enrollment barriers). Thus, as of November 1994 approximately 21,000 more new eligibles than anticipated had signed up, but the number of traditional Medicaid eligibles fell about 23,000 short, primarily because of fewer Aid to Families with Dependent Children (AFDC) recipients than projected. This is consistent with other recent evidence that suggests that decoupling Medicaid from welfare can reduce reliance on welfare.[10]

Eligibility turnover is a major concern in many of the states because it limits a plan's ability to amortize initially high marketing costs and new enrollees' care costs over time. Extensive eligibility turnover also is inconsistent with a managed care model that focuses on prevention, early treatment, and continuity of care. Guaranteed eligibility is used less extensively than it could be because of concerns about its impact on cost. Minnesota, under its recently approved 1115 waiver, will use a "one-month rolling eligibility period" to address the problem of short-term eligibility turnover because of failure to meet administrative requirements.

Eligibility turnover also can occur when new and old eligibility processes are not completely coordinated, causing those who lose eligibility for Medicaid through AFDC to be disenrolled rather than being converted to other available options. This appears to have occurred at times under the Oregon Health Plan and possibly also under TennCare.

Oversight

The experience in all five states shows that effective oversight is essential. Each of the states, however, uses a different model, sometimes for historical reasons.

Under TennCare, new organizations formed rapidly and could be authorized by TennCare as preferred provider organizations (PPOs) rather than going through the state health maintenance organization (HMO) licensure process. Yet TennCare's process for overseeing these plans was not well developed in the first year. For example, marketing policies were not published during the first year, and few policies or procedures were put in writing. To respond to these and other problems, Tennessee recently increased the authority of the insurance department over PPOs.[11] Similarly, California is phasing out its independent contracting with primary care case management programs regulated by the Medi-Cal agency, in favor of HMO licensure mechanisms regulated by the state's Department of Corporations. In contrast, Oregon has a long history with regulating Medicaid managed care through the Medicaid program rather than through more general HMO licensure, which in Oregon is restricted to federally qualified HMOs.

Oversight requires state resources and staff. In California the lack of sufficient staff to oversee plans was cited by plan administrators and outsiders as creating serious constraints on implementation. In New York problems arose because administrative functions are fragmented and decentralized, which added to administrative costs and created confusion for health plans.[12]

None of the states had sufficient data to routinely monitor either baseline care patterns and access or the effects of the initiative; this is also a failing of traditional Medicaid. Virtually no state had information on care patterns and access to care for the uninsured before they were eligible for the program. Medicaid data could be used to monitor changes in care patterns and access for those who are continuously eligible, but states must manipulate eligibility, claims, and provider participation files to provide relevant information. This is not often done. Few states could tell us with statistics where Medicaid enrollees received care prior to the initiative. Maintaining data systems under managed care and capitation also is problematic, since claims are not submitted to the state.

Sacramento illustrates dramatically how data shortcomings influence policy development and evaluation. Virtually all stakeholders agreed that while initial implementation of managed care was rocky, the key issue is whether access to care improves. Unfortunately, the commission to assess the initiative is stymied by the lack of systematic information evaluating or even describing care patterns and access before the initiative. Some, for example, argue *ex post facto* that access to care was reasonably good before the initiative, at least for the average child or pregnant woman enrolled in Medicaid. But no one has data on this issue, at least not in a usable form.

Delivery and Coordination

Managed care strategies require states to develop policies and procedures on (1) which managed care plans are eligible to participate; (2) which requirements these plans need to meet; (3) which benefits they should be required to provide, and which should be "carved out" and paid for separately on a fee-for-service basis; (4) what the rates should be and how they should be established; and (5) how, if at all, safety-net providers should be explicitly included in the initiative. All of these policies influence the delivery of care under the initiative. Exhibit 3 summarizes key features of each state's approach.

Structure of Delivery Systems

The five states' approaches vary but tend to be built around mandatory enrollment models using fully capitated plans where possible. Either full or partial capitation is used in each state for virtually all contracting between the state and health plans. Partial capitation or noncapitated models seem to be used mainly when an infrastructure in an area (especially a rural area) cannot support full capitation or when the available providers are poorly positioned to support the risk. Oregon has the most explicit policy of this type. The state ultimately wants to use only fully capitated plans, and it has assessed its ability to do this, by county. If the state decided that insufficient capacity existed in fully capitated plans, it used a mix of fully and partially capitated plans or (in very isolated rural counties) primary care case management models. Oregon has relied on fully capitated plans much more than was originally expected, in part because new plans formed for the initiative, and some commercial plans viewed it as a way to expand their base in rural areas.

Exhibit 3 Medicaid Managed Care Features of Each State Initiative

	California	Minnesota	New York	Oregon	Tennessee
Statewide focus					
Planned	Yes	Yes	Yes	Yes	Yes
During visit	Limited counties	Many counties	Some counties	Yes	Yes
Mandatory enrollment	Yes[a]	Yes[b]	No[c]	Yes	Yes
Managed care structure					
Capitated plans	Full and partial	Full only	Full and partial	Mostly full	Full only, but risk status unclear for some plans
Eligible without state HMO license (Medicaid approval)	Yes, but being phased out	No, with minor exceptions	Yes	Yes	Yes
Benefit package	Selected carve-outs (Sacramento)	Full Medicaid package	Negotiated carve-outs, open access to selected preventive services	Priority list, initial carve-out of mental health and chemical dependency	Carve-out of long-term care and Medicare crossover benefits
Rate setting	Plan-specific negotiated rates with demographic adjusters; cap at 95 percent of FFS (Sacramento)	Regional rates with demographic adjusters (cap at 95 percent of FFS); adjustment for plans with teaching or disproportionate-share hospital	Regional caps (95 percent) on FFS negotiated rates for demographic groups; plan-specific negotiated rates	Actuarially based rates with assumed managed care savings; area and eligibility group adjustment; retrospective maternity/newborn adjustment	Statewide rates with demographic adjustments and offset; after withhold, payments are about two-thirds the estimated amount

Source: Authors' research.
Note: FFS is fee-for-service.
[a]Currently only in Sacramento and in a limited number of other counties, but this is a key feature of the California initiatives being phased in.
[b]In several counties, but many in the state (especially in rural areas) remain in fee-for-service.
[c]Pending 1115 waiver application would modify this. Enrollment is now mandatory in one small demonstration project.

The form of managed care used in each state reflects characteristics unique to its managed care infrastructure, the providers available in low-income areas, and the state's prior experience. In Minnesota, for example, HMO penetration in urban areas is very high, and there is a well-developed HMO regulatory infrastructure. Thus, the state can require plans to obtain an HMO license to participate in the Medicaid managed care program. California could do the same thing, although historically it has used a variety of managed care plans. In contrast, New York, which has a heterogeneous population and a generally limited managed care infrastructure, relies on a much greater mix of managed care models.

Capitation Rates and Risk Adjustment

States' approaches to setting capitation rates vary. Three states set rates uniformly for all plans in an area, while two negotiate with plans. In most cases, the amount paid is restricted to a maximum of some percentage of fee-for-service experience. Although capitation rates are said to be below commercial rates in all of the states, the rates in Oregon and Minnesota are much less controversial with plans than those in Tennessee are, as the rates there are considerably below the historical fee-for-service experience. However, there is concern, at least in Oregon, about whether the states will be able to sustain the rates over time.

Risk adjustment is key to setting equitable rates, since the Medicaid population is diverse and plan costs may vary considerably, depending upon their enrollees. Risk adjustment facilitates equitable compensation when plans serve more expensive populations and protects against windfall gains by health plans when a healthier population is enrolled. Unfortunately, although risk adjustment is important, little is known about how to do it practically.[13] The study states use relatively simple methods of adjustment: demographic, eligibility category, and geographic variables. Some states place more emphasis than others on the actuarial soundness of rates and the equity of the incentives. Oregon, for example, had an outside actuarial firm develop its rates. Different rates are set across a variety of geographic regions, and the state uses a creative approach to improve equity across plans with different maternity experience. Minnesota adjusts payments for what it perceives to be a more costly case-mix in some safety-net plans. In contrast, Tennessee uses a single statewide rate for demographic groups that reflects only about two-thirds of anticipated fee-for-service costs.[14]

Benefits and Carve-Outs

Some benefits can be excluded (or carved out) from the managed care plan's capitation rate, allowing enrollees to seek these services fee-for-service through traditional Medicaid. Minnesota and Oregon seem less likely to carve out benefits for persons enrolled in managed care. Because care is provided to persons, not conditions, any carving out of benefits can, at least in theory, create problems with coordination and burden-shifting. Yet not all plans and their providers, especially those with limited Medicaid experience, offer the full range of benefits and services typical of Medicaid. Carving these out can provide enrollees with access to providers who are more experienced with specific health problems or needs. We could not determine from the information available whether particular approaches work consistently better than others.

Oregon's effort to structure its benefit package through a formal priority-setting process has garnered considerable national interest. Our interviews suggest that health plans do not have major problems with the prioritized list of covered services. Some providers find it valuable; others report confusion as to what is covered. Contributing to the acceptance of the list are (1) the provider-led and "consultative" way in which it was developed, (2) the level at which the cutoff is set, (3) the fact that the state provides a benefit hotline staffed by registered nurses and runs a monthly meeting of plan medical directors to address coverage questions, and (4) the willingness of the state and health plans to be flexible in responding to physicians' concerns. For example, the state moved treatment of hernias in children under age eighteen "above the line" on the priority list in response to providers' concerns. Anecdotal evidence suggests that some "below-the-line" services continue to be provided for nonmedical reasons. For example, some providers perform nonmedically indicated circumcisions in response to cultural or religious norms. Other services—especially when they are viewed as inappropriate, need to be scheduled, or are expensive—are most likely not provided.

Enabling Services and Medicaid

States vary in the extensiveness and form of their requirements for "enabling" services such as translation, outreach, and transportation. For example, California requires new enrollees to be assessed within 120 days, whereas Oregon has no such requirement and generally tries to avoid what it views as micromanaging plans. Some plans see a philosophical conflict between a single standard of care (which they prefer) and structuring services around the needs of particular payer populations. Plans that place more emphasis on providing such enabling services perceive that they are at a disadvantage relative to their competitors that do not emphasize such services. Plans in Minnesota say that now, after years of experience, they appreciate the specific care issues associated with certain Medicaid groups. One plan provides cellular phones to high-risk pregnant women who do not have telephones at home. Another subsidizes tuition for child enrollees to attend an asthma camp.

Cost Sharing

TennCare has the most expansive eligibility definitions but also uses the most extensive cost sharing for those who are not traditionally eligible for Medicaid. Enrollees above the poverty level are supposed to pay premiums on a sliding scale, although these were not often collected in the program's first year because of administrative problems. TennCare requires enrollees with incomes above poverty to pay deductibles and coinsurance. Recently, Tennessee also proposed cost sharing for enrollees below the poverty level who are not otherwise eligible for Medicaid, although this was not federally approved. TennCare adjusts the plan's capitation rates downward to reflect anticipated recoveries from cost sharing. However, some plans absorb these costs.

Deductibles seem to be particularly problematic. They can serve as barriers to persons who need maintenance drugs because low-income beneficiaries cannot pay the up-front cost of the deductible. At least one plan paid for drugs, even if the deductible was not met, because it feared the costs of not doing so.

Participation by Commercial HMOs

The extent to which commercial HMOs are involved in Medicaid managed care initiatives varies by state. All commercial plans in Oregon have participated; plan participation in California is more mixed. Both Minnesota and New York show that making participation in Medicaid financially advantageous to plans increases Medicaid participation by commercial HMOs that once were reluctant to enter the market. Medicaid participation is made more attractive by making it a condition for other kinds of eligibility, such as participation in the state employees' plan, or for desired exceptions, such as various taxes or surcharges.

Although the states vary in whether they require managed care plans to be licensed as HMOs, none relies exclusively on commercial plans. All five states contracted to some extent with plans formed primarily in response to the particular state initiative or to previous Medicaid managed care initiatives, for at least two reasons. First, traditional providers for low-income persons wanted to continue in this role, and some formed their own managed care plans to do so. Second, new plans were important to generate sufficient capacity, particularly when commercial plans were not interested in aggressively expanding to pursue the Medicaid market.

Transitional Issues

TennCare tried to move rapidly from traditional Medicaid to managed care. Experience suggests that this is difficult to do, especially when there is only a limited managed care infrastructure and little time to plan. Tennessee was unable to change in so short a period to a system of well-organized, effectively configured managed care plans. Provider networks in the first year were not fully developed. For example, a plan could have in its network a hospital with a plan-affiliated surgeon but no anesthesiologist. Alternatively, the structure of the network could result in referrals to specialists who were far from an enrollee's residence.[15] Phone systems for patients were often inadequate; as a result, responses were delayed, or patients were connected with persons who were not familiar with the TennCare population. We heard reports of difficulties with drug formularies and exceptions processes; it is not clear whether this was because they were poorly developed, because physicians did not understand them, or because pharmacists resented them.

In addition, many patients continued to use their previous providers either because they did not know what plan they were in (state notifications were late), were dissatisfied with the plan to which they were assigned, or did not understand the system. The second-largest plan did not have a billing system that was even partly operational until mid-1994.[16] Participating providers were not paid or were paid lump sums that they could not associate with services, leaving them dissatisfied, especially those who were paid fee-for-service.

Health Care System Effects

Access to Care

The states' experience highlights the fact that Medicaid initiatives affect persons who are already insured or covered by Medicaid in a different way than they affect persons who gain coverage through a new initiative. The former have the most to lose (especially if benefits and access are already relatively good), and the latter, the most to gain. Although Oregon lacks data on these issues, most stakeholders perceive the effects of Phase I to be generally positive because the uninsured are better off, and those previously receiving Medicaid are essentially in the same position. In fact, some previous enrollees gained through minor expansion and coordination of benefits despite confusion associated with the transition. Surveys in Tennessee show similar patterns, but both groups had a less positive experience overall, probably because of the disruption and confusion in TennCare's first year.[17] In Minnesota innovative features such as loaner telephones are perceived as having improved access for those who already were covered.

Most concerns we heard about care were more likely to focus on the chronically ill and those with special needs than on the average enrollee. Persons become eligible for Medicaid because of either low income or sickness and disability. The latter group, generally adults, is more likely to have special needs, chronic illnesses, or other problems that cause them to function less effectively in traditional, mainstream care systems. Research suggests that those in poor health are more vulnerable to delivery system problems or disruptions associated with the start of a new initiative. Unfortunately, most techniques for monitoring and evaluation focus more on averages than on distributions. Thus, they are not particularly sensitive to measuring effects that apply only to a subpopulation.

The states' experience also indicates that managed care on its own will not remedy access problems related to provider shortages, especially in the short run. For example, low provider supply constrained the development and adequacy of managed care networks in rural and some inner-city areas of Tennessee. This generated access problems even as the initiative prompted the state to expand the authority and supply of nurse practitioners.

Safety-Net Providers and the Uninsured

Participation in a state's Medicaid managed care program does not seem to be a good proxy for safety-net protection, a concept related to but distinct from the effects on access. Most hospitals and community health centers had some affiliation with managed care plans, whether or not this was formally required, but state initiatives typically modified disproportionate-share funding and cost-based payments to federally qualified health centers and at times disrupted the flow of patients.

Some safety-net providers were in a stronger position than others to respond more actively to their state's program. A plan based around the public hospital system in Minneapolis is thriving. However, the Memphis public hospital has been severely stressed by TennCare, which led to a major reduction in Medicaid revenues. Some providers, especially those that are experienced, are large, and have established plans, appear likely to survive and grow. Access to capital and expertise is a constraining factor for some safety-net systems.

The size and role of the safety net also vary across communities. Stress on the safety net is more likely to have a negative effect in cities such as Los Angeles, New York, and Memphis, which historically have relied on large public systems, than in communities such as Sacramento and Orange County, where the safety net is much more limited.

The most serious concern is that a weakening of the safety net will reduce standby protection for those who remain uninsured or become so if the state's initiative fails. This is especially a concern to the extent that public subsidies for such services are being independently reduced by other changes in federal, state, or municipal policies. This may not be a Medicaid or managed care responsibility, but it is an important public policy concern.

When coverage is expanded, but not universally, funding once used for cross-subsidization is now used to support eligibility expansion.

Thus, safety-net providers are less able to tap such sources as disproportionate-share hospital payments and cost-based payments to federally qualified health centers to cover indigent care. In theory, the result should be positive to the extent that state initiatives reduce the number of uninsured persons and demand for uncompensated and subsidized care. However, some providers said that the volume of such care has not changed, probably because the demand for such services has been greater than the supply. Thus, improved access for the newly covered comes at the expense of those who remain uninsured.

Other Spillover Effects

In many states Medicaid is the largest purchaser of health care, or second largest after the state employee plan. By forcing a managed care strategy, TennCare generated systemwide activity, such as the purchase of physician practices, that is typical only in more advanced managed care markets. In Oregon commercial plans participated, because they viewed the statewide Oregon Health Plan as a vehicle for developing managed care networks in rural areas. Minnesota's initiative has had similar effects. Thus, one potential spillover effect in these three states is growth of the commercial managed care sector, especially where managed care penetration once was low.

Conclusions and Lessons

Conclusions

The conclusions from the five states we studied contain both positive and negative messages. States such as Minnesota and Oregon have moved a large share of their low-income populations into relatively well-designed managed care programs. Other states, such as Tennessee, have had major problems, at least in the early stages of implementation. Still others, such as California and New York, illustrate how long and complex the implementation process can be, particularly in large and diverse states. Both positive and negative effects on access to care appear likely in all five states. Thus, it is particularly disturbing that so few of the states had good baseline data on access, to judge whether the effort was worth it, both for persons already covered by Medicaid and the newly enrolled. In a previous study we suggested that a national Medicaid survey generating timely, state-specific estimates is feasible and should be implemented.[18] This is an important issue, whether or not managed care exists.

The five states we studied illustrate sharply the diversity in population, managed care infrastructure, provider networks, and state infrastructure across the states. A program that works well in California may not work well in New York. The same program also will probably not work equally well in all of the different areas within a state. States also vary in political climate and styles in ways that influence both what is viable and the effects of change. It is hard to imagine, for example, that the process of consensus and consultation used in Oregon to establish its priority list would work as well in New York, which is considerably larger and more diverse and has a combative political style.

Lessons from the States

Although our study illustrates why states need to tailor approaches to their unique environments, it also suggests that there are things that any state needs to consider in developing effective initiatives for low-income persons. In brief, we draw ten lessons about how states can increase their potential success in restructuring Medicaid with managed care for low-income populations.

(1) Invest in an effective enrollment process that anticipates confusion and questions. This includes well-designed written materials geared toward low-income populations, a toll-free telephone number with the capacity to address a large volume of questions, and some way to provide individual counseling in person.

(2) Emphasize education about the system for both enrollees and providers. This is important both when previous managed care experience is limited and in established systems to address changes and resolve new problems.

(3) Build a well-developed oversight system to minimize problems and monitor performance. Without this, marketing abuses and miscommunication are inevitable. Both access and quality standards for plans are important, particularly for new plans. The time and resources needed to establish an oversight system should not be underestimated.

(4) Build managed care strategies that are sensitive to the configuration of existing plans and providers and to the experience they have had in accepting risk for medical delivery, particularly for low-income populations. Before transferring risk to a provider, assess their administrative capacity and their ability to absorb risk.

(5) Allow sufficient time for implementation and system development, so that any controversy, confusion, and potentially serious access problems may be addressed in the transition. Substantial lead time is needed to develop effective procedures, oversight, and education. States that are considering very rapid time frames, perhaps to avoid political opposition (as in Tennessee) or to address serious budget constraints, must recognize the controversy, confusion, and short-term transition-related problems that will arise with rapid implementation.

(6) Invest in administrative structures and assume that these will cost, rather than save, money, at least in the short term. New systems and administrative demands are generated by managed care. States typically will not be able to offset these with other administrative cost savings.

(7) Pay special attention to policies and systems for the chronically ill. This population is particularly vulnerable to the effects of managed care because such persons are likely to have special health care needs. New types of systems may be needed for chronically ill persons and other subgroups of the Medicaid population that have special needs.

(8) Set rates that are sensitive to the populations enrolled in managed care plans and the costs associated with treating them. The adequacy of the rates affects which plans participate and whether care is comparable to that received by others. Because the Medicaid population is diverse, risk adjusters that modify payments to plans based on the health care needs of and the expected costs for enrollees are needed to encourage equity and to avoid windfall gains.

(9) Minimize extensive and rapid eligibility turnover. Eligibility turnover and managed care do not mix well. The "on again/off again" cycle of eligibility under Medicaid adds to administrative costs and makes it hard for health plans to provide continuity of care.

(10) Set objectives that are realistic. Financing a Medicaid managed care program does not by itself resolve the access problems created by an insufficient or poorly distributed supply of providers. In creating a benefit package, it is important not to impose unnecessary barriers to care. It is unrealistic to expect Medicaid managed care alone to generate enough savings to cover all of a state's uninsured residents. An adequately financed safety net is critical to maintaining access for those who remain uninsured.

In sum, establishing effective managed care programs for low-income populations requires work and time. A variety of diverse factors, policies, and procedures will influence outcomes. In short, the success of the iniative is "in the details" and depends on both the commitment and the financing available to support them.

Acknowledgments

All views are solely those of the authors and do not necessarily reflect the views of Mathematica Policy Research, The Henry J. Kaiser Family Foundation, or The Commonwealth Fund. Barbara Lyons, at the Kaiser Family Foundation, oversaw this project for the sponsors. Diane Rowland, Kaiser senior vice-president, deserves special recognition for developing this project and providing guidance. Karen Scott Collins,

Cathy Schoen, and Lois Simon of The Commonwealth Fund and Marsha Lillie-Blanton of Kaiser were active participants. At Mathematica Policy Research, Marilyn Rymer Ellwood contributed to the Minnesota case study and served as a reviewer of this paper and the associated case studies. Hilary Frazer was a project analyst and coauthor of the Tennessee case study. Daryl Hall edited the manuscript; and DeWayne Davis, Kathleen Donaldson, and other staff at Mathematica lent secretarial and administrative support, for which the authors are grateful.

Notes

1. Health Care Financing Administration, Office of Managed Care, *Medicaid Managed Care Enrollment Report*, U.S. Department of Health and Human Services Summary Statistics (Washington: DHHS, 30 June 1994).
2. D. Rowland and K. Hanson, "Medicaid: Moving to Managed Care," *Health Affairs* (Fall 1996): 150–52.
3. U.S. General Accounting Office, *Medicaid: States Turn to Managed Care to Improve Access and Control Costs*, GAO/HRD 93-86 (Washington: GAO, March 1993).
4. California and New York are large states where initiatives are being phased in through collaboration with localities. We spent more time in these states (five days) and focused more on specific markets—Sacramento, Los Angeles, and Orange Counties in California and New York City and Albany/Rensselaer in New York.
5. M. Gold et al., "Behind the Curve: A Critical Assessment of How Little Is Known about Arrangements between Managed Care Plans and Physicians," *Medical Care Research and Review* (September 1995): 307–41.
6. J. Holahan et al., "Insuring the Poor through Section 1115 Medicaid Waivers," *Health Affairs* (Spring 1995): 200–17.
7. M. Gold, K. Chu, and B. Lyons, *Managed Care and Low-Income Populations: A Case Study of Managed Care in Oregon* (Report of The Henry J. Kaiser Family Foundation and The Commonwealth Fund, Washington, D.C., July 1995): M. Gold, H. Frazer, and C. Schoen, *Managed Care and Low-Income Populations: A Case Study of Managed Care in Tennessee* (Report of The Henry J. Kaiser Family Foundation and The Commonwealth Fund, Washington, D.C., July 1995); M. Sparer and K. Chu, *Managed Care and Low-Income Populations: A Case Study of Managed Care in New York* (forthcoming); M. Sparer, M. Ellwood, and C. Schoen, *Managed Care and Low-Income Populations: A Case Study of Managed Care in Minnesota* (Report of The Henry J. Kaiser Family Foundation and The Commonwealth Fund, November 1995); and M. Sparer, M. Gold, and L. Simon, *Managed Care and Low-Income Populations: A Case Study of Managed Care in California* (Report of The Henry J. Kaiser Family Foundation and The Commonwealth Fund, May 1996).
8. When MinnesotaCare converts to managed care, they plan to have a mail-in selection process because that is how the enrollment process is carried out. Some are concerned that this could lead to problems.
9. GAO, *Medicaid: States Turn to Managed Care.*
10. R. Moffitt and B. Wolfe, "The Effect of the Medicaid Program on Welfare

Participation in Labor Supply," *Review of Economics and Statistics* (November 1992): 615–26.

11. B. Snyder and E. Cromer, "TennCare Faces Rehab," *Nashville Banner*, 27 January 1995, A1, A16.
12. Since our visit, the state has attempted to address the issue by consolidating state commercial and Medicaid managed care oversight in a newly created Office of Managed Care within the state Department of Health.
13. Physician Payment Review Commission, "Risk Adjustment," in *Annual Report to Congress, 1994* (Washington: PPRC, 1994), 135–58.
14. This estimate is for initial capitation rates once the "withhold" is considered. The withhold reflects on offset held in reserve by the state to protect against losses.
15. To some extent, this reflects the low participation rates of some specialists, such as orthopedists, who were said to be boycotting the program, and general shortages of physicians, especially in inner-city and rural areas.
16. This plan had historically capitated its primary care providers, many of which were community health centers that viewed the capitation rates as considerably better than they could obtain through other plans paying fee-for-service. This plan also puts a priority on expediting payment to capitated providers, especially those whose circumstances made cash flow more critical.
17. W. F. Fox and W. Lyons, "A Survey to Determine Insurance Status of Tennessee Residents" (Report prepared for the Tennessee Department of Finance and Administration, 25 August 1995).
18. M. Gold et al., "Design and Feasibility of a National Medicaid Access Survey with State-Specific Estimates," *Medical Care Research and Review* (September 1995): 409–30.

CHAPTER

12

REFORMING STATE MEDICAID PROGRAMS: FIRST-YEAR IMPLEMENTATION EXPERIENCES FROM THREE STATES

Judith Wooldridge, Leighton Ku, Teresa Coughlin, Lisa Dubay, Marilyn Ellwood, Shruti Rajan, and Sheila Hoag

IN THE early 1990s, states made healthcare reform a high priority in response to escalating Medicaid costs and increasing numbers of people without health insurance. More and more states began to reform their Medicaid programs through demonstrations authorized by Section 1115 of the Social Security Act. These demonstration programs, which require federal approval, give states great flexibility to modify Medicaid. Most demonstration states aim to control costs through mandatory managed care and to expand eligibility to reduce the number of uninsured people. Before 1993, only Arizona had a comprehensive Section 1115 demonstration. By late 1996, ten states had implemented comprehensive Section 1115 demonstrations, five more applications had been approved, and nine others were under review by the Health Care Financing Administration (HCFA).

Originally published by Mathematica Policy Research, Inc. A later version of this chapter appears in *Managed Care for the Public Good*, edited by S. Davidson and S. Sommers, forthcoming from Jossey-Bass. Inc.

Section 1115 demonstrations make major changes in the way healthcare for the poor is financed and delivered. Consequently, many important policy questions arise: How do the shift to managed care and the expansion of coverage to new groups affect access to care and quality of care? How do these changes affect the structure of the healthcare delivery system? What can we learn from how these programs are implemented and financed? What is their ability to control costs?

This publication summarizes the first annual report of a five-year evaluation to assess implementation of five Section 1115 demonstrations and impacts on covered beneficiaries. The evaluation is sponsored by HCFA and is being conducted by Mathematica Policy Research, Inc., and its subcontractor, the Urban Institute. The demonstrations, which are implementing managed care statewide, include (1) Hawaii's QUEST, (2) Rhode Island's RIte Care, (3) Tennessee's TennCare, (4) Oklahoma's SoonerCare, and (5) the Maryland Medicaid Section 1115 Health Care Reform Demonstration. This report focuses on implementation during 1994 in Hawaii, Rhode Island, and Tennessee, which have expanded eligibility to include some uninsured low-income people. Oklahoma implemented its program in 1996 and Maryland will implement its program in 1997, too late for inclusion here.

Findings in Brief

Other states, as well as managed care organizations (MCOs), providers, consumers, and the federal government, may find the following key findings on startup experiences useful:

- States can implement major Medicaid program changes in a short period.
- More time is needed for the planning and implementation phase.
- States can expand Medicaid managed care rapidly, although it is too early to assess the implications for quality of care and MCOs' long-term financial stability.
- States need more administrative resources during startup.
- Procedures for enrolling pregnant women and newborns may need to be modified under managed care.
- Consumers need more education about managed care.
- Safety net providers may need special support.
- Budget problems may undermine expansions.
- Controversy can be resolved through increased communication.
- Despite startup problems, these demonstrations survived political changes.

Before the Demonstrations

The three states applied for Section 1115 demonstrations for similar reasons:

- Medicaid costs had been increasing, and they wanted to control costs and improve the cost-effectiveness of their programs.
- They were concerned about reducing the uninsured population.
- They wanted to take advantage of the administration's support of expedited demonstration approvals.

Immediate Motivations Differed

However, their immediate motivations differed. In Hawaii, QUEST was designed to integrate three state insurance programs. The state had been moving toward universal health insurance long before QUEST and had the lowest level of uninsured people in the nation. So, Hawaii focused on slowing growth in Medicaid costs by enrolling participants in MCOs. It also focused on increasing federal matching of state expenditures by integrating its General Assistance program and the State Health Insurance Program (SHIP), a program for low-income uninsured people, with the Medicaid program for nonelderly and nondisabled people. The goal of program integration was to provide seamless coverage, with consistent eligibility criteria and benefits, and to ensure that the two state programs could receive federal matching funds.

Rhode Island's program goals grew out of concerns about primary care access problems in the Medicaid program, illustrated by the high proportion of expenditures on inpatient hospital stays and excessive use of emergency rooms for primary care. Additionally, increases in unemployment resulted in increases in the number of people without health insurance.

Tennessee, which was anticipating the end of the state's hospital tax in 1993 (the basis for disproportionate-share hospital funding), believed new taxes were politically infeasible, and needed a way to solve its budget crisis. Furthermore, 16 percent of people under age 65 in the state lacked health insurance, and the state was eager to expand insurance coverage for this group.

Before the demonstrations, the health service delivery systems in the three states varied considerably. These contrasting markets influenced state program development, approaches to capitation rate setting, and ease of implementation. Managed care penetration in Hawaii and Rhode Island was above the national average, at 23 percent and 26 percent of the insured population enrolled in health maintenance organizations (HMOs), respectively. By contrast, Tennessee had little managed care penetration; only 6 percent of the insured population was enrolled in HMOs. However, managed care was a small part of the Medicaid program in all three states (four percent or fewer of Medicaid enrollees were voluntarily enrolled in HMOs). Hospital bed supply was greatest in Tennessee, which had a high proportion of beds per person and low occupancy rates, and lowest in Hawaii, which had a low proportion of beds per person and high occupancy rates. In Tennessee, Medicaid payments to physicians were relatively generous, as a result of increases in the 1980s to improve access. By contrast, physician payments in Rhode Island were very low, and one demonstration program goal was to improve Medicaid physician payments and participation. A unique feature in Rhode Island was that community health centers served one-quarter or more of Medicaid recipients.

The Programs

The three states designed their programs rapidly (see Table 1). They received demonstration approval within 5 months after applying and implemented their programs between 6 weeks later (Tennessee) and 12 months later (Hawaii).

All three demonstrations introduced statewide managed care during 1994, covering all or part of the traditional Medicaid population as well as new populations that were previously ineligible (see Table 2). Tennessee's program was the largest and most inclusive, and Rhode Island's the smallest and least inclusive. All three programs required people in the expansion group with incomes above a threshold to pay part of their costs. In Tennessee, the threshold was family incomes above 100 percent of the poverty level; in Hawaii and Rhode Island, it was family incomes above 133 percent of the poverty level (or above 185 percent of the poverty level for pregnant women and infants).

The demonstrations maintained or expanded the benefits provided under Medicaid. TennCare eliminated Medicaid limits on physician services, outpatient visits, home health visits, and prescriptions. It also added adult psychiatric inpatient coverage. Although QUEST covered the same benefits as Medicaid, these benefits were more generous than those provided by SHIP. RIte Care added a comprehensive package of family planning benefits for 2 years to women who would otherwise have become ineligible for Medicaid 60 days postpartum. It also added nonemergency transportation, interpreter services, childbirth education, parenting education, nutrition counseling, and smoking cessation classes.

Participants in all three states had to choose an MCO when they enrolled in the demonstration. In Tennessee and Hawaii, initial program

Table 1 Length of Time Between Application and Implementation

State	Application Submitted	Application Approved	Program Implemented
Hawaii	April 19, 1993	July 16, 1993	August 1, 1994
Tennessee	June 16, 1993	November 18, 1993	January 1, 1994
Rhode Island	July 20, 1993	November 4, 1993	August 1, 1994

Table 2 Eligibility, Coverage, and Enrollment

State	Medicaid Groups Included	Expansion Group Included	Enrollment After One Year
Hawaii (QUEST)[a]	AFDC-related and poverty-related groups	Nonelderly, nondisabled uninsured people with incomes under 300 percent of the federal poverty level[b]	157,000
Rhode Island (RIte Care)	AFDC-related and poverty-related groups	Uninsured children under age 6 and pregnant women with family incomes under 250 percent of the federal poverty level	70,000
Tennessee (TennCare)	All groups except qualified Medicare-only beneficiaries	Uninsured people (with subsidies up to 400 percent of the poverty level) and medically uninsurable people	1,251,000

[a]In 1996, Hawaii restructured the QUEST program to reduce participation and expenditures greatly.
[b]Most of the newly eligible population was already covered under state General Assistance and SHIP.

enrollment was by mail, with no counseling provided, and everyone in the covered Medicaid population was enrolled in managed care all at once. Rhode Island's process was more personalized; the state tried to counsel Medicaid participants in person, and enrolled them in RIte Care during a 12-month period.

Although the process varied, all three states contracted with enough MCOs in different areas so that all participants had a choice between at least two MCOs (see Table 3). All MCOs received capitation payments from the state to serve the enrolled populations.

Hawaii and Rhode Island requested proposals from MCOs, and then negotiated capitation rates with each one individually. Both states contracted with five HMOs (one of which was formed by federally qualified health centers [FQHCs]). Hawaii also contracted with two dental MCOs and two behavioral health MCOs. In Tennessee, there

Table 3 Managed Care Contracting

State	Number of MCOs	Number of Newly Formed MCOs	FQHCs Formed an HMO?	Number of Statewide MCOs
Hawaii	5	1	Yes	1
Rhode Island	5	1	Yes	5
Tennessee	12[a]	5[b]	No	2[c]

[a]Five of the MCOs were PPOs.
[b]Three of the five new MCOs were sponsored by teaching hospitals.
[c]In 1996, a third MCO was offered statewide.

was no formal request for proposals from MCOs. The state drew up two standard contracts (one for HMOs and one for preferred provider organizations—PPOs). Seven HMOs and five PPOs signed these non-negotiable contracts. Tennessee paid the same capitation rates to all MCOs (although rates varied by member characteristics).

During the first year, capitation rates per member, per month, averaged $115 in Rhode Island and $188 in Hawaii (Hawaii's rate included dental coverage). Tennessee set an average payment rate and then discounted that rate to include expected savings from managed care and to share with providers the savings accruing from reduced numbers of uninsured people. After discounting, the payments averaged about $101 per member, per month, during the first 6 months of TennCare.

In Tennessee, the five PPOs have until 1997 to implement primary care gatekeeper arrangements, so many enrollees and providers are not yet subject to standard managed care practices. (These PPOs are simply limited provider networks; they do not allow members to use out-of-plan providers.) In the other two states, primary care gatekeepers are required. Tennessee also allowed MCOs more freedom than the other states to market to enrollees. For example, MCOs could market door-to-door and, with permission, in welfare offices where people apply for Medicaid.

A condition of demonstration approval was that it be budget neutral to the federal government during the five-year demonstration period (see Table 4). To varying degrees, each state assumed it could slow growth in Medicaid program costs and use some of the savings to serve more people. Tennessee and Hawaii ended their disproportionate-share payments to hospitals, freeing up federal funds for program expansion. Hawaii and Rhode Island assumed that they would have served women and children covered under Section 1902(r)(2) provisions in the absence of the demonstrations. This assumption allowed them to increase their

Table 4 Budget Neutrality

State	In tial 5-Year Budget (Millions)	Expected Federal Savings (Millions)	Expected State Savings (Millions)
Rhode Island	$708	$1.3	$1.1
Hawaii	$1,291	$5.4	$429
Tennessee	$19,600	$3,200	$1,600

"baseline" costs against which budget neutrality was measured. Tennessee planned the largest expansion and needed the greatest relative savings per person to finance it. Although Hawaii had to stretch its federal dollars to serve more people, it also hoped to save some more state funds from the SHIP program to support expansion. Rhode Island planned the smallest expansion. Moreover, because all of the expansion group could have been eligible for Medicaid under section 1902(r)(2) provisions, Rhode Island's program did not depend on savings from managed care to finance the expansion group. The state budgets and expected savings were as follows.

Hawaii expected to save state funds through incorporating state programs (SHIP and General Assistance) in the QUEST program and getting federal matching payments. RIte Care financed its demonstration by keeping the current Medicaid budget intact and appropriating an additional $6.5 million to cover the expanded population and the administration of RIte Care. In addition, some Department of Health program funds were shifted to RIte Care. Both states assumed that the program would receive funds from enrollee premiums and copayments.

To finance the state share of the TennCare budget ($8 billion), Tennessee planned to draw on a variety of sources, most of which were eligible for federal matching payments. These sources included the state general fund, other state health programs, certified public expenditures (basically, uncompensated care costs in public hospitals for TennCare-eligible persons not enrolled), premium payments from enrollees, a nursing home tax, and local government subsidies for indigent care. The state also included the costs of provider charity care in its budget (these costs were not federally matched). Capitation payments to MCOs were reduced to reflect the provider charity contribution.

Program Administration

The administration of the three programs differed. In Hawaii, the Med-QUEST division of the Department of Human Services assumed some of the responsibilities of the Department of Health, which had administered SHIP. The Med-QUEST Division also took primary responsibility for QUEST enrollment functions, which welfare staff had previously handled. This required the division to hire and train workers to assess eligibility and enroll participants into MCOs. RIte Care made the largest structural change; it is run by the Office of Managed Care, which was initially staffed jointly by the Department of Health and the Department of Human Services, as well as an outside contractor. An executive committee made up of the directors of the Departments of Health, Human Services, and Administration, as well as a representative of the governor, oversaw the Office of Managed Care in the first year. RIte Care is now operated by the Department of Human Services. In Tennessee, the Medicaid Bureau was renamed the TennCare Bureau. The state also added an eligibility determination contractor for the newly covered uninsured and uninsurable groups.

Implementation Experience

Although it is too early to determine the impacts of these three demonstrations on beneficiaries, we can draw the following conclusions about program implementation.

Programs were designed quickly, providing limited opportunities for consultation with stakeholders. Opportunities for input to program design were limited in all three states because of the speed with which the demonstration applications were developed and submitted. To some degree, this caused problems in all three states. In Tennessee, interested groups had opportunities to meet with the governor before the demonstration application was submitted for approval, but their comments were largely ignored since they were opposed to key program elements. Physicians became angry when the state ignored their views, and the state's medical association tried to block TennCare through legal action. MCOs were able to review drafts of the MCO contract, and some consumer groups met with the state biweekly from June to December 1993. However, the first public hearings on TennCare took place in 1995, one year after TennCare began. In Hawaii, there was also little opportunity for public input. Physician groups objected both to the process and the focus on managed care, and legislators threatened to block implementation. In Rhode Island there appeared to be little provider concern about the move to managed care, except among FQHCs, but consumers and their organizations criticized the state for not involving them more in the design. As a result, RIte Care staff made many efforts to involve consumer advocates during implementation planning and the first year of operations. At the national level, the National Association of Community Health Centers sued HCFA to stop implementation of Section 1115 demonstrations.

Program startup was troubled. All three states had implementation problems at startup, although the amount of confusion varied with the size of the program, the speed of implementation, and the scope of the changes. Enrollment-related problems occurred in all three states. There were delays between application and MCO enrollment, MCOs could not reconcile discrepancies between their membership records and the state's, consumers encountered problems or were confused about how to enroll in the program or select MCOs or physicians, providers could not always tell which MCO their patients were enrolled in, and enrollment of pregnant women and newborns was not always smooth.

The TennCare program enrolled three-quarters of a million people into MCOs on January 1, 1994. Administrative problems accompanied this considerable achievement. These problems were exacerbated by the brevity of the period between program approval and implementation, and the lack of managed care experience in the state. Despite hard work by state and MCO staff, the necessary eligibility and claims processing systems were not working smoothly on January 1, 1994. In addition to confusion about enrollment, the state was not ready to oversee MCOs. Moreover, some MCOs ran into provider network problems. The largest TennCare MCO (Blue Cross) initially lost one-third of its physician network because physicians objected to the MCO's requirement that they accept TennCare patients if they continued to accept state employees. This situation led to difficulties getting access to some specialists. Throughout the first 18 months, the second largest TennCare MCO (Access MedPlus) had major problems paying provider claims and required close monitoring by and help from the state.

Hawaii's much smaller program was also challenged by the volume of eligibility applications it had to handle at the start of QUEST and the inexperience of the staff handling this function. Because of the ensuing application backlogs, applicants had to wait more than a month to get an appointment for eligibility determination. The state had anticipated a wait of only 10 days, during which it would pay fee-for-service for services applicants received. The prolonged delay led to problems for the state in deciding how to provide coverage during the waiting period. Furthermore, many beneficiaries had to change physicians unnecessarily.

Rhode Island was criticized for implementing RIte Care before everything was ready. Even though enrollment into managed care was phased in during a 12-month period, the state's eligibility system still had problems, causing confusion for providers and consumers. RIte Care placed new demands on the state's Medicaid Management Information System (MMIS), which had only been implemented in December 1993. Furthermore, because the HMO formed by the FQHCs was not licensed when RIte Care began, it requested a delay in RIte Care implementation. Instead, the state allowed enrollees choosing this plan to remain in fee-for-service Medicaid until the plan received its license. The HMO believed this had a negative effect on its enrollment. Other HMOs considered this an unfair advantage, and one threatened to sue the state.

States were able to attract MCOs and retain their participation. Despite states' limited experience with Medicaid managed care, they were able to contract with capitated managed care plans quickly. Each state included new MCOs, some formed by FQHCs, others by teaching hospitals. MCO operations appear to have been reasonably smooth in Hawaii and Rhode Island. Some MCOs in Tennessee were not fully developed at startup, however, because of the brief planning period, the lack of managed care experience, and the absence of a strong state licensing mechanism for MCOs.

All of the initial MCOs were still operating 12 months after startup (18 months in Tennessee), but we are unable to predict their long-term viability at this point. While the Rhode Island MCOs did not provide details, they indicated losing money in the first year, though none was insolvent as a result. The state intended to change the MCOs' contracts in Year 2 to improve consumer access to services. Provider reimbursements for pregnancy care and delivery have already increased. In Tennessee, none of the MCOs reported making much money in the first year, and some reported losses. Eighteen months after startup, the state increased capitation rates by 9.5 percent rather than the 5 percent increase scheduled in the contracts. The MCO contracts were renewed after 18 months with stiffer penalties for failure to report accurate encounter data to the state and diverse additional requirements to provide ongoing managed care education. In contrast, all MCOs in Hawaii appeared to make money during the first year. The state renegotiated capitation rates after one year, reducing them slightly. As QUEST started its second year, the state also capped enrollment in the largest plan to ensure adequate enrollment in the other plans (so that the other plans would stay viable).

Provider payments relative to Medicaid varied across the three states. MCOs set provider payment methods and amounts, subject to the capitation payment rates the state paid. In Hawaii, payments appeared to be about the same as under Medicaid. In Rhode Island, payments to primary care physicians appeared to be higher, as intended. With the exception of primary care physicians in some plans, Tennessee providers reported lower payment rates than under Medicaid.

In Hawaii, program payment levels did not appear to change much from Medicaid rates. It was too early for hospitals to determine how QUEST had affected them, although there were no dramatic initial effects. Payments to hospitals by MCOs often included disproportionate-share hospital supplements.

RIte Care intended to improve primary care physician participation by increasing payment rates, and early signs are that it has been successful, although there were initial concerns about participation in parts of the state. Hospitals felt it was too early to assess RIte Care's impacts on their finances, but all 15 hospitals in the state were participating in it. After extended debate, the state decided that MCOs have to pay hospitals for emergency room screening (also an important issue in the other two states).

Tennessee providers' reports of low payments by MCOs are consistent with the deeply discounted capitation payment to MCOs. To assist providers in the transition to managed care, Tennessee provided supplemental provider payments during the first year. Nevertheless, cash flow worsened under TennCare (a small sample of hospitals reported that the days in net accounts receivable doubled under TennCare, compared to Medicaid). Major changes in the amounts providers are paid under TennCare have led to concerns about and actions to sustain the viability of some safety net providers. Most notably, the Regional Medical Center in Memphis ("The Med") received a special payment of $12 million in 1995 to assist its transition to managed care and to ensure continued access for vulnerable populations.

FQHCs lost cost-based reimbursement in these programs, which was a serious problem for them. As a result of FQHC pressure, Rhode Island pays a supplemental fee of $10 per member, per month, to FQHCs for each participant who selects that FQHC as a primary care site. The supplement was intended to assist FQHCs in the transition to managed care. Hawaii also provided a temporary FQHC supplement.

Providers had to adjust and experienced some administrative problems. All three demonstrations required new MCOs to develop healthcare provider networks rapidly. They also required providers to adapt their clinical and administrative practices as the Medicaid program changed from largely fee-for-service to managed care. All types of providers in all three states complained about the lack of managed care education for consumers, who did not understand their obligations to use primary care gatekeepers or conditions under which they should use emergency rooms.

Providers in all three states were critical of administrative problems (especially uncertainty about patient eligibility). In Hawaii and

Tennessee, primary care physicians spoke of difficulties in making referrals to specialists because of low specialist participation. Hawaii's physicians were also concerned about disruption of patient relationships when MCOs arbitrarily assigned patients to physicians regardless of their choices. These physicians lost a lot of old patients but gained many new ones. In Tennessee, providers complained of slow payments and frequent payment denials by MCOs. But, within 15 months of TennCare implementation, some facility-based providers had begun to use their market power to act on problems, such as lack of timely payment. All providers indicated that administrative problems with payments were at least as problematic as low payments.

In Rhode Island, participation in a commercial HMO contracting to serve RIte Care enrollees obligated physicians to take part in the demonstration. This requirement, known as mainstreaming, apparently caused few problems for physicians. In Tennessee, the same requirement in the Blue Cross provider network upset physicians considerably. Physician participation in QUEST was entirely voluntary.

Low-income consumers appeared satisfied with the demonstrations, although disabled and chronically ill consumers were less satisfied. In focus groups, disabled and chronically ill consumers appeared slightly less satisfied with the programs than low-income consumers, because of greater concerns about access to specialists and emergency care. (This may have been true under fee-for-service too.) The relatively low rates of plan switching (10 percent or less) during the first open enrollment period support these reports. Despite their overall satisfaction, consumers in all three states identified problems with the eligibility and enrollment processes (some had not understood initially that they were supposed to choose an MCO and a primary care physician, and some had delays in receiving care because of enrollment problems). RIte Care consumers were especially pleased with the greater choice of places to receive care than under Medicaid (some had transferred from clinics to private doctors) and the removal of the stigma associated with being on Medicaid. (However, some Rhode Island physicians were concerned that consumers switching from FQHCs to private practitioners might not receive all the support services they needed.) By contrast, Hawaii and Tennessee consumers complained about physician choice (in Hawaii, consumers objected to losing their previous doctors and dentists, even when the provider participated in the plan and was requested by the consumer). Tennessee consumers mentioned problems with prescription drug coverage and access to primary care physicians and dentists. RIte Care participants said that restrictions on emergency room access left them puzzled about what constituted a genuine emergency.

Tennessee and Hawaii had budget problems in the first year. Tennessee was unable to raise all of the budgeted state funds during the first year of TennCare and thus could not receive the maximum federal matching payment allowed. Because of these problems, the state closed enrollment in the program for the uninsured at the end of 1994 to everyone except people losing Medicaid eligibility and medically uninsurable people; enrollment had not reopened as of December 1996.

QUEST participation was 40 percent higher than initially planned, partly because of unexpected program popularity and partly because of a statewide recession, leading to serious budget problems. In 1995 and 1996, the state took increasingly stern measures to rein in costs by restricting eligibility and lowering capitation payments to MCOs.

In the first year, Rhode Island appeared to underspend its per member, per month, targets. It enrolled only 1,000 people in its expansion group, one-tenth of the expected number. The implications are still being worked out, but the underspending may be due to different demographic characteristics in the enrolled population than projected. It could also mean that capitation payments were set too low, as MCO representatives have claimed.

The state monitoring process for MCOs was still being developed. States are responsible for monitoring MCOs to ensure that they fulfill their contracts. Quality improvement monitoring was still in the developmental stage in Hawaii and Tennessee. These states concentrated on more basic operational problems during the first year than Rhode Island, which had well-developed state quality improvement standards. To monitor plan performance, the states need accurate encounter data (which are also required for the evaluation). Eighteen months after startup, none of the states had produced final encounter data for the first year, which limited their ability to monitor MCO performance during startup.

The states are modifying program administration and MCO requirements in response to problems. Because of implementation problems, states are modifying both program administration and MCO requirements, although they have retained basic program structures. In addition to restricting program eligibility, the division of Med-QUEST in Hawaii made two important administrative changes: It developed a special unit for expediting certification of pregnant women, and it arranged to station eligibility workers at FQHCs. By the end of the first year, Hawaii had greatly reduced the waiting time between application and enrollment. In Rhode Island, the state moved the Office of Managed Care into the Department of Human Services to facilitate RIte Care administration, and it took steps to expedite enrollment of newborns, which had been problematic. It also made or plans to make several operational changes in response to first-year experiences, including requiring MCOs to pay for an emergency room screening that determines whether a visit is an emergency. In early 1995, the new governor of Tennessee transferred the TennCare Bureau from the Health Department to the Department of Finance and Administration to reflect de facto reporting lines. He also added an assistant commissioner and supporting staff to the Department of Commerce and Insurance to strengthen oversight of TennCare MCOs. Eighteen months after TennCare began, the state made an unscheduled increase in the capitation rate, in response to criticisms that the rate was too low, and added terms to MCO contracts to improve encounter data reporting and ongoing managed care education.

Startup Lessons

A number of constituencies can learn from the startup of the Section 1115 demonstrations in Hawaii, Rhode Island, and Tennessee. These constituencies include the federal government, the participating states, other states that may be planning Section 1115 demonstrations, MCOs, providers, and consumers. The lessons below, drawn from startup experience, may help these constituencies understand their options and the most efficient ways of meeting their goals.

States can implement major changes in a short period. The three demonstration states implemented major changes in a year or less. These changes resulted from the combined efforts of state and federal agencies, MCOs, healthcare providers, and advocates. In varying degrees, each state provided health insurance to new groups that would otherwise have remained uninsured.

More time is needed for planning and implementation. In Tennessee, an array of problems resulted from rapid implementation. Both Hawaii and Rhode Island took about a year after approval to implement their programs and still encountered difficulties, albeit less severe ones than Tennessee's. Consumers are more confused when managed care enrollment occurs statewide all on one day (as in Hawaii and Tennessee). Although Rhode Island's rolling implementation schedule also had shortcomings, it did not tax staff capacity to the same extent.

States can expand Medicaid managed care rapidly, although it is too early to assess the implications for quality of care and MCOs' long-term financial stability. An initial evaluation question was whether existing MCOs would participate or whether new MCOs would be formed to participate, because these states had limited Medicaid managed care experience. None of the states had difficulty getting plans to participate, and some new MCOs were developed explicitly for the programs. Some of the new MCOs, such as those owned by federally qualified health centers and Medicaid-only plans, could not have been formed under standard federal rules (though they could operate for up to three years under Medicaid 1915(b) waivers). The MCOs that served the most patients used network-style managed care. They were eventually able to form both urban and rural networks, although access problems occurred initially in some areas and physician specialties (some of which continue). The longer planning periods in Hawaii and Rhode Island, and Rhode Island's strong state licensure requirements, appeared to ease the transition to managed care. The lack of managed care infrastructure in Tennessee seems to have created problems, suggesting that states need to review MCOs' readiness before startup and consider limiting their enrollment until they prove they can operate smoothly. It is too early to assess MCOs' quality of care or long-term financial stability.

States need more administrative resources during startup. In the short term, states may require more (and different) staff to implement managed care demonstrations than they do to manage fee-for-service Medicaid programs. All the states initially had staff shortages, especially in enrollment and consumer relations. States used consultants constructively to help design and manage program elements, such as managed care contracting and capitation rates, thus adding expertise that was not available internally. From the start, states need to develop automated data systems to track enrollment in MCOs. States may have underestimated the necessity for the types and amounts of resources needed to monitor MCOs. In states with little managed care experience, MCO startup problems can be serious and long-lasting. Rhode Island, which had the strongest managed care market and the most developed HMO licensure requirements, had far fewer initial MCO problems than Tennessee.

Procedures for enrolling pregnant women and newborns may need to be modified under managed care. All three states encountered snags in enrolling one or both of these groups in managed care, which threaten access to care. All states have improved the process by which newborns are assigned to the same MCO as the mother, and Hawaii added a unit to expedite certification of pregnant women.

Consumers need more education about managed care. Enrollees often did not understand their choices among MCOs or how managed care worked. Only Rhode Island made any serious attempts at patient education in the first year, but even there, providers felt that more ongoing education was needed. Unbiased enrollment counseling is critical when a program starts and word-of-mouth advice within the community is scant. At a minimum, states should have accurate directories of participating physicians available to help enrollees select MCOs. Ongoing education is needed to explain managed care practices, such as how to use primary care gatekeepers and when to use the emergency room.

Safety net providers may need special support. Experiences in Tennessee suggest that, if states want the safety net hospitals to continue to serve vulnerable populations, they may need to make special arrangements to help them in the transition to managed care. Experiences of some FQHCs in all three states indicate that their ability to continue to serve the remaining uninsured people may be compromised by lower payments, even when states make supplementary payments.

Budget problems may undermine expansions. Both Tennessee and Hawaii suffered unanticipated budget problems. Tennessee was unable to raise enough funds for the state share of the budget. It was forced to curtail enrollment of the uninsured after one year and to make a number of budget adjustments in the first and second years. Hawaii's participation level was much higher than expected, forcing program cutbacks in the second and third years.

Controversy can be resolved through increased communication. In all three states, startup was accompanied by controversy. Conditions appeared more stable and less controversial by the end of the first year (18 months in Tennessee). Key factors in the improvements were flexibility in solving problems and increased communication among the state, MCOs, healthcare providers, other stakeholders, and consumers.

Despite startup problems, these demonstrations survived political changes. These types of programs are not abandoned easily after startup. In all three states, new governors have been elected (two from the opposing party). They have made no move to dismantle the programs but have committed their support to them and, in some cases, have made important administrative improvements.

About the Study

Data for this report were collected from documents, focus groups, and interviews with key persons in each state. Interviews with state officials, staff of MCOs, providers, legislators, and advocacy organizations, as well as focus groups with consumers and physicians, took place during two one-week visits to each of the states in mid-1995. Documents were provided by HCFA, the states, MCOs, providers, and others.

CHAPTER

13

QUALITY ASSURANCE FOR MEDICAID MANAGED CARE

Suzanne Felt-Lisk and Robert St. Peter

THE QUALITY Assurance Reform Initiative (QARI) system, developed in 1991, is now the only model of a comprehensive, state-based system for ensuring and improving quality of care in Medicaid managed care. As Medicaid managed care enrollment continues to grow rapidly, the results of the three-state demonstration of the QARI system are particularly important, given the system's comprehensive nature in the context of limited federal and uneven state requirements related to quality of care. In this report, we summarize findings from the evaluation of the QARI demonstration and their implications for policy.

Federal regulations for Medicaid managed care, though more extensive than for fee-for-service Medicaid, simply require states to provide for an annual, external review of quality of care in health plans serving Medicaid beneficiaries, require such plans to have a quality-assurance program, and require states and these plans to have a process for addressing enrollee grievances.[1] Most states have additional requirements, either as part of the Medicaid program or as part of state licensure for health maintenance organizations (HMOs), though these requirements vary widely.[2] Given this regulatory context, along with accelerating growth in

From *Health Affairs* 16 (3): 248–252.

Medicaid managed care and isolated reports of abuses where oversight was lacking, the Health Care Financing Administration (HCFA) and others believed additional guidance was needed.

Working with the National Academy for State Health Policy, medical directors of health plans, states, and others, HCFA developed guidelines for the QARI system. Through a competitive process, three states—Minnesota, Ohio, and Washington—were selected to participate in a demonstration to test the guidelines. Here, we discuss the results of a three-and-one-half year evaluation of that demonstration. Mathematica Policy Research, Inc., conducted the evaluation under a grant from The Henry J. Kaiser Family Foundation.

The QARI system calls for health plans to have internal quality-assurance programs and for states to set, and monitor compliance with, standards for an acceptable program. QARI emphasizes quality measurement, continuous quality improvement, and involvement of health plans and Medicaid beneficiaries in quality oversight.[3]

The Demonstration and Evaluation

The three demonstration states implemented the QARI system in very different state environments. Washington's Medicaid managed care program was small before QARI, with 35,000 enrollees (6 percent of all beneficiaries) and almost no quality oversight process in place. Ohio and Minnesota were similar in having larger programs (159,000 and 97,000 enrollees, respectively) and existing quality-oversight processes, but they differed in that Minnesota's program was mandatory in the context of a mature commercial managed care market, whereas Ohio's program was mostly voluntary and operated in a less mature commercial market.[4]

In evaluating the QARI demonstration we found that QARI was feasible to implement, but it required several years and substantial resources. We also identified specific ways to refine QARI and to better support states' and plans' implementation of the system. This report summarizes findings for policymakers on how well QARI protects quality.[5] The evaluation findings are based largely on annual site visits to the three states in 1993, 1994, and 1995 and review of related documents. In addition, a diverse set of health plans (three plans in each state) was selected for in-depth case studies. The week-long annual site visits included interviews with state Medicaid program staff and management, staff in other state agencies with related responsibilities, health plan representatives, staff at the external review entity, and representatives of Medicaid beneficiaries.

Results

Substantial changes were made in each state over the course of the demonstration, both in state systems for quality oversight and improvement (Exhibit 1) and in health plans' quality-improvement programs. These changes resulted in a more cooperative, coordinated environment for quality improvement and a stronger voice for Medicaid beneficiaries; better quality-improvement programs in health plans; and better knowledge about health plans' performance on quality measures across several clinical areas of concern.

Coordination

The QARI demonstration contributed to a more coordinated and cooperative environment for states and plans to address quality-improvement issues. QARI did so by reinforcing the states' decisions to move from a more regulatory approach toward a partnership approach with health plans and by providing a reason for states and plans to meet and share information over an extended period. Although there were numerous glitches in this partnership process (for example, because of meetings led by state staff lacking strong facilitation skills), there were benefits too: State staff were better educated on the status of health plans' information systems and quality-improvement programs, and there was better communication between state staff and health plans about the usefulness and interpretation of quality measures and results of reviews.

We found that coordination was key for health plans concerned with the burden of multiple overlapping reviews and requests. The three states worked to coordinate their requests and reviews within their states and increased this focus as the demonstration progressed. One state coordinated its Medicaid agency's requests for information on quality during the health plan contracting process with other state contracting requirements. One state conducted an abbreviated "look-behind" review of a plan's quality-improvement program when the plan had recently been accredited by the National Committee for Quality Assurance (NCQA). Two of the states were planning to include some Health Plan Employer Data and Information Set (HEDIS) or Medicaid HEDIS quality indicators in the next round of reviews, rather than developing many new measures. The states were hoping to achieve more coordination of requests and reviews in the future. Turf issues and different perspectives among state agencies were barriers to more complete coordination during the demonstration period.

Exhibit 1 Overview of State System Changes under the Quality Assurance Reform Initiative (QARI)[a]

Framework	Standards for Plans' Internal Quality Programs	Focused Studies	External Review
Washington			
New unit created with six staff at end of demonstration Enrollee satisfaction survey conducted and complaint system redesigned Site visits conducted by state staff to monitor implementation of QARI Coordinated contracting process established between Medicaid and basic health plan agencies	Standards incorporated into contracting process, with recognition that new plans will not fully meet all standards immediately	Focused studies implemented and repeated Health plan input sought to help to shape next round of studies Follow-up on results is at discretion of health plans; we noted some responses[b]	Review organization made responsible for focused studies, including their design (except for one study)
Minnesota			
Number of state staff with responsibility for quality improvement increased to five Satisfaction survey conducted jointly with others; results widely disseminated Ongoing quality advisory committee in place	Requirements continue to follow the outline of QARI without its details Plans agreed to work toward implementing most of the QARI standards with accompanying detail	Focused studies implemented in collaboration with plans Plans required to explain their response to areas identified as weak	Review organization collaborated with state and plans
Ohio			
Notable shift in staff's view from regulatory oversight without outside involvement to quality improvement with input from health plans and others Deemed status policy prepared so that NCQA-accredited plans would not be subject to duplicate review	Standards incorporated into regulation but add little to prior regulations	Focused studies implemented in collaboration with plans Plans required to take corrective action where "key" items are identified as weak	Review organization revised and implemented studies designed by state and plans

Source: Mathematica Policy Research analysis of site visit interviews and documentation collected annually in 1993, 1994, and late 1995.

[a]Changes are noted relative to the year prior to beginning QARI; in some cases a state may have had a particular policy in the more distant past that was not considered if not implemented just prior to QARI.

[b]Since the demonstration period, Washington staffers have worked to tighten their approach to follow-up and have met with each plan to discuss how it will follow up on the study results.

Medicaid Enrollees

Medicaid managed care enrollees have a stronger voice in the states' systems than they did before QARI because of the implementation of beneficiary satisfaction surveys in all three states and an improved complaint system in one state. QARI also influenced HMOs to pay more attention to the experience of their Medicaid enrollees as a distinct population and encouraged plans to compare Medicaid-specific information with that of other enrollment groups. The demonstration supports the need for population-specific analysis, since measures such as immunization rates for the Medicaid population were substantially below those for the overall population in the plans we visited and statewide rates.

Quality-Improvement Programs

QARI succeeded in better aligning the quality-improvement programs of the Medicaid-serving plans with industry standards. Although plans with less sophisticated programs were generally not able to close the gap with commercial plans, their efforts to establish internal quality programs and comply with the QARI standards moved them in the right direction.

The QARI component calling for states to monitor health plans' compliance with standards for internal quality improvement fell seriously short of providing a comprehensive approach for evaluating such programs. States tended to rely on a checklist approach to documenting compliance with their standards but did little to assess overall effectiveness of the programs.

For example, two plans rated highly by a state's review differed substantially in their programs' ability to identify problems. Quality monitoring and improvement efforts in the plan with a relatively well-functioning program (Plan A) included participating in a monitoring system that provided monthly indicators on a wide variety of clinical measures by payer. Plan A had used these data to identify adverse events for asthma as a problem area and then contracted for intensive case management for asthma patients with a specialized firm. The plan also had identified the preterm birth rate for Medicaid enrollees as a problem and thus instituted an intensive prenatal education program that included nurse visits. In contrast, Plan B analyzed the characteristics of asthma patients by age group, counted the number of hysterectomies (thirty-four) and reviewed those charts for quality issues, and calculated the cesarean-section rate and the rate of C-section complications and reviewed those eight charts for quality problems. A plan physician suggested these focus areas.

Given these activities—which meet state requirements and QARI guidelines read narrowly—Plan B could not give a reasonable example of how its system had worked to identify problems and improve quality for its members. This and other similar examples led us to conclude that QARI standards on state monitoring should be revised—or reviewer guidelines developed—that would assist states in monitoring more effectively. For example, rather than emphasizing the number of quality studies that a plan conducted or a plan's compliance with each phrase of state requirements alone, the monitoring could focus on how its system as a whole has worked to (1) identify and assess areas needing improvement and then focus on areas deemed important for the plan's population, (2) address these areas, and (3) follow up to track improvement.

Health Plan Performance

Focused studies provided states with a useful but blunt tool for monitoring changes in the quality of care statewide and, when properly designed, among individual plans. A total of seventeen such studies were conducted during the demonstration and covered seven clinical areas of concern: immunizations, asthma, prenatal care, asthma-related diseases, diabetes, emergency care, and well-child screenings under the Early and Periodic Screening, Diagnosis, and Treatment (EPSDT) program. The states worked with health plans and external review organizations to design the studies, which included many specific performance indicators in addition to the relatively small number of indicators specified by QARI for pregnancy and immunization.[6]

All of the demonstration states now have baseline information on the quality of care delivered to Medicaid enrollees, which covers several clinical areas of concern for this population. Most of the statewide studies were successful in identifying areas that needed quality improvement and areas in which plans were performing well. This information prompted or reinforced support for new quality-improvement initiatives by health plans; if successfully implemented, the initiatives should result in higher-quality care.

The focused studies also highlighted Medicaid enrollees, an emphasis that otherwise would have been missing from many of the plans' ongoing quality-improvement projects. For plans with less sophisticated quality-assurance programs, their participation in the focused studies gave them some of the experience needed to begin to use this approach in quality-improvement initiatives that were unrelated to QARI. Perhaps most important, the sharing of information from these studies among plans and their providers created the potential to change providers' or clients' behavior, thus improving the quality of care. Assessing the effect of this information sharing, however, would require a longer time frame and additional data for analysis.

Study Limitations

During the demonstration period several important limitations of the focused studies reduced their potential to improve quality. These included (1) the absence of benchmarks or comparable data on fee-for-service enrollees; (2) the significant lag in reporting results from the studies, which diminished their usefulness to clinicians and plans; and (3) the sampling and design features of some of the studies, which limited the usefulness or the credibility of the resulting data. For example, results for a plan that were based on sample sizes of five or ten medical charts, as we found in some studies, do not support a state's request for a health plan to take corrective action.

Conclusion

Results from the evaluation generally support the conceptual framework of QARI as an effective system for monitoring and improving the quality of care for Medicaid managed care enrollees. However, delays and implementation problems weakened the demonstration's expected impact on quality. States may be able to avoid similar implementation problems by reviewing the lessons from the demonstration.[7] HCFA can assist states in integrating new quality initiatives into the QARI framework by updating and refining national QARI guidelines so that they better suggest effective monitoring techniques, incorporate HEDIS 3.0 measures, and encourage states to take advantage of the NCQA accreditation process. The demonstration experience also confirms the importance of planning and having adequate lead time for introducing Medicaid managed care.[8] Both states and plans found that it took several years and significant resources to develop quality-assurance and improvement systems where they previously did not exist.

QARI has enhanced the ability of state agencies and health plans to identify and address quality-improvement issues, motivating system changes in their infrastructure and operations. These changes have great potential to spur continued improvements in quality of care over time. The effects, however, were not equal among all participants. The demonstration most benefited the state with a less developed quality-assurance structure in place at the beginning of the demonstration. It also had a more positive effect on plans with less sophisticated quality-assurance programs or programs needing major revisions. Conversely, plans that applied for NCQA accreditation improved their programs substantially during the demonstration, but QARI contributed far less to these improvements than the accreditation process did.

Thus, QARI worked alongside a number of other initiatives that were prompted by private purchasers to enhance the quality of managed care. The development of HEDIS 3.0 performance measures and the increasing prevalence of NCQA accreditation among commercial plans should lessen the effort required to implement a QARI-type quality-improvement system, but they do not reduce the need for such a system. QARI's greatest promise within the Medicaid context is to encourage the development of quality-improvement systems in states and plans where they are as yet undeveloped. As such, QARI provides a useful protection for Medicaid managed care enrollees.

Acknowledgments

The views presented here are solely the authors' and do not necessarily reflect those of Mathematica Policy Research or The Henry J. Kaiser Family Foundation (KFF). Marsha Lillie-Blanton, formerly of KFF and now at the U. S. General Accounting Office, oversaw this project for KFF and provided valuable comments on the evaluation report on which this report is based. Marsha Gold of Mathematica designed the evaluation, directed it in the beginning, and provided valuable comments on an earlier version of this report.

Notes

1. *Social Security Act,* sec. 1902(a)(30)(C); and 42 CFR 434.53.
2. Physician Payment Review Commission, *Annual Report to Congress* (Washington: PPRC, 1995), 339–69.
3. Health Care Financing Administration, *A Health Care Quality Improvement System for Medicaid Managed Care: A Guide for States* (Washington: U.S. Department of Health and Human Services, July 1993).
4. HMO penetration for the privately insured population was 16 percent in Ohio and 33 percent in Minnesota in 1991. M. Gold and S. Felt, "Reconciling Practice and Theory: Challenges in Monitoring Medicaid Managed-Care Quality," *Health Care Financing Review* (Summer 1995): 85–105.
5. S. Felt-Lisk and R. St. Peter, *The Quality Assurance Reform Initiative (QARI) Demonstration for Medicaid Managed Care Final Evaluation Report, Volume I: Summary Report,* and *Volume II: Technical Report* (Washington: The Henry J. Kaiser Family Foundation, November 1996).
6. In the future, the states are planning to incorporate some HEDIS measures. However, HEDIS, unlike the QARI system, does not provide a framework or process for targeting areas of particular concern, analyzing the data that are collected, and following up on problem areas.
7. See *The Quality Assurance Reform Initiative (QARI) Demonstration for Medicaid Managed Care Final Evaluation Report.* Appendix E lists the lessons.
8. M. Gold, M. Sparer, and K. Chu, "Medicaid Managed Care: Lessons from Five States," *Health Affairs* (Fall 1996): 153–66.

CHAPTER

14

MEDICAID MANAGED CARE ENCOUNTER DATA: WHAT, WHY, AND WHERE NEXT?

Embry M. Howell

Introduction

Managed care is increasingly becoming a preferred administrative vehicle for States to control their Medicaid budgets and assure access to and coordination of services. Managed care now serves 23 percent of the Medicaid population. As reported by the Kaiser Commission on the Future of Medicaid (1995), enrollment in some form of managed care grew from 4.8 million Medicaid enrollees to 7.8 million in a single year—1993–94. This rapid growth is likely to continue with some of the larger States such as California and New York forecasting large expansions in 1996. Numerous States now have waivers from traditional Medicaid rules (known as 1115 or 1915b waivers) that allow for such expansion.

Most of the statewide waivers require enrollment in some form of capitated plan, rather than the primary-care case-management form of managed care. One consequence of the shift to capitation is that the FFS billing mechanism that has generated much of the administrative data used in policy planning and research no longer exists, at least not universally nor for all Medicaid services. States and HCFA have struggled with how best to replace FFS billing data with other comparable

From *Health Care Financing Review* 17 (4): 87–95. It is reprinted here without change.

information on Medicaid enrollees in capitated managed care plans. Both levels of government face the tradeoffs between their need for data to manage the program efficiently and assure that beneficiaries are well served, versus a desire to reduce the administrative burden on the plans which contract with the program.

Some recent studies have shown that the ability of plans to produce encounter data is often limited. For example, the Group Health Association of America (1994) found in its survey of 330 health maintenance organizations (HMOs) that a substantial proportion (more than 10 percent) did not currently have the ability to report patient characteristics or diagnosis for a hospital encounter and that data capabilities for reporting ambulatory encounters were even weaker. A Mathematica Policy Research study for the Physician Payment Review Commission (Gold et al., 1995) provides further insight on the reasons that data have been problematic in managed care. Problems arise most often when the data the plan collects are not automatically generated by the plan's payment system.

Though most HMOs that pay physicians on other than an FFS basis require encounter data, only a minority of plans with such requirements say that the required data are almost always submitted by providers. Clearly a plan cannot itself comply with a State's encounter data requirements if its providers do not send in encounter records. Another study of aggregate reporting showed similar problems, with some plans being unable to report aggregate measures of ambulatory care use because of the lack of such information in their administrative database (Aizer, Felt, and Nelson, 1996). Thus the structure of an encounter data system must include, at the most basic level, the provider, then the plan, then the State, and finally the Federal Government (should it choose to require Medicaid encounter data, which—to date—it only requires of some 1115 waiver States).

This article provides an overview of the types of encounter data currently being required of plans, and the problems and issues with providing and analyzing such data. It is based on information provided by HCFA and nine of the States which have had some of the earliest experience with obtaining encounter data as a substitute for FFS billing data. These States are Arizona, California, Hawaii, Maryland, Minnesota, New York, Rhode Island, Tennessee, and Washington. From them, we reviewed documentation of State data requirements, and we spoke with individuals about their experiences during the past few years as they struggled to implement useful reporting systems (Table 1). We also spoke with individuals in States (e.g., Massachusetts) which have chosen to require aggregate reports from plans as an alternative to encounter data.

Table 1 State Encounter Data Contacts

State	Agency	Title
Arizona	Arizona Health Care Cost Containment System	Operations Manager
California	Department of Health and Human Services	Chief of Medical Care Statistics
Hawaii	Department of Health	Director of Encounter Data System
Maryland	Department of Health and Mental Hygiene	Director, Policy and Health Statistics Administration
New York	Department of Health	Research Scientist, Managed Care Research Unit
Rhode Island	Health Department	Branch Chief, Health Statistics
Tennessee	TennCare Bureau	Director of Information Services and Director of Operations
Washington	Department of Social and Health Services	Data Specialist/Medical Assistance Administrator
Minnesota	Department of Human Services	Consultant

Source: Howell, E., Mathematica Policy Research, Inc., 1996.

Together these States had a little more than 50 percent of the Medicaid beneficiaries in managed care in June 1994 (Kaiser Commission on the Future of Medicaid, 1995). Some of the States have had a relatively long experience, dating back to the early 1980s, with developing reporting systems for Medicaid managed care enrollees.

Why Do HCFA and States Need Encounter Data?

Plans understandably have been skeptical of the need for vast volumes of data to be accumulated at the State or Federal level. Such skepticism has increased in States which have required encounter data but have not developed the management information systems and internal analytic expertise needed to analyze the data. There is a growing recognition, expressed by almost all the States with which we spoke, that only when data are used and used regularly will the effort to produce and submit data be worthwhile.

States have not often routinely used their encounter data in the past, because managed care has been a small part of the program in most States until now. Also, States that did collect data lacked a clear concept of how they planned to use them, and consequently lacked concrete plans for analysis and reporting. The precursor FFS billing data have often been used for reporting expenditures, a use that is not directly relevant for encounter data, because State expenditures for capitated plans are defined by premiums. (However, utilization variables such as hospitalizations can be used to create FFS proxy measures.)

We spoke with many individuals about the reasons they felt it was important or necessary to routinely collect encounter data. The data needs they expressed fell into the following categories:

- Accountability: utilization, access, and quality analysis.
- Ratesetting and risk adjustment.
- Studies of small, high-policy-interest populations.
- Community-wide studies.
- Other research and evaluation studies.

Developing broad utilization, access, and quality measures is the most common use of encounter data. Under capitation, plans are held accountable by the State for providing or arranging all medically necessary care funded by the benefit package for a defined population. State and Federal governments need to assure that patients are getting the care that they need. Though oversight of this issue occurs in a variety of ways (e.g., external reviews, onsite inspection, consumer complaints and grievances), administrative data are a useful tool for broad tracking and profiling to identify potential problem areas. These measures include, for example, rates of the use of preventive services, hospitalization (including readmissions), and selected surgical procedures.

Many of these measures are included in State aggregate reporting requirements and form the basis for some sections of the Medicaid Health Plan Employer Data and Information Set (HEDIS), which specifies a variety of aggregate reports that States might require plans to submit (National Committee for Quality Assurance, 1995). Critics of required encounter data reporting point out that many such utilization-access-quality measures can be obtained from aggregate reports. Also, many States and plans have found that administrative data lack some of the clinical detail needed for oversight, thus making medical record review and surveys necessary. Thus, States and HCFA must make a compelling case regarding why they need encounter data to develop such measures.

Often this case is based on the Federal and State need for more flexibility than is provided by routine aggregate reports. Although a certain format may be useful at the time when a report is developed, it is likely that another format may be desired subsequently. For example, mental health services for young adolescents may become an important policy topic, whereas the age breakdowns for aggregate reports may group individuals 10–19 years of age. Plans should consider that it may be in their long-run interest to provide encounter data, rather than to repeatedly respond to modifications in State or Federal aggregate reporting requirements.

FFS billing data have long been used for ratesetting or for developing risk adjustors to rates. In the past, States have developed capitation rates by a relatively simple approach of developing age-sex-eligibility group cells and averaging Medicaid FFS expenditures within each cell. An alternative is to accept bids from plans for specific categories of enrollees. Regardless of the method, there can be problems if plans with enrollees that are in poorer-than-average health either choose not to participate or suffer large losses under Medicaid managed care. Plans whose networks are made up primarily of traditional safety net providers to the Medicaid population (such as affiliations of community clinics or public hospitals) may be particularly vulnerable. Thus it is to the advantage of both the States and the plans to have the fairest rate possible.

Although the state-of-the-art for developing risk-adjusted rates is still developing, there are many research projects underway to refine such approaches. Some of the most promising, such as Ambulatory Care Groups, are based on using FFS billing or encounter data to adjust payments by the diagnostic mix of a plan's panel of patients (Physician Payment Review Commission, 1995). States which have almost all enrollees in capitated plans lose the ability to test and ultimately use such approaches unless they require encounter data.

Another way to reimburse plans separately for high-cost outliers is through reinsurance, which is a retrospective approach that may accomplish a similar purpose to prospective risk adjustment. A plan that enrolls a high-risk Medicaid population might be allowed to retrospectively receive increased reimbursement for its high-cost population. Detailed encounter data will facilitate a State's ability to use reinsurance, because the State would not otherwise have sufficient information on the distribution of utilization of certain high-cost services (e.g., hospitalizations) in order to evaluate plans' claims.

Related to this outlier issue is a more general need to frequently study small, high-policy-interest populations. A small percentage of Medicaid beneficiaries account for a large share of costs. These individuals, who tend to be sicker and more vulnerable, are the most likely to be affected by the health system, both positively and negatively. However, because of their small numbers, it may be hard to detect problems for these individuals from aggregate data only. More detailed encounter data may be important in allowing States to fulfill their fiduciary and oversight role for these populations. The experience of HCFA and the States with FFS billing data is illustrative of this need. Early in the Medicaid program, simple aggregate reports were frequently sufficient for both HCFA and the States' needs. Surveillance and Utilization Review Subsystem (SURS) and Management Analysis and Reporting Subsystem (MARS) reports were required for certification of the State's Medicaid Management Information System and were often used by the States for internal reporting. A uniform report from the States to HCFA, the HCFA-2082 report, served many of HCFA's management needs. However, as the program grew and as certain high-cost populations became of greater interest (examples include persons with acquired immunodeficiency syndrome, pregnant women, and the mental health and substance abuse population), these reports no longer sufficed to answer questions from State or Federal legislatures or other policymakers. State and Federal analysts then began using the detailed person-level data derived from FFS billing to answer questions regarding use of services and expenditures for such groups. The detailed data were needed in order to refine analyses based on specific diagnoses or specific services.

Another related issue that requires encounter data is the frequent need to assess the health of whole communities or other geographic areas. A State might want to compare utilization of all Medicaid enrollees in a county or ZIP Code, or for all services provided within a given geographic area. The analysis might identify geographically based access problems in order to help the States and HCFA decide whether certain hospital or health plan services are essential to a particular geographic area. To do such a study, the analyst would need the encounter data for all individuals who lived in an area (or who provided services in an area), based on patient or provider address. Aggregate reports from plans would not generally be sufficient. Studying Medicaid enrollees' care at the community level may also facilitate cooperative identification of areas for improvement across plans. Problems that cut across health plans may be best addressed through such cooperative efforts.

Although not all-encompassing, the prior examples are illustrations of the many ways in which States, HCFA, and other policy analysts could typically use encounter data. However, such data will only be useful if they are relatively complete and an accurate representation of the care plans are providing.

What Is an Encounter?

Some of the struggle to develop successful Medicaid managed care reporting systems has to do with the lack of agreement about what is the proper "unit of analysis" for reporting. When the unit of analysis is the plan, States might request aggregate reports on all of the Medicaid enrollees a plan served in a particular reporting period. Almost all States require some type of aggregate reports either on a monthly, quarterly, or annual basis.

Another possible unit of analysis is the individual enrollee. This form of analysis is particularly attractive because managed care aims to promote accountability for care to defined populations. Plans could be requested to report aggregate counts of services or other summary data on each Medicaid enrollee in the plan on a monthly or annual basis. We did not find any States that are requiring this type of reporting, although States potentially can construct such records from encounter data.

Finally, and most commonly, States may require records for each encounter, or a subset of encounters. We found somewhat varying, but generally similar, definitions for an encounter. One person gave the following definition: "An encounter is a bundle of services provided to one client by one provider in one time period." Using this definition, if an individual patient went to two different providers in a day, they would have two encounter records. Such definitions can become difficult to operationalize when, for example, a provider is actually a hospital outpatient department with multiple clinics or a multi-specialty group practice. In such circumstances, the number of encounter records will probably depend on how the State enrolls providers and assigns unique provider identifiers. Other areas that can lead to variations include, for example, such non-ambulatory services as hospital and nursing home care. We found that most States include such services and define a separate bundle of services (e.g.; the hospital stay) as an encounter. Also, very often pharmacy services are included with an individual prescription being called an encounter. In all cases which we examined, the definitions of encounters, as operationalized in the States' data requirements, approximate closely the unit of analysis for their preexisting Medicaid FFS billing system.

What Variables Are Collected on Each Encounter?

There has been a period of evolution at both HCFA and in each of the States regarding the list of variables and other reporting specifications for their encounter data, and much of the experience is very recent. One State described a period early in their attempts to obtain encounter data in which they simply asked plans to submit data "within the parameters of our computer system." Similarly, HCFA in its original terms and conditions of approval of statewide managed care 1115 waivers has required that encounter data be collected, but has not specified the content or definition of variables. Not surprisingly, plans have often had extreme difficulty complying with such unspecified requirements. States with more experience have now learned that very precise definitions of files—including lists of variables and variable definitions—and precise submission specifications are needed. Also, they have learned that plans need ongoing training and technical assistance, especially early in the development of the system. Finally, there needs to be intensive, ongoing editing of the data as they come in, and feedback to the plans on the quality of the data. Many States define and circulate the edit specifications, along with the error tolerances for each variable.

Working mostly independently of each other, HCFA, and other payers, each State with which we spoke had developed a variable list for what is to be included in its encounter data set. During the same recent period, 1993–95, a parallel effort was underway at HCFA to define a uniform encounter data set (known as McData) for both the Medicare and Medicaid programs. The draft McData variable list was sent on September 17, 1995, to 1,000 individuals and organizations for review and comments. HCFA received about 200 responses. About 40 percent of these responses were from plans. They expect the final data set will be substantially similar to the draft version. In a survey sent out with the specifications, HCFA found that 93 percent of the 200 respondents felt that it was appropriate to have a national standard encounter data set.

In addition to the standardization that will probably result from the McData effort, several States and HCFA have built on the efforts of the National Uniform Claim Form Committee, which developed the HCFA-1500 billing form for ambulatory services, and the National Uniform Billing Committee, which developed the UB92 hospital billing form, as well as the American National Standards Institute (ANSI), which has developed standards for electronic submission of the HCFA-1500 and UB92 forms. Indeed, the push for standardization is a major impetus for the HCFA McData effort.

Table 2 shows the draft McData encounter data set and some other examples of variables that occur on State encounter data sets. It shows that most of the McData variables are required by almost all of the nine States.

The variables in this typical encounter data set include the identity, and sometimes other characteristics, of the individual receiving the care (i.e., the Medicaid enrollee) and the individual or institution providing the care. The reason that the characteristics of enrollees or providers are not always required is that some States plan to obtain those characteristics from their enrollment or provider reference files. (This could be more difficult at the Federal level, because HCFA might not have ready access to those files, which are often complex in structure and less uniform across States. States could also have difficulty matching to the reference files if identifiers submitted by plans have errors.) The encounter data set also includes selected information about the service provided including the date or dates of service, the procedure code, which tells which service was provided, and the diagnosis or diagnoses, describing the condition that required the care. Different types of services (for example, hospital, outpatient, pharmacy and dentistry) will require somewhat different variables, and often the States use different file formats for different types of encounter records.

Some States have very rigorous edits that are applied to data as it comes in. Examples include edits to assure that all codes are valid, that numeric data are present where required, and that dates are in logical sequence. States generally specify submission schedules and tolerances which may vary for different categories of variables (e.g., 95 percent of primary diagnoses should be present and within valid range).

Enforcing Encounter Data Collection

States report both carrots and sticks that may or may not be included in plan contracts to enforce the submission of complete and accurate

Table 2 Encounter Data Requirements by State

Item	Arizona	California	Hawaii	Maryland	Minnesota	New York	Rhode Island	Tennessee	Washington	Number of States
McData Variables										
Enrollee ID Number	X	X	X	X	X	X	X	X	X	9
Enrollee Name*	—	X	—	X	—	—	X	X	X	5
Plan ID	X	X	X	X	X	X	X	X	X	9
Provider ID	X	X	X	X	X	X	X	X	X	9
Provider Location*	X	X	X	—	—	—	—	—	—	3
Place of Service	X	X	X	X	X	—	X	—	X	7
Specialty/Provider Type*	—	X	—	X	—	X	X	X	—	5
Date of Service	X	X	X	X	X	X	X	X	X	9
Diagnoses	Ambulatory: 1 Hospital: 2	3	Ambulatory: 1 Hospital: 9	2	Ambulatory: 1 Hospital: 9	Ambulatory: 4 Hospital: 1	Ambulatory: 7 Hospital: 11	9	1	9
Procedure Codes	X	X	X	X	X	X	X	X	X	9
EPSDT Indicator	X	—	—	X	X	X	—	—	X	5
Patient Status	X	X	X	X	X	X	X	X	—	8
Revenue Codes	X	X	—	—	X	—	X	X	X	6
National Drug Code	Long-Term Care Plans	X	X	X	X	X	Aggregate Data	X	X	7
Dental Quadrant/ Tooth Number	—	X	X	X	—	X	—	—	—	4
Other Examples of Required Variables										
Birthdate*	—	X	X	—	—	—	—	X	X	4
Sex*	—	X	X	—	—	—	—	X	—	3
Quantity	X	X	X	X	X	X	X	—	—	7
Days Supply	—	X	—	X	X	X	—	—	—	4
Admission Type	X	—	X	X	X	—	—	X	—	5
DRG	—	—	—	X	—	X	X	—	X	4
Family Planning Indicator	—	X	—	—	X	X	—	—	—	3
Newborn Birthweight	—	—	—	—	—	—	X	—	X	2

Source: Howell, E., Mathematica Policy Research, Inc., 1996.
Notes: ID is identification. EPSDT is early and periodic screening, diagnosis, and testing. DRG is diagnosis-related group.
*Fields could be derived from enrollment or provider files.

data. There may be financial penalties for late submission (e.g., a percent reduction in the capitation fee). Alternatively, timely submittors of valid data may be allowed to expand Medicaid enrollment more rapidly.

Most States and HCFA report substantial ambivalence about how tough such enforcement should be, because they are anxious to have plans participate in managed care and recognize that the data requirements are burdensome. As mentioned, many plans do not yet have well-developed internal systems that can generate encounter data completely and consistently. Also, Medicaid often is only one of a number of diverse parties making data requirements of a plan. If reporting requirements are poorly conceived, the State could drive away the plans that it most wishes to attract (e.g., those with substantial commercial populations). Consequently, there may be interagency conflicts within State or Federal government, with data and research officials being strongly in favor of encounter data, and managed care program officials being more sympathetic to plan difficulties. Although most States recognize that their clout in requiring data has increased considerably over earlier years when Medicaid HMO enrollments were lower, most States remain in a cooperative, rather than combative, mode and hope that this cooperative approach will lead to better data over time.

It is important to note that encounter data systems are still in a developmental stage in all the States we talked to, with the exception of Arizona, which has been working on their system for a decade. Although some other States have a long history of contracting with HMOs (e.g., California, Minnesota, and New York), their major expansions into Medicaid managed care have only recently forced them into serious development of their encounter data systems.

The lack of internal staff capacity is one major impediment to development of an operational encounter data system. All of the steps previously outlined (e.g., developing specifications, providing technical assistance to plans, editing the data, providing feedback, and using the data) are time consuming and require staff and resources that many financially strapped States do not currently have. States are particularly challenged now since most will—at least in the short term—need to continue to maintain the administrative structure for FFS billing. HCFA has provided some help through the recent development of a technical assistance document to States (McCall, 1995). There is also a technical assistance contract to assist 1115 waiver States with the development of their encounter data. However, this type of assistance is late to arrive, is limited in scope, and will not be sufficient. All levels of organizations involved in the effort to develop workable encounter data—providers, the plans, the States, and HCFA—will need to obtain (either directly or through contract or both) the expertise to develop such systems.

Pitfalls in Collecting and Analyzing Encounter Data

In order to make the encounter data that many plans and States will be struggling to provide and analyze most useful, it is important to consider some of the lessons learned from experience with such efforts with FFS billing data, and from recent experience with encounter data. These include the following:

- Regular communication among providers, plans, States, and HCFA is essential. Feedback and discussion of results will assure that data problems are examined and resolved.
- States must have clear specifications for required data, and must not change those specifications very often.
- When data are received, States must carefully review and edit the data. In addition to range edits, they should examine frequency distributions and outliers. Edits used for FFS billing data may not be appropriate.
- Developing useful encounter data is a time-consuming, labor-intensive effort. Attempting to develop a system without the proper resources to do so at the plan, State, or Federal level will lead to questionable results. Putting resources into such efforts early will prevent problems later.
- Finally, even though the system appears to function smoothly, it is important to keep examining and refining the data as they come in.

These lessons apply to all levels of an encounter data system. A plan must follow such steps as it relates to its providers. Similarly, a State needs to address the same issues in relating to participating plans. And finally HCFA, to the extent that it receives data from States on a mandatory or voluntary basis, will need to develop a similar approach to data cleaning and analysis.

Acknowledgments

I appreciate the assistance of Rick Friedman at HCFA and of representatives from the States cited in the article. Several reviewers at Mathematica Policy Research also provided very helpful comments.

References

Aizer, A., Felt, S., and Nelson, L.: *Experience in Collecting Selected HEDIS 2.0 Measures for the Medicaid Population.* Henry J. Kaiser Family Foundation. Washington, DC. May 1996.

Gold, M., Hurley, R., Lake, T., et al.: A National Survey of the Arrangements Managed Care Plans Make with Physicians: Results from a 1994 Survey of Managed Care Plans. *New England Journal of Medicine* 333: 1678–1683, December 21, 1995.

Group Health Association of America: *HMO Industry Profile.* Washington, DC. November 1994.

Kaiser Commission on the Future of Medicaid: *Medicaid and Managed Care.* Washington, DC. June 1995.

McCall, N.: Collection and Use of Encounter Data in a Capitated Managed Care Program. In Horvath, J., and Kaye, N., eds.: *Medicaid Managed Care: A Guide for States.* Portland, ME. National Academy for State Health Policy, 1995.

National Committee for Quality Assurance: *Medicaid HEDIS.* Washington, DC. December 1995.

Physician Payment Review Commission: *Annual Report to Congress,* 1995. Washington, DC. 1995.

PART

4

CROSS-CUTTING ISSUES EMERGING FOR PUBLIC POLICY AND RESEARCH

Introduction: Anticipating the Future and Asking the Right Questions

Managed care, once considered an "alternative delivery system," is rapidly dominating acute medical care in this country. As a result, distinguishing issues related to managed care from those related to the healthcare system as a whole is becoming increasingly difficult. The implications of this change are potentially profound, and we are still struggling to define and understand them.

The final part of this book addresses some of the broader issues raised by the changing role of managed care in our health system. The first article, "Association Leaders Speak Out on Health System Change," describes how the changes in the healthcare system were viewed nationally by health association leaders in late 1995 to early 1996. Virtually all believed that major system change was inevitable, bringing with it a transition to new market dynamics and new structures for financing and organizing healthcare that could fundamentally alter the way the healthcare system functions. While the transition to managed care is not the only change under way, it is a major one that has come to symbolize other broader shifts in the healthcare market. The scope of these dynamics and the pressures they could create are illustrated in the next article, "Effects of the Growth of Managed Care on Academic Medical Centers and Graduate Medical Education." Based on case studies of the San Diego, Minneapolis, and Washington, D.C., markets, the article focuses on understanding how managed care changes the financing available to and demands on the academic medical centers that train our nation's health work force.

The next two articles address questions related to designing the information infrastructure for the healthcare system of the future, which is becoming increasingly important as the healthcare system changes with the growth of managed care and related trends. In "Shifting the Paradigm: Monitoring Access in Medicare Managed Care," the authors consider changes in the way access occurs in managed care and how this influences the way it needs to be conceptualized. They also look at what the shift to managed care implies for measures and data sources needed to monitor access. Although focused on Medicare, the analysis is broadly applicable to the general population. Similar issues are considered from a somewhat different perspective in "Surveying Consumer Satisfaction to Assess Managed-Care Quality: Current Practices." This article synthesizes existing work to develop survey-based measures of consumer satisfaction as a quality measure of managed care plans' performance. As summarized in the article's postscript, work in this area continues to have high priority, with initiatives being launched in both the public and private sectors.

The final article in the book, "The Design of the Community Tracking Study," summarizes one important current effort to monitor and assess health system change. Though not focused exclusively on managed care, this nationally representative study, with funding from The Robert Wood Johnson Foundation, provides an important opportunity to gain insights into what the shift to managed care as well as other trends mean for the healthcare system and those served by it. Studies like this and others under way are critical: A consistent theme that emerges in virtually all studies covered in this anthology is that the ramifications of current marketplace change are far-reaching. The existing research can inform, but it also illustrates how many more questions remain and how hard it will be to answer them.

References

Moon, M. 1996. *Medicare Now and in the Future*, 2nd ed. Washington, DC: Urban Institute Press.

Rowland, D., J. Feder, B. Lyons, and A. Salganicoff. 1992. *Medicaid at the Crossroads*. Baltimore, MD: Kaiser Commission on the Future of Medicaid.

CHAPTER

15

ASSOCIATION LEADERS SPEAK OUT ON HEALTH SYSTEM CHANGE

Janet M. Corrigan and Paul B. Ginsburg

TO MOST observers the recent pace of U.S. health system change is staggering, despite differences across communities in the paths and speed of change and differences in the impact of change on various health care constituencies.[1] As part of its effort to monitor and analyze health system change, the Center for Studying Health System Change conducted interviews with leaders of fifteen national professional organizations and trade associations.[2] We selected these persons for two reasons: They have broad exposure to both national and regional developments in the health care industry; and they are well positioned to provide in-depth knowledge of the ways in which their constituencies are being affected by and responding to health system change.

In this paper we first discuss the prevailing attitudes of association leaders toward the changes under way in the health care system and the efforts of various constituencies to influence or adapt to change. We then discuss problem areas that will likely place pressure on the health care system and the divergent views expressed by the respondents regarding the long-term direction and impact of health system change.

From *Health Affairs* 16 (1): 150–157. It is reprinted here without change.

The Process of Change: Common Themes

Virtually all of the leaders we interviewed recognized that major health system change was inevitable, and most believed that it was long overdue. They viewed large private purchasers as having played a particularly important role in igniting many changes through their efforts to slow the rate of increase in health care premiums. But some of these leaders pointed to fundamental changes in medical practice and technology, such as the burgeoning medical knowledge base and increasingly sophisticated clinical information systems, as important forces in precipitating and shaping change over the long run.

Most emphasized that the health care system is in transition. Some viewed the coming few years as a period of experimentation with new market dynamics and new financing and organizational structures. Many also were mindful of the geographic diversity of health system change and believed that one should not assume that local markets will reach some common destination.

Nearly all of the leaders saw both positive and negative aspects of change. Many noted the progress being made in "cutting fat out of the system." Although they all recognized the potential to build better systems to coordinate and manage care and to support clinical decision making, some viewed the glass as half empty (not much has happened yet) and others as half full (progress is being made).

On the other hand, the interviewees expressed concern that the rapid and chaotic pace of change has created a situation that is easy to exploit. Several cited the "siphoning off of dollars" by investor-owned organizations and said they expected that these organizations will leave health care "when they can no longer make money except through the denial of needed care."

The association leaders were mindful that the current changes in the health care industry will not resolve, and may even exacerbate, certain fundamental problems—most notably, the growing number of uninsured persons and the lack of adequate support for public health services. Others noted that current changes are likely to give rise to new problems, such as erosion of the "foundation of medical practice" (doctor/patient relationships, professional collegiality, and ethics) and a general loss of consumer confidence. There was a sense that changes have been driven by purchasers and that, for the most part, consumers have yet to feel any impact.[3]

Despite their uncertainty about the future and concern about potential crises, the majority supported letting the dynamics of the competitive marketplace operate. This stemmed in part from the conclusion that recent attempts to establish federal policy were an abysmal failure and that near-term future efforts were unlikely to be more successful.

Impact on Constituencies

There was little agreement among the leaders we interviewed as to the impact of health system change on various constituencies and even less about the roles that constituencies will assume in response to change. We provide a sample of the views.

Private Purchasers

Although virtually all of the respondents credited private purchasers with pushing change forward, they mostly were referring to a relatively small but influential subset of employers: national Fortune 500 companies. These large employers wield much purchasing power and have shown their willingness to switch plans in their quest for more "value for the dollar." Small and medium-size employers, which generally serve local markets, have been less active but are becoming increasingly organized within local business coalitions, many of which have sizable purchasing power.

There is much geographic variation in the influence, preferences, and demands of employers, in part because of the distribution of national/regional versus local employer groups. The former were described as seeking standardization of health benefits across sites, economies of scale in health benefits administration, and maximum leveraging of purchasing power by negotiating with large national insurers and health plans that serve all or most of the communities in which their employees reside. Local coalitions embrace a somewhat different model that seeks to bring together all purchasers in a community, both public and private, and that emphasizes community-based health improvement initiatives.

The leaders held divergent views on employers' role in promoting quality. Some expressed frustration that despite repeated attempts, employers still are unable to obtain comparative data on health plan performance for a particular set of conditions and outcomes. Others questioned the depth of employers' commitment to quality, noting that surveys and focus groups have found that employers look at information on quality "only if the price [plan premium] is right." In the words of one respondent, the "rhetoric does not match the behavior," and as a result, "there is a lot of dissonance between health plans and employers."

Insurers and Health Plans

Among association leaders, there was much enthusiasm about the potential value of managed care. As one of them observed, "Managing health care is the great American contribution to health care worldwide. Properly conceived, it is a big improvement." Most of the leaders recognized that a lot of work needs to be done to achieve this potential. According to one of the respondents, "most plans are still at the stage of trying to eliminate hospitalizations."

Some of the leaders referred to the "new market dynamics" that are encouraging investment in infrastructure, especially automated information systems. As managed care market share has increased in some communities, there is "less opportunity to make money from churning [engaging in practices that encourage very sick enrollees to disenroll from a managed care plan], so emphasis has shifted to retaining enrollees as long as possible and keeping them well." In addition, employers' demands for outcomes data require much more sophisticated information systems.

There was general recognition among our participants of the importance of providing consumers with a choice of products (health maintenance organizations [HMOs], preferred provider organizations [PPOs], point-of-service plans, and conventional insurance), which in turn afford consumers some choice of physicians. Employers' and consumers' demands for choice have encouraged many plans to develop three options—HMO, PPO, and point-of-service products. Most of the respondents see these three products as permanent offerings, although some anticipate a leveling off in the growth of PPOs. In the words of one respondent, you can "only squeeze so much out of discounted payment." Another noted that the issue of choice of physicians may be "overblown," since even "under indemnity most people just go to the specialist they are referred to by their primary care provider."

Many leaders pointed out the challenge that the managed care industry faces in developing stable, productive relationships with physicians. Growing tension between these groups has sparked various responses. For example, some plans are trying to build bridges by bringing physicians into the "investor loop" as shareholders, in the hope of building commitment, loyalty, and common goals. Many group practices have tried to establish networks that are large enough and have the appropriate multispecialty mix to assume total financial risk and provide most or all of the care needed by enrollees.

Hospitals

The term *health system change* elicited comments about both the trend toward horizontal integration and downsizing of hospitals, which began in the 1970s, and the implications of marked growth in managed care, a more recent phenomenon. The respondents found it difficult to characterize the effects of change on the hospital industry as a whole, stressing that there is much diversity by region and type of hospital.

In their discussion of horizontal integration, many of the leaders cited the dramatic growth of Columbia/HCA and raised questions and concerns about the long-term implications of the corporation's activities. Columbia/HCA has engendered "enormous fear in the not-for-profit hospital world," according to one respondent. This fear stems in part from growing recognition that Columbia/HCA is a formidable competitor with access to capital and major economies of scale. There also is concern that Columbia/HCA will continue to acquire not-for-profit hospitals, especially now that it is developing a more hierarchical management structure that focuses on the operation of hospital networks rather than individual hospitals. If Columbia/HCA enters the insurance and managed care business, as many speculate it will, it may encourage use of Columbia/HCA hospitals through contracting arrangements and/or seek deeper and deeper discounts for services provided by non-Columbia/HCA hospitals.

Many of the leaders noted the efforts of some hospitals to assume a more central role in the provision of managed care products. A few spoke positively about experiments with various models of organized care delivery. Some of these models designate a primary care provider to serve in a coordinating role for a group of institutional and individual providers; other, more "virtual" models rely on automated information systems to serve as the "glue" for coordinated decision making among providers who practice in different community settings.

Other leaders were pessimistic about hospitals' chances of becoming more than "inpatient facilities," pointing out that hospitals are not viewed as desirable partners. They have very high fixed costs and, in the words of one respondent, represent "systems that no longer meet the needs of patients." Participants also noted that some health plans that have owned or operated hospitals are divesting themselves of these institutions, and physician groups that are seeking partners might look to physician management or information systems companies instead of hospitals.

Academic Medical Centers (AMCs)

More than any other constituency, AMCs were singled out as facing very difficult decisions pertaining to their core functions (education, research, and patient care). The increase in managed care, accompanied by more competitive markets, has made it difficult for AMCs to use patient revenues to cross-subsidize the education and research functions and to subsidize patient care for the uninsured. Some managed care arrangements have disrupted the flow of patients to AMCs, threatening the patient base required to carry out research and education. And, as noted by one respondent, the ongoing tightening of policies applicable to Medicare's direct and indirect medical education payments "seems to be making life even more difficult for AMCs, at a time when they are already under extreme pressure."

A closer relationship between managed care organizations and AMCs was seen as inevitable by many of the association leaders. However, some viewed recent acquisitions and partnership agreements as very promising, while others felt that such arrangements will raise fundamental questions concerning AMCs' mission and role. In the words of one interviewee, "There is no market interest in the teaching and research functions." Over the long run, as profit margins decline, AMCs owned by for-profit organizations are likely to confront more and more barriers to fulfilling their mission. Other leaders cited the need to explicitly recognize that the teaching and research functions performed by AMCs benefit society and that these "social goods" will succumb to market pressures unless ways are found to uncouple their support from patient care revenues.

Physician Groups and Other Providers

Most of the interviewees believed that the continued movement of physicians into group practice, especially multispeciality group practice, is inevitable. Larger group practices generally have greater resources to invest in building more sophisticated infrastructures, such as clinical information systems, and they benefit from economies of scale. Others point to growth in managed care as the factor that drives providers to seek group practice settings. "There is growing resentment of the intrusive aspects of many managed care arrangements," one participant noted, and this is driving physicians into larger group practices capable of directly assuming financial risk and internalizing functions such as credentialing and quality/utilization review. Still others noted that some of the recent mergers and acquisitions involving group practices probably result from physicians' "cashing out" on the assumption that their practice is worth more now than it will be in the future.

The leaders differed in their expectations of the long-term success of various health plan models. Some anticipated continued rapid growth in loosely structured products offered through individual practice associations (IPAs), noting that consumers seem to want a broad choice of providers. Others believed that multispecialty group practices are strategically positioned to develop the most successful managed care products. According to one interviewee, "The shift from buying on price to buying on quality is coming soon, and a unique product will be needed to succeed."

Some of the leaders observed that practice management companies are playing a growing role in health system change, especially in parts of the country where physicians practice in small groups. They bring sophisticated management and information systems, access to capital, and expertise in contracting with managed care plans. Although the benefits of physician management organizations and other entrepreneurial efforts were noted by several respondents, one leader stressed the importance of promoting "economically linked" practices that encourage physicians to "get in the boat and row with their oars in the same direction."

Most of the respondents believed that managed care and competition have had measurable effects on physician practice. Many cited the positive contributions of care management tools and techniques, such as practice guidelines and provider profiling, to "cutting fat out of the system" and reducing undesired variability in practice styles. However, some expressed concern that unless these processes are "internalized" in physician practice, they will fail to achieve their full potential and will produce negative side effects, such as resentment among physicians and "weakening of the bonds between doctors and patients." Another concern was the disruption of established patient referral patterns because of managed care organizations' physician credentialing and hospital contracting decisions.

The leaders also addressed the use of capitation payments (at the level of individual physicians or small groups) and other compensation systems that link remuneration to the use of fewer resources. One interviewee said, "Financial incentives to undertreat have far more serious ramifications for patients than the financial incentives to overtreat that are inherent in fee-for-service medicine." On the positive side, one leader noted that capitation payments often allow physicians and provider groups greater flexibility in treating patients and create fewer practice constraints. But there were serious doubts among many association leaders about whether capitation payments will survive the test of time.

The Pressure Points

Although each constituency represented by our group of leaders has its own set of concerns, the common concerns that surfaced in the interviews included the growing numbers of uninsured and underinsured persons; the inability of current financing and delivery models to adequately address the needs of the elderly and disabled; and erosion of public confidence in the system. A number of the association leaders viewed the current period as "the calm before the storm."

The Uninsured and Underinsured

Nearly all of the respondents cited the growing uninsured population as a problem that is likely to get worse before it gets better and that may become a crisis by the year 2000. Some voiced concern that this issue, more than any other, might precipitate large-scale public intervention. One leader, who was supportive of a competitive market approach, said, "We are very mindful that the uninsured issue can come back and bushwhack us politically at a later date."

Most of the respondents viewed government as responsible for helping those who do not have insurance, but they held very different views about how government should intervene. Suggestions included issuing vouchers to the uninsured to allow them to join private health plans; expanding Medicaid eligibility; encouraging the formation of purchasing alliances to reduce the cost of insurance to small groups and the size of the uninsured pool; and allowing those under age sixty-five to participate in Medicare at their own expense.

There was general recognition that system changes could have the unintended consequence of closing traditional doors of access for the uninsured. Although many anticipate that most safety-net providers (for example, community health centers and inner-city hospitals) will either sponsor or contract with existing managed care plans, competitive pressures will make it increasingly difficult for these providers to serve the uninsured through cross-subsidies from Medicaid, Medicare, or private-pay patients. Physicians and other providers are increasingly pressured to increase productivity under managed care and are less likely to devote a portion of their practice time to charity care.

The Elderly and Disabled

The leaders questioned the ability of managed care organizations to gear up to meet the needs of the elderly and disabled. Although managed care systems are effective in controlling Medicaid costs associated with Aid to Families with Dependent Children (AFDC) eligibility, the majority of Medicaid expenditures are for those with long-term disabilities, and few of these persons are enrolled in managed care. According to our participants, Medicare risk contracts have been limited in the number of health plans participating and the percentage of Medicare enrollees choosing managed care.

When asked to explain their concerns about moving the elderly and disabled populations into managed care, the leaders focused on two areas. First, methods of risk adjusting capitation payments to prepaid health plans are inadequate (in the words of one leader, "a huge problem"). Second, effective care management for these populations requires a complex system of multidisciplinary services coordinated over extended periods of time.

Erosion of Confidence

Less concrete than other concerns, but equally disconcerting to most of the interviewees, is the potential for erosion of public confidence in the health care system. There was strong sentiment expressed among these leaders that negative comments reported in the general press are contributing to heightened public concern about access to and quality of care. One respondent observed that "the negative accounts in the press about managed care are so pervasive, they almost appear to be orchestrated." Another referred to this problem as a "well-organized system of bashing."

Regarding potential effects of diminished public confidence, one leader said: "Horror stories lead to lots of state legislation, such as any-willing-provider and patient protection acts, and the long-term effects of these legislative efforts are unknown." Another commented that "the demonization of managed care may really slow down efforts that could be very beneficial to the patient community."

The Destination

There was far greater agreement among the leaders about the process of change and its near-term effects than there was about the likely destination of change. Association leaders have differing opinions about dominant players in the future organization and delivery of health care and about future roles for consumers and the public sector.

Dominant Players

Most of the leaders viewed "the pendulum" as having swung in a direction that favors the development of large national health care organizations. In discussing the future, most spoke of forces that will accommodate smaller-market players and will attenuate the growth of large companies. There was little support for the view that the nation would become a "Land of the Giants." Several forces were cited.

First, experience in other industries has demonstrated time and again that there are limits to scale. Said one interviewee, "Health care is going through the consolidation that other industries did in the seventies and eighties. But look at AT&T; it is now divesting and becoming a niche player."

Second, there are many successful local or niche players, and as one leader said, "Many communities like their local plans." Opportunities abound for smaller players to join with information systems companies, management service organizations, and other companies to gain access to capital and specialized expertise and achieve economies of scale.

Third, the increased organization of local physicians and hospitals into multispecialty groups, physician/hospital networks and organizations, and other entities capable of accepting financial risk and care delivery responsibilities is likely to impede the dominance of national firms.

Fourth, direct contracting by employers could strengthen the role of local, provider-sponsored plans because "both purchasers and physicians believe that health plans take too much money out of the system." Others viewed direct contracting as an experiment that is likely to fail, pointing out that direct contracting requires employers to take on some administrative responsibilities that plans now perform, precisely at a time when many employers are seeking to reduce their benefits administration burden and move away from micromanagement of health firms.

Fifth, there is a revitalization of the role of the community. "There is growing recognition that many issues just don't get addressed if you have health plans focusing only on their currently enrolled population and assuming that the average length of enrollment is two to three years," one leader said. Many national plans are getting more involved in local communities to attempt to serve them better.

In summary, some leaders anticipated that provider-sponsored plans will be the dominant players of the future. Most said they envision a health care industry characterized by much diversity, both across and within communities, and by health plans of "all stripes."

Consumers and the Public Sector

The leaders identified two forces that might affect the future direction and pace of change: consumers and the public sector. Although there was much uncertainty about the role that these groups will play, the leaders agreed that the health care system is embarking on a new "experiment"—a period in which consumers will have more information about health and the health care system and greater financial incentives to maximize use of this information. More information on healthy lifestyles, diseases and conditions, and health care treatments is reaching consumers through newspapers, radio, television, and the Internet. The availability of report cards on health plans, hospitals, and physicians is encouraging better-informed decision making. In addition, private purchasers are encouraging greater consumer responsibility for their health and health care use through greater cost sharing and participation in choosing a health plan.

Although most of the leaders viewed these new roles for consumers positively, they were skeptical about the likelihood of a significant impact on the health care system in the near term and uncertain about long-term effects as well. Several respondents spoke about the potential for consumers to play a more active role in the diagnosis and treatment of their conditions, and the prospect evoked mixed reactions. On the positive side, some of the leaders believed that greater consumer knowledge and participation in decisions should lead to better outcomes. One interviewee noted, "We are a long way from having informed consumers, and before we do, we will need a physician community that is willing to accept consumers as decisionmakers." On the negative side, more information in the hands of consumers may fuel the "litigious nature of society," and practice guidelines may increasingly be used to protect physicians from litigious patients. The increased availability of information means greater public access to both correct and incorrect information, and the latter can do great harm.

There were divergent views on the potential role that report cards might play in ensuring quality of care. At one end of the spectrum were one or two leaders who viewed comparable performance data as a replacement for ineffective regulatory and accreditation processes. At the other end were one or two who felt strongly that "more information for consumers won't mean less need for public-sector oversight and accountability."

The majority of interviewees were doubtful that report cards would play much of a role in ensuring accountability, at least in the short run. According to one, "Report cards are a great idea, but [I am] not sure you can get enough 'vote with your feet' that the health plans will get the message." Most of the respondents expressed frustration with current report card efforts. The two concerns cited most frequently were that the focus of most of these efforts is on hospitals and health plans, whereas consumers are interested in physicians; and that the types of performance measures selected to date are not measures of outcomes, but rather, measures of enrollee satisfaction and the medical care process.

Little consensus emerged about the likely future role of government. The leaders were pessimistic about fashioning an effective public-sector role to address the growing number of uninsured persons. In the words of one health system leader, "1993–1995 was a big setback in a public policy sense." Interest-group pressure on the current legislative process tends to result in legislation that "has something in it for everybody" but fails to embody a coherent policy strategy.

Concluding Thoughts

For nearly all health care care industry constituencies, the new marketplace precludes a "business-as usual" attitude, but there was strong sentiment among these leaders that there are many opportunities for those who are willing to assume new roles and responsibilities and, most importantly, who are open to new partnerships. Many respondents not only are assisting their constituencies in responding to change but also are leading their own organizations through major restructuring. About one-third of the leaders indicated that their organization or association had recently undergone or has been seriously considering major changes in its governance structure or membership composition.

Most of the association leaders perceived a rough road ahead for quite a few years. Although none of them expressed grave concern or alarm, there was broad recognition that the marketplace changes under way fail to address some fundamental issues—in particular, the growing uninsured population—and that the way in which these issues are resolved may greatly alter the course of change.

We found it sobering that this particular group of leaders, representing organizations that devote considerable attention to shaping federal policy, was keenly aware of the pivotal role that private-sector employers have played in health system change and that most attributed this role to the failure of public-sector reform initiatives. Many expressed concern about the possibility that future public policy directions at both the federal and state levels will diverge from the direction forged by current private-sector initiatives, which might produce a health care environment that is characterized by conflicting pressures and incentives.

Notes

1. See, for example, P. B. Ginsburg, "The RWJF Community Snapshots Study: Introductions and Overview," *Health Affairs* (Summer 1996): 7–20.
2. The interviews were conducted between October 1995 and February 1996. Each interview was conducted by a team of two or three researchers, who followed a core protocol, and added questions based on respondents' knowledge and responses to questions. The lead interviewer (Paul Ginsburg) was the same for all fifteen interviews, and a second researcher (Janet Corrigan) participated in thirteen interviews. Other researchers involved in the interviews were Peter Cunningham, Joy Grossman, Peter Kemper, and Linda Kohn of the Center for Studying Health System Change; Robert St. Peter of the center and Mathematica Policy Research; and Stephen Long and Susan Marquis of RAND.
3. These opinions are consistent with findings of a recent national consumer survey. J. R. Knickman et al., "Tracking Consumers' Reactions to the Changing Health Care System: Early Indicators," *Health Affairs* (Summer 1996): 21–48.

CHAPTER

16

EFFECTS OF THE GROWTH OF MANAGED CARE ON ACADEMIC MEDICAL CENTERS AND GRADUATE MEDICAL EDUCATION

Marsha R. Gold

IN THIS article, I present insights into how the proliferation of competitive health care financing and service delivery systems based on managed care affect the financial support available to academic medical centers (AMCs), especially to their programs in graduate medical education (GME). These insights are based largely on case studies and a review of the literature, conducted in mid-1994[1] and funded by the Public Health Service, that I carried out with the support of others at Mathematica Policy Research (MPR), an independent public policy research firm located in Washington, D.C.

We conducted the case studies in the health care markets of San Diego, California, Minneapolis–St. Paul, Minnesota, and Washington, D.C. While qualitative and inherently subjective, the findings of these studies are valuable sources of information and insight because they are timely and capture dimensions poorly reflected in the more formal available data, especially considering that health care markets everywhere are in a period of rapid change.

Specifically, our findings, which I discuss in detail later in this article, provide information related to four major questions:

1. Are managed care plans willing to pay a premium to AMCs in competitive markets?
2. To the extent that AMCs are more expensive than alternative providers because of their teaching responsibilities, how much of these expenses have traditionally been paid through patient care revenues of various third-party payers?
3. How are AMCs faring now, and to what extent have they been adversely affected by the growth of competitive systems?
4. How is the proliferation of competitive systems affecting graduate medical education?

Methods and Case-Study Sites

Study Challenges and How We Addressed Them

The issues of concern to this study are not easily addressed through existing research or extant national statistical systems. First, few systems are timely enough to capture changes in the health care system, which are rapidly occurring in the marketplace. Second, existing data systems are not typically comprehensive or detailed enough to incorporate analysis that accounts for the role of the variety of entities that make up AMCs and determine the financing of GME and the AMC as a whole. In particular, data systems are better at capturing information about the teaching hospital than at capturing the contributions of the faculty practice plan or other revenue sources (e.g., research, medical school) to AMCs and their training functions. Third, even if the systems were comprehensive, it would be hard to analyze training costs, since AMCs provide a complex set of joint products involving teaching, research, and patient care.

Academic medical centers vary considerably in their organizational and financial structures, but all have developed elaborate systems of cross-subsidies. This makes analysis difficult, as does the historical decentralization of decision-making power to the departmental level, at least within the medical school. In most cases (Medicare being a major exception), patient care is paid for with an aggregate sum that does not explicitly identify a share to support training. Even if it did, AMCs have considerable freedom to determine how revenues are used and economies achieved. Thus, the indirect medical education payments do not necessarily show the indirect costs of GME at hospitals and, conversely, a reduction in support for GME would not necessarily translate into reductions in training when alternatives for generating equivalent savings could be more appealing.

Given these challenges, we based our study around case studies of AMCs in three markets so that we could obtain timely information about the issues of concern. These case studies involved primary data collection based both on interviews conducted on-site and on the review of documents. For the most part, my reports of these cases reflect the situation in 1994, although I made selective updates for major changes that I am aware of. A context for these case studies was created with information derived from an initial review of the literature and existing data sources and from a recently completed national statistical analysis of these issues.[2]

Approach to the Case Studies

The degree of penetration of managed care and competitive systems varies from market to market across the country. We focused the case studies on markets most affected by trends related to managed care and thus most likely to provide insight about how other AMCs could be affected by the proliferation of competitive systems.

Two of the three markets are recognized leaders in managed care development: San Diego and Minneapolis–St. Paul. The third—Washington, D.C.—has a less developed but evolving managed care system, leading us to conclude that the market might provide an instructive point of comparison. Because it is located in the nation's capital, we sense that its institutions would be more familiar to federal policymakers and legislators, possibly making our findings more meaningful to them. In addition, we had contacts in all three markets who would facilitate the process of arranging interviews. This was particularly crucial, since we needed access to a broad range of relatively senior individuals to discuss potentially sensitive issues. We also had a very constrained time frame in which to work, since the interviews had to be arranged and conducted over only two to three months during the summer. (The Office of the Assistant Secretary of Health at the U.S. Department of Health and Human Services wished to be able to use the study to address issues pending in health reform, potentially to be considered during that legislative session.)

Each site visit lasted from three to four days. The types of organizations included in the cases varied in the different markets, reflecting each market's unique features. In all cases, our objective—which we succeeded in meeting—was to interview the leaders and key staff at the AMC(s) (including the teaching hospital, faculty practice plan, and medical school), at least one potentially competing hospital or health system with a large tertiary care base, and two or more managed care plans in the market. This approach, along with the use of common questions and attention to the same issues, allowed conclusions to be cross-validated and to be made based on the inputs of several alternative perspectives. The same individual, an experienced senior health policy researcher on the MPR staff, made all of the three site visits.

The Three Case-Study Markets

The three markets we studied—San Diego, Minneapolis–St. Paul, and Washington, D.C.—are all heavily influenced by managed care. San Diego comes closest to the classic market, with the rapid evolution of competitive systems largely driven by the private sector. Minneapolis–St. Paul, like San Diego, is a very mature and competitive managed care market, but there is greater support within the market for collaborative policy development to address public policy concerns such as health promotion and quality enhancement. The business community is also central to the evolution of the Minneapolis market through its role as a purchaser. While less mature than the other two markets, the managed care market in Washington is reasonably well developed. Also, many perceive that competition is becoming even more intense now, and a shake-out is likely.

The structures and roles of AMCs also vary across the markets. In San Diego, there is a single dominant AMC [the University of California at San Diego (UCSD) Medical Center], accounting for most of the residencies, which in turn are relatively concentrated in a few hospitals. In Minneapolis–St. Paul, there is a single dominant AMC (the Health Sciences Center of the University of Minnesota), but residencies are more dispersed among a number of hospitals, and there is emerging competition from the Mayo Medical Center. While the Center is located outside the metropolitan area and serves as a national and regional referral center, it is increasing its role in the Minneapolis–St. Paul market. Washington's GME and health care system constitute the most complex of the three markets—because of both its size and the involvement of three major political jurisdictions (Virginia, Maryland, and the District of Columbia). In Washington, we therefore studied two of the three AMCs, George Washington University Medical Center, and Georgetown University Medical Center. (Howard University's AMC was studied only peripherally because of resource constraints and because it has an atypical financing stream related to its role in training minority physicians.) Unlike the AMCs at the UCSD and the University of Minnesota, Washington's two studied AMCs are private and do not generally receive public support.

In all three markets, the AMCs we studied are well respected but are not among the top-ranked, most prestigious few in the nation. While it is not possible to generalize to all AMCs on the basis of only three cases, we perceive that the major findings and conclusions from these are relevant to a large segment of AMCs nationwide.

San Diego

San Diego has a mature managed care market whose health care system has been rapidly consolidating. The key distinction between coverage in the marketplace is between capitated plans [health maintenance organizations (HMOs) and related forms] and all other forms of coverage. While the managed care market includes numerous HMOs, the delivery system has been consolidating into a small number of entities (three or four) that actually manage and assume risk for care under contract to HMOs. Within the market, there appears to be consensus that there are too many hospital beds, too many specialists, and, possibly, too many physicians overall.

San Diego is unusual for a market of its size in terms of its relatively short history with teaching programs. The UCSD School of Medicine enrolled its first class in 1968. That school has a strong base in the medical sciences and a heavy emphasis on specialty training, and ranks high in clinical research, which accounts for half of the medical school's expenditures. State funds represent the most flexible, but dwindling, share of the school's support (14%). The UCSD AMC's major teaching hospital was previously the county hospital, and though other providers are involved, this AMC still sees itself as a major provider of care for the uninsured and the Medi-Cal population.

The AMC's approximately 500 residents (approved by the Accreditation Council for Graduate Medical Education, or ACGME) basically rotate, as appropriate, through the two Center hospitals and the Veterans Administration Hospital. Pediatric residencies are provided in conjunction with Children's Hospital. Residencies outside the UCSD AMC's system are limited in San Diego. State legislation has been proposed to increase the proportion of residencies devoted to primary care, which is pressuring the entire University of California system to place greater emphasis on primary care training.

Minneapolis–St. Paul

Minneapolis–St. Paul has a mature managed care market whose health system has also rapidly consolidated. There are two main competing systems, formed through mergers, though purchasers' concerns over this consolidation are likely to result in change. The two systems, along with Blue Cross and Blue Shield, account for 80% of the total Minnesota managed care market. Price competition has been heating up in the market, though it is not as intense as in San Diego. Premiums, for example, were expected to rise by only 3–4% when we visited, with some groups holding steady.

The Health Sciences Center of the University of Minnesota (UM) is the dominant AMC in the market. This AMC has about a thousand residents, followed by the Mayo Medical Center (with about the same number, but fewer full-time positions). Hennepin County Health Center has an independent program with under 200 residents. Compared with the other AMCs we studied, the UM's AMC trains a larger share of primary care physicians, reflecting both the entry of students from the two-year program at the University of Minnesota, Duluth, and a rural physician associate program. Fifty percent of this AMC's medical school graduates are said to enter primary care residencies.

The Mayo Medical Center emphasizes specialty training—only 20% of the residencies are in obstetrics, pediatrics, internal medicine, or family practice. It also is distinctive in that its decision making is centralized within the system; physicians are salaried and have set clinical responsibilities. The state of Minnesota has been a leader in state health reform efforts, prompting many of those involved in health care to position themselves for a system with much greater statewide emphasis on managed care. The University of Minnesota draws 50% of its revenue from patients who live outside the ten-county metropolitan area, 30% percent from those in other areas of the state, 13% from those in the four-state region, and 6% from those who live elsewhere.

Washington, D.C.

Washington, D.C., is a rapidly evolving managed care market where counts of penetration are complicated by the three political jurisdictions that constitute the market for this area. The market is heavily influenced by the federal government. There are numerous large providers and health plans, but none is clearly dominant, and the system is less consolidated than are those in the other two markets. The market is heavily influenced by its three diverse geopolitical jurisdictions and by natural boundaries such as the Potomac River, all of which influence care-seeking behavior.

Georgetown University (GU) Medical Center has a larger medical school and set of residencies than does George Washington University (GWU) Medical Center (521 versus 378 residents). In the absence of state support, both depend on clinical revenue. The GWU AMC has considerably less research revenue and thus is particularly dependent on clinical revenue. Both of these AMCs differ from others we studied in their use of open faculties, which draws members from the community. The GWU AMC is unique in that it has an HMO owned and controlled by the university. The HMO was originally established for training purposes and is still very involved in training. (After the site visit, GWU announced its intention of divesting itself of both the teaching hospital and the HMO. As of July 1996, no arrangements had been made.)

The Washington market includes Maryland, the state with the only remaining all-payer hospital-rate–setting system. Both AMCs are in the District of Columbia. Because Maryland's system highly limits discounting, we were told that this gives District hospitals greater flexibility in negotiating rates even though average rates for District hospitals are higher than those in Maryland.

Findings

1. Are Managed Care Plans Willing to Pay a Premium to AMCs Under Competitive Systems?

a. Managed care plans generally negotiate with AMCs rates that are competitive with those paid for similar services offered by other providers.

In the three markets we visited, managed care plans did not perceive themselves as paying a premium (or much of one) to AMCs unless the services were not available elsewhere; the AMCs understood this. The widely held view was that the market, primarily purchasers, is largely price-driven and does not support such a premium. Some plans indicated they might pay more for better quality or for treatment of severely ill patients, but few believed that such justification for such higher payments could be readily documented.

b. When a "premium" is paid, it is generally small, perhaps on the order of 5–10% and is generally justified on the basis of patient mix or other factors.

When the UCSD AMC developed a plan for containing costs to reduce the disparity between its rates and those of competitors, it assumed that it could compete if it reduced its rates from 35% higher than those of community hospitals to only 10–15% higher (adjusted for case mix and severity). However, just two years later, it is now less certain about the ability to sustain this differential.

One plan that mainly serves national accounts and thus needs coverage in the San Diego market pays the UCSD's AMC for hospital services at a rate it said is competitive with that paid for similar services to non-AMC providers. The AMC receives some special treatment from the plan for high-cost cases and selected tertiary services. The UCSD AMC's medical group was able to effectively make the case with this plan that it experienced adverse selection, and so it negotiated for all rates to be about 10% higher than they would have been to other providers. In Minneapolis, one payer adjusts its rates into 35 diagnosis-related-group (DRG)–like categories, so there is some implicit premium for higher costs associated with particular case mixes. However, one AMC noted that the adjustment did not always generate the full face value of the rates. In Washington, one plan noted that it sought to negotiate for broad packages of services, and so it might pay more for one service if this allowed it to bundle a broad set of services, thus expediting an HMO's ability to deliver care.

An exception to the rule in payment parity is any specialized tertiary service for which there is little competition. For example, there may be no discounting of burn services. However, as one plan noted, these kinds of specialized services account for a very small share of an HMO's premium (e.g., 7%).

While some plans adjust rates for case mix, the representatives of the AMCs we spoke with perceived that their tertiary settings led to adverse case mixes that were not adequately accounted for in rate setting. For example, a small but expensive number of patients needing specialized services might have been referred to the AMC. On the other hand, at least one interviewee noted that there are many ways in which AMCs might "game" the system to increase revenues.

c. AMCs are the sole providers for only a few tertiary services in the markets we studied, and managed care plans thus typically have choices in contracting.

In most cases, there are well-respected competitor hospitals that have affiliated physician staff who were often trained by the AMCs in the market. As one interviewee noted, "We trained our competition." In Washington, for example, Georgetown's AMC has a long-established affiliation with Fairfax Hospital for training a variety of specialists. Fairfax is part of the ANOVA Health System, an emerging dominant player in the northern Virginia managed care market, and it offers extensive tertiary services, many of which are staffed by and compete with physicians trained through the Georgetown affiliation. In San Diego, for example, the UCSD AMC's strong research orientation has led to some turnover among faculty more interested in clinical care. Having left the university, many of these faculty have established competing programs with other competing systems.

While obviously crude and based on broad DRG-based classifications, an analysis of the San Diego market highlights how care is likely to be dispersed across diverse providers even for relatively specialized services. (We obtained the analysis from one of the competing health systems in the area.) The analysis indicates that in the first half of 1993, the UCSD AMC accounted for only 7% of cardiovascular surgery, 24% of gastrointestinal surgery, 22% of tertiary oncology, and 22% of tertiary trauma services provided in the local market.

2. To the Extent That AMCs Are More Expensive Than Alternative Providers Because of Their Teaching Responsibilities, How Much of These Expenses Has Traditionally Been Paid through Patient Care Revenues of Various Third-Party Payers?

Some GME costs have traditionally been offset by third-party revenue from charge- or cost-based payers, but these sources are becoming less available in highly competitive or even less competitive markets.

a. The AMCs we visited typically saw some net cost to training, though, at best, only the direct costs could be quantified.

The structure of the typical AMC makes it hard to analyze training costs. Because much of training occurs through the provision of patient care, it also is difficult, if not impossible, to separate precisely training costs from patient care costs.

At the medical school level, training costs tend to be financed through a combination of state support (for public institutions) and clinical revenues generated by the faculty; research funding makes a limited contribution. Hospitals fund the bulk of the costs of residents largely from clinical income and from some limited support provided by the faculty (e.g., from their practice incomes or from research grants). The respective roles of the medical school and the hospital in financing, however, vary across the AMCs, thus complicating the calculation of direct costs. For example, at the UCSD Center, faculty salaries are paid directly by the school of medicine, but this is not true at some other AMCs. In Minnesota, residents are paid through the medical school even though most funds come from the hospital. None of the AMCs we visited had estimates for the indirect costs of medical education, such as lost productivity, extra testing, and duplication of services, though they perceive these costs to be important. For example, one AMC administrator cited a combination of various revenue streams [e.g., Medicare's Direct Medical Education (DME) and Indirect Medical Education (IME) payments] as the source of his estimates of GME costs.

Training costs vary with the stage of training. We were told that medical students (especially in the clinical years) are more expensive than residents, who become less expensive over time—their costs may balance out over a three-year period. For example, the GWU Health Plan (the GWU Center's HMO) estimated that training residents requires 20–25% more space and 20–25% more personnel than would be needed otherwise, and that residents reduce productivity by 25–33%. However, the expense of teaching is viewed as proportional to residents' experience, with the health plan losing money on a first-year resident, breaking even the second year, and generating a surplus in the third.

Because residents provide services that others would otherwise need to provide, it is not clear, on a net basis, how they affect costs. At the UCSD Center, for example, a decline in general surgery residents led to less coverage of the emergency room and orthopedics, and to a request to add a physician assistant. If there are fewer residents, there is potential for the faculty workload to change because faculty may be required to work more hours, which may or may not be desirable. Reduction in the number of residents is not the only factor affecting faculty workloads. We heard at UCSD, for example, that faculty are "working harder for fewer dollars." This was not only an effect of competition but also a response to reductions in state funding, the economy, and greater competition for research funds.

We also found differences of opinion about how large these cost differentials for training inefficiencies were or had to be. One managed care plan, for example, questioned why physicians should not be trained to practice in the cost-effective style that would be expected of them in the future.

> *b. Our literature review indicates that explicit payment for GME is restricted primarily to Medicare and some Medicaid payers even though these functions are subsidized indirectly by charge-based payers—a declining share of the market.*

Through the Medicare program, the government is the largest single explicit payer of GME costs. Considering direct and indirect payments, we estimate that the government contribution accounted for approximately 2% of total spending for hospital care and 9% of Medicare prospective payment system (PPS) payments in 1991. In 1989, 23 of the 37 states using PPS methods in their Medicaid programs also included an adjustment for teaching. However, to the extent that Medicaid rates are below cost (as they typically are), they provide little GME support even if they explicitly recognize the function. Medicaid (and to some extent, Medicare) support is potentially further reduced by the shift to managed care that has become increasingly rapid since the time of our study. While some Blue Cross and Blue Shield plans historically paid for GME because they used cost-based rates, few do so now.

Historically, private payers have supported GME indirectly because their revenues have been used to underwrite the costs of the AMC. This has been particularly true for charge-based payers that offer traditional indemnity products. However, these payers now represent a declining share of the market and, in today's market, even these payers are changing their payment methods in response to competition. For example, the UCSD Center's medical group estimated that traditional indemnity plans now pay 60% of charges compared to 80% previously—and they now account for only 8% of revenue. In contrast, one large preferred provider organization (PPO) pays 55–60% of charges, and a capitated plan pays 50%. However, the latter also generates more business. Medicare has reduced its payments from 50% to 42% of charges, and Medicaid pays on 26%. The comparison against charges provides a consistent metric for comparing payers but may understate each payer's contribution to cost. For example, the Prospective Payment Assessment Commission estimates that in 1993 Medicare hospital payments were 96% of costs nationwide. These proportions vary substantially by type of hospital and state.[3] Medicare, for example, pays 97–98% of costs in major teaching hospitals.

These patterns by payer suggest that the level of payment, rather than the explicit recognition of training costs, determines support for GME. From our case studies, it is clear that today's market has reduced the availability of traditional charge-based revenue, both because the role of traditional indemnity insurance in the market is smaller and because the market allows less of a premium to be paid. To the extent that managed care has replaced traditional insurance, AMCs receive lower rates. It is not clear whether they are lower than those of Medicare and Medicaid, and whether they vary by state or institution. One AMC in Minnesota estimates that if costs equal 70% of charges, then Medicare pays 65–70%; Medicaid, 64%; managed care, 50–75%; and more lucrative payers (e.g., workers' compensation), 80%.

Another factor that will affect the "premium" paid by managed care is the form of payment. For example, discounted per diems are common at the UCSD Center, but length of stay has been dropping substantially, and so revenues have shrunk.

c. *Medicare is viewed as an important source of funding for training, but relatively little attention has been given to how the shift to capitation could affect the distribution of these payments.*

When Medicare calculates capitation rates for risk-based plans, it attempts to approximate, though not always successfully, what the costs would have been for comparable individuals treated in the same market under fee-for-service systems. This "AAPCC" is the capitation rate paid to managed care plans, adjusted for case mix based on demographic factors. GME payments under Medicare are included in the cost base used to establish the "USPCC" or national estimates of Medicare per capita costs. Area differences in GME are accounted for by the "geographic adjuster," a five-year rolling average comparing county Medicare costs with the national average and generating the AAPCC. This method is budget-neutral with respect to federal payments for GME in the national market so long as managed care plans using Medicare make the same average use of AMCs as do physicians as a whole who are using Medicare to provide fee-for-service medicine. We have no evidence as to whether this assumption holds. However, what is most relevant to the study is the fact that once GME funds are included in capitation payments, there is no guarantee they will go to AMCs. That is, these funds could be distributed among all the hospitals rather than being targeted at AMCs.

The representatives of the AMCs and managed care plans we interviewed generally indicated that managed care plans pay AMCs based on negotiated rates, not Medicare rates. Thus, Medicare's subsidy to support indirect and direct payments for graduate medical education does not necessarily pass through to specific AMCs. Given other study findings, this suggests that if managed care grows within the Medicare program, the result will be less targeting of GME support to specific AMCs based on Medicare's criteria. The impact of this imbalance will depend on how managed care's total rates and payments compare with those of Medicare. That is, it is possible that managed care plans pay no premium to AMCs but could still pay rates higher than those of Medicare.

3. How Are AMCs Faring Now, and to What Extent Have They Been Adversely Affected by the Growth of Competitive Systems?

AMCs have not experienced major short-term adverse effects as a result of the growth of managed care, but they are concerned about, and are working to position themselves for, the future.

a. *A recent national study shows that the hospital margins of academic health centers (AHCs) have improved relative to other large hospitals despite the growth of managed care, largely because they have limited cost growth and protected collection rates.*

In his 1994 analysis of the financial experiences of AHCs from 1984 (when Medicare PPS was implemented) to 1991–92, Hadley found that AHC hospitals' margins actually increased over the period, while those of other large hospitals decreased even though HMO enrollments grew in many of the markets where the AHCs are located.[2] This occurred because AHCs limited their cost growth and protected their "collection rates" (i.e., deductions from gross charges) better than did other hospitals. He concludes that "the primary implication for the future is that AHC hospitals, even with their substantial missions of care to the poor, medical education, community service, and medical research, will take measures to preserve their financial viability when external changes . . . alter the economic environment in which they operate." While this study covers only the period ending 1991–92, the general conclusions are consistent with our observations in the three case study sites. That is, for the AMCs we studied, our results generally do not indicate that AMCs' financial positions had eroded as of mid-1994 and confirm that AMCs have taken some steps to contain costs.

b. AMCs are making efforts to position themselves for a future that they assume will involve more managed care, but depending on their forms and histories, they face disadvantages in doing so.

Most of the AMCs we visited are responding to the need for more competitive pricing by instituting broad-based cost-reduction strategies. The AMCs were able to make these reductions without greatly changing service mix, though they expect they may need to eliminate or reduce certain unprofitable services in the future. In some cases, the savings were obtained by cutting replacement reserves, a strategy that results in only short-term savings (assuming a need to eventually replace capital).

The perception is that some AMCs might not survive, though those we visited are more confident. The more important issue for them is how much they would be changed and whether they would remain distinctive. Most are working to increase the numbers of their covered lives, generally through diverse managed care arrangements designed to bring in more people and to create a better mix of primary and specialty care by increasing affiliations with primary care providers. Most efforts focus on enhancing the ability to compete for routine referral and inpatient services that make up most inpatient care ("bread and butter" services) and are the most competitive services in the market. Tertiary care appears to make up a small percentage of services at AMCs, and in any case, it is hard for AMCs to survive only on these services.

An institution's competitive position, among other things, is affected by the following: (1) its public or private status; (2) whether it has an open or closed panel; (3) its history of managed care contracting; (4) whether it has its own managed care plan; and (5) how it is viewed by community providers and health plans.

Public institutions have the advantage of flexible funding sources to support training, though these sources have been diminishing as percentages of medical school revenues, and they are more important to faculty support and undergraduate training than to the expense of residents. Private institutions are more flexible in terms of contracting and responding to the environment. For example, the need for state approval delayed for many years the construction of a new hospital in La Jolla in the San Diego area and seriously affected both the UCSD AMC's ability to position itself and the ultimate value of the facility itself. Lack of capital to negotiate arrangements with practices is regarded by that AMC as one of the major impediments to succeeding in building a network in collaboration with community physicians. It cites competitors who are said to have $40 to $50 million they can use to "buy" practices.

Whether an AMC has an open or closed medical staff (i.e., whether community-based physicians have admitting privileges) also affects its position. Only the Washington AMCs have open faculties, though the UCSD's AMC is attempting to develop one. AMCs with closed medical staffs do not typically have strong feeder systems and therefore may have smaller patient bases. This becomes especially important when length of stay is declining and when competition is keenest for "bread and butter" services. The UCSD's AMC, for example, originally had a study that calculated that a patient base of 220,000 would be sufficient to support its needs, but later calculated a figure that was twice as high, given the changes in hospital use patterns in the market. Several representatives of HMOs we interviewed in the Washington market noted that an important factor in their contracting was the ability of their physicians to provide care to hospitalized patients, which would appear to be a disadvantage for closed medical staffs.

Historical managed care arrangements that affect AMCs in an evolving health care market constitute another factor that affects strategy. In Minneapolis–St. Paul, for example, many managed care arrangements were developed years ago when the University of Minnesota was less interested in affiliation, and Group Health, Inc. (GHI—the earliest HMO) had problems finding institutions willing to grant privileges to its physicians. This history means that the University of Minnesota is a marginal player in the metropolitan managed care market and may find it hard to reenter the market, at least within the Minneapolis–St. Paul metropolitan area. In Washington, Georgetown's AMC has had a long affiliation with Kaiser, possibly because the plan was originated at the university. On the other hand, although the AMC at George Washington has had a long history with Group Health Association (GHA), the plan was acquired by Humana. And even plans that seek stability have shown that they are willing to change provider arrangements if they are not working out.

The fact that an AMC has its own managed care plan could help or hurt it. It provides a natural feeder base for specialized referrals and hospital services and a set of experiences with managed care. However, having such a plan could also constrain an institution's competitive response and potentially discourage competing plans from affiliating with it. For example, George Washington has its own HMO, which accounts for about half of its managed care revenue, while Georgetown's has tended to rely on contracts with existing HMOs, though it is now sponsoring an employee PPO and considering how it should evolve. Because of their role in tertiary care, AMCs are also concerned that they retain a variety of managed care contracts. AMCs such as the one at the University of Minnesota are working to position themselves to achieve both these objectives.

Finally, many AMCs we visited are at a disadvantage because of the tensions between "town" and "gown." Many AMCs are viewed as being specialty-dominated, historically arrogant, and not customer-driven. While many are making major efforts to change, their histories affect how they are viewed by community physicians and competing institutions, which obviously have their own interests at heart. Another complaint we heard from community providers is that AMC faculty are unresponsive in handling referrals and often fail to return the patient to the referring physician or notify the physician of the treatment. On the other hand, this faculty behavior does not appear to be inevitable, since one HMO cited customer orientation as an important reason for becoming more involved with a particular AMC. And another noted that in today's competitive market, physicians may be attracted to AMCs because they perceive that AMCs will not skimp on quality.

4. How Is the Growth of Competitive Systems Affecting Graduate Medical Education?

The growth of competitive systems is generating pressure to change GME, but the system is slow in responding, and there are many barriers and issues associated with a transition to primary care and ambulatory-care-based training.

a. Managed care plans perceive that AMCs are training the wrong physicians, in the wrong specialties, and in the wrong settings.

The HMOs perceive a much greater need for primary care training in settings that reflect the current market and delivery system. There appears to be some interest in having managed care plans serve as training sites for primary care physicians and, possibly, having them underwrite some of these costs, especially to the extent that the plans gain by increasing recruitment. (This varies considerably by market and plan.) In San Diego, the Sharp system established its own family medicine department to help it recruit providers in a market it perceived as turning out inadequate numbers of primary care physicians, since it perceived the local AMC as being unwilling to change.

While our limited study provides no firm indication of the interests among managed care plans on a national level in serving as training sites, the fact that they perceive new physicians as poorly trained for the managed care setting has been documented in other broad-based studies, including a recent one involving site visits to 23 HMOs.[5]

On the other hand, AMCs are uncertain about the interests of managed care plans. One AMC administrator articulated the concern that managed care is a marginal buyer that is cannibalizing the system, causing dislocation, and not willing to pay anything for the next generation of physicians beyond what would support its narrow self-interest.

b. The domination of specialties in AMCs has evolved as a result of a variety of strong incentives, and there are both pressures for and obstacles to change.

Well-established financial incentives appear to have "succeeded." They favored procedure- and specialty-oriented care, more care rather than less, and the development of more complex service infrastructures even where existing competing services might be underutilized. In the markets we visited, the AMCs are churning out specialists who, in turn, want to train more specialists. Faculty, for example, gain an advantage from trainees who might enhance their ability to pursue research interests and devote less time to clinical care, especially for patients seen outside the faculty practice plan. Faculty can also gain prestige from having residents and fellows in their specialties and subspecialties. But, in turn, these specialists are often hired in the community, leaving the AMC with few distinctive services, since they "trained the competition." Despite some erosion, departmental power bases are still very strong, and procedure-oriented specialties and those departments that have strong research bases are stronger still because their greater revenues allow them to sponsor more residency programs. While competitive pressures are forcing some reassessment, the threat of legislation on residency mix (i.e., the Isenberg bill) was probably a greater influence than competition on the residency mix of the UCSD's AMC.

On the other hand, interviewees perceived that specialty incomes are declining relative to those of primary care physicians, and for some specialties (e.g., radiology), there may be no new positions in highly saturated markets. It is unclear how much of this can be attributed to oversupply and competition versus the effects of the growing use of resource-based relative value scales. In our visits, we saw growth in family medicine residencies but not major shifts in the specialty orientations of the AMCs we visited. In general, the changes in residencies at the time of our visits appeared to be small and at the margins. However, we did see dynamics that might lead to such shifts and some changes in faculty mix.

c. *The shift to ambulatory care delivery as well as to competitive systems is encouraging more training in ambulatory care settings, but there are obstacles to creating effective programs as well as differences of opinion about what this training should involve and what role AMCs should play.*

At UCSD's AMC, a major incentive for training in ambulatory care is that the typical length of stay has dropped so low that the patient is not hospitalized long enough to support training needs. Yet, this type of training, according to observers in several markets, is more demanding than inpatient training. The ambulatory care setting is more decentralized, making supervision more difficult; also, finding space in which residents can observe is an issue. We heard different reports on how well patients would accept care from trainees, both in general terms and in more specific ones, such as the inefficiencies and greater lengths of time associated with such care. Some informants suggested that a patient's reaction could depend on how the attending physician or organization presents the situation. When physicians are paid on a financial basis that results in reduced income for inefficiencies (e.g., capitation), they may be less willing, we were told, to have a resident join them in office care even though they may be very willing otherwise to serve as an "attending" (with its associated status) at the hospital. Establishing payment offsets for these effects is hard when residency training funds flow through hospitals, which might legitimately question the use of such payments in non-hospital settings. But providing them to medical schools could increase the potential for further encouraging specialty training.

Beyond the economics, there appear to be strong differences of opinion about how ambulatory care training should be structured. Among the AMCs we studied, there was concern about the possibility of returning to the "pre-Flexnerian" era of apprenticeships, along with a perception that community-based providers, including some managed care plans, do not understand what GME teaching requires. Managed care plans perceive these problems to be less extensive, and they are often receptive to the idea that AMCs would coordinate and facilitate training using an approach that one plan termed "teaching the teachers."

d. Our cases highlighted potential conflicts between national, state, and market needs and their influences on the workforce.

AMCs view a strong intellectual and scientific base as essential to training. If specialty training is to be reduced, it may make sense to concentrate such training in certain locations. Individual markets, however, are unlikely to support current levels of specialty training, since the beneficiaries of the resulting training programs would flow beyond the market to the region or even the nation as a whole. States have a similar view. For example, reform in Minnesota is focused on the GME needs for the state, generating concerns among AMCs such as the Mayo Clinic that regard their missions as more national. Most of the AMCs we visited had at least regional markets for their trainees, and some were national. There also is a problem if a local market does not provide enough patients to support a particular type of service, perhaps because patients are dispersed throughout competing systems. This could be more likely in a managed care environment.

Unfortunately, tensions in a managed care environment between local and national objectives create a dilemma. Our analysis suggests that market forces alone may not necessarily result in the appropriate level, mix, or concentration of specialty training. Managed care will push for fewer specialists, but the built-in incentives of AMCs are likely to generate pressure for more specialists and fewer primary care physicians than the market wants. Yet virtually none of those AMCs or HMOs we studied wished to see the federal government specify which types of residents should be trained, and we assume even fewer AMCs would support federal action to identify a select group of AMCs to turn out any requisite number of "superspecialists."

In addition, some medical educators wonder if it is realistic or effective to assume that physicians should have a generalist orientation. They either challenge the view that generalists could know enough to be the most cost-effective providers, or they wonder whether nurses might not be a better choice for the intended function.

Finally, it should be stated that although support for pooled funding for GME is widespread, there are different opinions about the form it should take. Among managed care plans, there is greater interest in tying support to the setting of training rather than just to hospitals or medical schools.

Conclusions

Our study suggests that the public policy issues associated with AMCs in a competitive environment are complex and tend to preclude "black and white" solutions. While AMCs are not currently in short-term crisis, there is some legitimate concern that their missions could be jeopardized by competitive forces and such forces' influences on the availability of funding and patients within AMCs. On the other hand, the health care environment has changed, and AMCs, among others, need to respond. In particular, they need to develop training that is appropriate to the shift in care to outpatient settings, the growth in managed care, and a greater concern for cost and cost-effectiveness. Not all AMCs or residency programs may be needed, and others will have to change.

From a public policy perspective, the key issue is how to preserve yet reform those AMCs that are important for the future so that they are well positioned for the missions they will need to accomplish. Financing of AMCs has a major effect on the scope and mix of their GME programs and on the locations of training. Policies to help AMCs make the transition to a competitive market need to be considered jointly with policies for GME. While states can play an important role in developing these policies, particularly when they provide fiscal support for training, the federal government will critically influence policies because of its support of GME through Medicare and its general influence in the market. In addition, some federal role in policy development would appear important, given the regional and national labor markets served by some AMCs and specific specialty training programs.

Our study also suggests future approaches for research on AMCs that may be constructive. One such approach is longitudinal monitoring to discern trends, using measures sensitive to important change, in the financial status of AMCs, and assess how these trends influence valued public policy objectives such as training, care for the poor, tertiary care, and provider supply, positively or negatively. Because of the time lags in available data and these data's limitations, this monitoring may require approaches similar to that used in our study, potentially following a series of markets over time.

A second approach that deserves attention is to assess the impact of any change in the traditional AMC mission. For example, if AMCs switch their service mix, how does this affect the levels of resources available in the community, access to care, the ability to train, and the content of training?

A third potential type of study is to identify organizational arrangements and models for ambulatory-care-based training and their associated strengths, weaknesses, costs, and financing implications. This could be followed with a national survey to identify the use of these models and the factors influencing their adoption.

Acknowledgments

The author is grateful for assistance from Dr. Julianne Howell of the UCSD Medical Center who, with the support of Michael Stringer at that Center, arranged the San Diego site visit and provided an orientation and other assistance. Greg Hart of the Health Sciences Center of the University of Minnesota played a similar role in Minneapolis. In D.C., Linda Fishman of the Association of American Medical Colleges facilitated access to local AMCs. Jack Hadley of Georgetown University provided advice on important issues and made available related nationwide analysis. At Mathematica Policy Research, Karyen Chu served as project manager for the study and prepared the literature synthesis. Embry Howell and Jack Hadley provided useful feedback on the report. Daryl Hall edited the manuscript. Dr. Brian Biles, then with the Public Health Service (PHS) and now with the Commonwealth Fund, conceived of the need for this project. Both Dan Erman and Kate Rickard of the PHS staff facilitated the execution of the study, which was supported by the PHS.

Notes

1. Chu K. Literature Review—Financing of Academic Medical Centers and Graduate Medical Education under Competitive Systems with Managed Care. Report to the Office of the Assistant Secretary for Health, U.S. Department of Health and Human Services. Washington, DC: Mathematica Policy Research, November 1994.
2. Hadley, J., and Gaskin, D. J. HMO market penetration and missions of academic health center hospitals. In: Korn, D., McLaughlin, C., and Osterweiss, M. (eds.). Academic Health Centers in the Managed Care Environment. Washington, DC: Association of Academic Health Centers, 1995.
3. Prospective Payment Assessment Commission. Medicare and the American Health System: Report to Congress, June 1995. Washington, DC: Government Printing Office, 1995: 60, tables 2–18.
4. Felt, S., Frazer, H., and Gold, M. HMO Primary Patterns and Processes: A Cross-site Analysis of 23 HMOs. (Report submitted to the Health Resources and Services Administration, U.S. Department of Health and Human Services.) Washington, DC: Mathematica Policy Research, December 1994.

CHAPTER

17

SHIFTING THE PARADIGM: MONITORING ACCESS IN MEDICARE MANAGED CARE

Elizabeth R. Docteur, David C. Colby, and Marsha Gold

Introduction

Managed care currently plays a small but growing role in the Medicare program. At the end of 1995, 10.7 percent of Medicare beneficiaries were enrolled in managed care plans (Physician Payment Review Commission, 1996). Enrollment is heavily concentrated in plans that are paid under a risk contract to deliver services in exchange for a fixed payment per enrollee.[1] Enrollment in those plans has increased more than 30 percent since 1994, and the proportion of beneficiaries who obtain medical care through capitated plans is expected to continue to increase. Such expectations are fostered both by the increasing proportion of enrollees with managed care experience and by growth in private health plan participation in the risk program. In addition, increased beneficiary enrollment would be anticipated under policy proposals to expand the range of health care delivery alternatives available under Medicare.[2] Proposals to do so have been endorsed recently by both the Administration and by Congress.

From *Health Care Financing Review* 17 (4): 5–21. It is reprinted here without change.

The growth of managed care presents a number of challenges for Medicare policy, not the least of which is how to continue to fulfill the program's responsibility to ensure beneficiaries' access to care. In this article, we consider the implications of Medicare managed care growth for efforts to monitor beneficiaries' access. Systems currently used for monitoring access need to be revised, and data and measures suitable for monitoring will need to be developed. Ultimately, under a Medicare program that offers a wide array of health care financing and delivery options, monitoring efforts will need to be unbiased for the mode of health care delivery.

Approach to Monitoring Access

Ongoing monitoring efforts provide information on Medicare beneficiaries' ability to obtain medical care. Annual reports on beneficiaries' access are produced by both HCFA and PPRC. These monitoring efforts were mandated by Congress to track the impact of the Medicare fee schedule (MFS) and to provide information for updating the conversion factor under the process for setting Volume Performance Standards (Health Care Financing Administration, 1995b; Physician Payment Review Commission, 1995). Therefore, by design, these efforts have focused on access in FFS Medicare.

Policy interest and the availability of beneficiary-level Medicare data have supported numerous studies using a variety of methods for analyzing beneficiaries' access to care in the traditional Medicare program. In this section, we describe the dominant theoretical approach to evaluating access that has guided past studies, and the measures and data that have been used in both one-time studies and ongoing efforts to monitor access.

Conceptual Framework

Aday, Andersen, and colleagues established the conceptual framework for most subsequent analyses of access to care (Andersen and Aday, 1978; Aday and Andersen, 1981). In these researchers' view, access is a function of three categories of variables: (1) predisposing factors, such as personal resources, education, race, and age; (2) enabling factors, such as the availability of providers in a community, and individual's insurance coverage, and existence of a regular source of care; and (3) finally, an individual's need for health care, as indicated by health status and symptoms.

Using this framework, the effects of these variables on access to care can be observed through measurement of health care services utilization. Studies of access have lent support to this framework by demonstrating variation in the use of services that could be explained by differences in health status, sociodemographic factors, and characteristics of the health care market.

Although most studies of access focus on utilization as a measure of realized access, some studies have taken a different approach. For some researchers, access is a relatively narrow concept. For example, some equate access with having a usual source of care (e.g., Berki and Ashcraft, 1979). Others take a more expansive view of access as a multidimensional concept. Penchansky and Thomas (1981), for instance, describe the dimensions of access as availability, accessibility, accommodation, affordability, and acceptability.[3]

Because these definitions and frameworks were developed in the context of a system in which health care financing and delivery were largely separate systems, a distinction between the concepts of access and quality could be made. Palmer, Clark, and Lawthers (1994) describe the relationship between access and quality, noting that the former concept has traditionally been defined as entry into the health care system. Quality, by contrast, has been considered to be more driven by an individual's experience within the system. This distinction is blurred, however, where financing and delivery systems are merged.

More recently, the Aday-Andersen access definition and framework were modified and adapted by the Institute of Medicine (IOM) (Millman, 1993). The IOM model expands upon Aday and Andersen's earlier work by linking use of services to outcomes. The IOM definition of access (adopted in this article) entails "the timely use of personal health services to achieve the best possible outcomes" (Millman, 1993). The revised framework (Figure 1) helps to make the important distinction between factors that are patient-related and those more associated with the health system. Evaluation of access under this model involves both health-status outcomes and the equity of access across groups.

Viewed this way, the distinction between access as system entry and quality as processes and outcomes of care is less distinct, with a unified framework showing their interrelationship. This integration, as we discuss later, is a very important building block for conceptualizing access in an environment where cost containment is of growing concern.

Measures

Various measures have been used to monitor access in the traditional FFS Medicare program. The choice of measures has been driven by the populations studied, the access barriers, and the available data.

Population-Based Utilization Rates

Utilization rates are among the most widely used measures of access to care. Many studies implicitly assume and some explicitly state that higher

Figure 1 Institute of Medicine Framework for Access

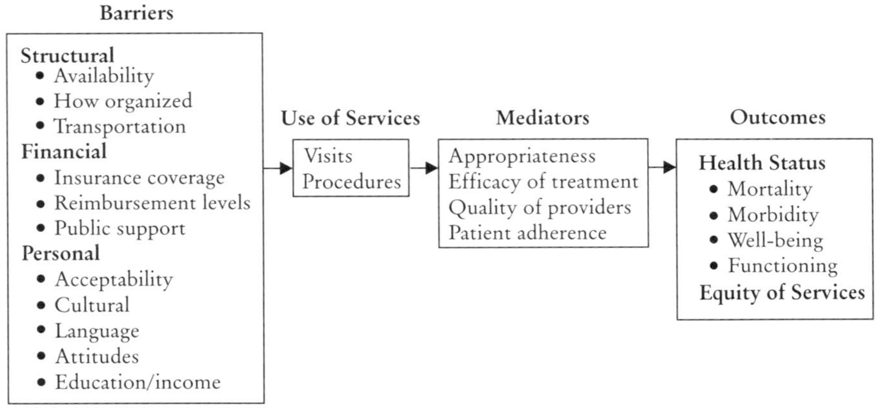

Source: Adapted with permission by the authors from a figure in Millman (1993). Courtesy of National Academy Press, Washington, DC.

utilization indicates better access. Other studies compare utilization rates for a specific service with established standards for use of that service. Either of these types of studies may entail contrasting the utilization of subgroups of beneficiaries or tracking trends in utilization over time.

Many different types of services have been assessed in studies of Medicare beneficiaries' access to care. Access to preventive services, for example, has been monitored by determining the proportion of beneficiaries receiving influenza immunizations (Health Care Financing Administration, 1995a). It is more difficult to analyze access to some other preventive or diagnostic services. For instance, diagnostic data are needed to make valid interpretations of utilization rates for Pap smears (Physician Payment Review Commission, 1994).

Beyond preventive care, other types of utilization have been studied in evaluations of access. Broad indicators of hospital use, such as length of stay and hospital charges, have been used in some studies, while other studies have focused on utilization of surgical and procedural services. Escarce and his colleagues, for instance, documented differences in utilization of such services by race (Escarce et al., 1993). As part of its monitoring efforts, PPRC (1995) analyzed a recent decline in cataract lens replacement surgery, noting that this decline could be explained in part by depletion of the pool of Medicare beneficiaries eligible for the procedure. The shortcoming of most of these use-based measures—

particularly the more aggregate ones—rests in the absence of information about the efficaciousness of the care addressed by the measures.

Measures of Appropriate Care

Measures of appropriate care go beyond utilization measures in that they compare information about the process of care that is provided or not provided to established medical standards. Application of these measures is constrained by limitations in the ability both to identify those patients in need of specific care and also to determine what care is appropriate to a given need.

It is possible, for instance, to identify the proportion of Medicare patients who fail to receive expected followup care. Researchers in one study that exemplifies this approach looked at nine medical diagnosis groups that required hospitalization and evaluated the probability, by race, of beneficiaries' receiving appropriate followup care after hospital discharge (Moy and Hogan, 1993).

Some such measures are now included in efforts to monitor beneficiaries' access (Physician Payment Review Commission, 1995). A set of 47 clinically based indicators of access to care was developed by RAND under a PPRC contract. By drawing on demographic and clinical information available in claims and enrollment databases, these indicators can be used to determine the rates at which appropriate care is provided.

Health Outcomes

Morbidity and mortality rates are commonly used outcomes indicators. But given that the consequences of inadequate or poor quality care may take years to become evident, these are not particularly useful measures for policy purposes. More timely measures of the outcomes of care can be created by identifying health conditions that could have been prevented had appropriate care been received as the need arose. These condition-specific outcomes measures may also provide better information regarding a specific health care delivery environment because they are more likely to be sensitive to care received in the short term. By contrast, the more global outcomes generally tend to be more heavily influenced by factors such as personal history and behavior, socioeconomic factors, and other factors operating independently of current health care delivery arrangements.

Sentinel health events, also known as ambulatory-care-sensitive conditions, are an extension of the public health practice of measuring standard morbidity and mortality rates. These events are defined as diseases, disabilities, and deaths that can be prevented, treated, or controlled with access to appropriate primary care. Such events serve as indicators of potential unmet need. For example, research studies using sentinel events have examined avoidable hospital conditions as indicators of poor access to primary care (Weissman, Gatsonis, and Epstein, 1992; Bindman et al., 1995).

Some outcomes measures that can be used for monitoring access in the Medicare program have been identified. For example, the set of clinically based measures developed by RAND for PPRC included a few measures of avoidable adverse outcomes. Among these were rates of non-elective hospital admissions for specific conditions, emergency department visits related to certain diagnoses, and readmissions following an initial hospitalization (Physician Payment Review Commission, 1995).

Provider Participation Measures

Because provider availability is thought to be an enabling factor in determining access, the extent of provider participation in the Medicare program has been used as an access measure in ongoing monitoring efforts.[4] Specific indicators that have been used include the ratio of physicians to beneficiaries, the number of physicians newly serving and ceasing to serve beneficiaries, and the concentration of patients among physicians serving beneficiaries (Physician Payment Review Commission, 1995).

Other Access Indicators

Other types of access indicators have also been used. Measures of the extent to which beneficiaries have trouble obtaining or delay seeking medical care, and the extent to which they have a particular physician or office as a usual source of care are considered direct measures of access. Measures of barriers to care, such as language or transportation problems, aid the ability to interpret these findings. Indirect access measures include beneficiary satisfaction with various aspects of their care and their ability to obtain care. Finally, descriptive measures on supplemental insurance coverage, out-of-pocket costs for health care, waiting times for appointments, sites of care, and distance traveled to care all provide information that can be used to assess beneficiaries' access. All of these measures serve as fairly gross indicators; however, they may be sensitive to important changes in access for particular groups.

Data

In monitoring Medicare beneficiaries' access, the various types of measures already discussed can be developed predominately from three routinely generated sources of data: claims, beneficiary surveys, and enrollment files. These data have served as a foundation for measuring access to care across a number of dimensions. Other data have been generated to supplement ongoing monitoring efforts, and these have been analyzed to provide insight on access questions.

Claims

In the traditional Medicare FFS program, claims that are submitted by providers for payment supply information on services, beneficiaries, and providers. Claims data have been used to track patterns of utilization in specific areas, to develop clinically based indicators of access, and to measure the extent of provider participation in the Medicare program.

Medicare has a standardized claims reporting system. Before the mid-1980s, each of 56 Medicare carriers had its own data system and coding conventions. Since then, Medicare has gradually developed a national system, first with the Part B Medicare Annual Data (BMAD) system, and now with the National Claims History File (NCHF). Since 1985, HCFA has required the use of Current Procedural Terminology codes for most physician services and has standardized the use of specialty, type of service, place of service, and modifier codes. With implementation of the MFS, the final standardization of Medicare data was achieved by eliminating most local procedure codes and by nationalizing payment policies. Data for other provider sectors are also available through the NCHF.

In addition to standardizing data elements, Medicare claims data are available in a relatively timely fashion. Under the NCHF, claims can be monitored on a flow basis, if desired.

Beneficiary Survey Data

Self-reported beneficiary data on access is routinely generated through the Medicare Current Beneficiary Survey (MCBS), a continuous survey of longitudinal design. The MCBS is a survey of about 12,000 beneficiaries sponsored by HCFA's Office of the Actuary. The MCBS was constructed to be representative of the Medicare population as a whole. The oldest-old and disabled beneficiaries under 65 years of age were oversampled to support analyses of these populations. To maintain the longitudinal panel, additional beneficiaries are added to replace those no longer in the sample because of death, emigration, or refusal to participate (Adler, 1994).

The survey and its supplements contain information on access, utilization of services, expenditures, health insurance coverage, health status, and physical functioning as well as demographic data. The access supplement survey is conducted yearly. It provides information on beneficiary satisfaction and perceived barriers to care as well as direct measures of access, such as waiting times for appointments and out-of-pocket costs.

Enrollment Data

A third source of data for monitoring access is enrollment records. From enrollment data, a denominator file has been developed that includes information on beneficiary eligibility, location of residence, and limited sociodemographic characteristics. This file makes it possible to compare utilization and outcomes rates across some subgroups of Medicare beneficiaries.

Monitoring Access of Vulnerable Populations

Monitoring efforts that focused on the impact of the MFS have tracked access for groups that were thought to be at risk for problems in obtaining care because population averages could cloak access problems for these groups. In general, the vulnerable populations chosen for targeted monitoring efforts were ones that had lower incomes and that had experienced discrimination. Subgroups that have been selected for targeted monitoring efforts include black beneficiaries, beneficiaries without supplemental insurance, and beneficiaries living in poverty areas (Health Care Financing Administration, 1995b; Physician Payment Review Commission, 1995).

Analyzing access of vulnerable populations serves a secondary purpose in that these groups might be expected to be among the first to experience any declines in access caused by MFS implementation. Such targeted monitoring efforts thus may provide an early warning to policymakers when access problems arise. Although ongoing monitoring efforts have not shown reductions in access for these groups, analyses have confirmed that these vulnerable populations continue to have poorer access than other beneficiaries. PPRC found that black beneficiaries and those who live in urban Health Professional Shortage Areas or urban poverty areas use fewer physician services and have poorer health outcomes (Physician Payment Review Commission, 1996). In addition, beneficiaries with low incomes, without supplemental insurance, or with functional disabilities that cause them to require assistance disproportionately report difficulty in obtaining medical care.

A limitation of currently used definitions of vulnerable subpopulations is that these definitions focus on broad characteristics that can be readily measured from available data. Others have defined vulnerability using clinically based or socially based criteria. For example, although her work was not specifically focused on the Medicare program, Aday (1993) theorized that those at risk for poor physical, psychological, or social health are those who have limited resources in terms of social status, social capital, and human capital. Her list of vulnerable populations includes those who are chronically ill, disabled, mentally ill, and homeless, among others. The issue of better defining vulnerable subpopulations will be a particularly important one as access-monitoring approaches are modified to reflect the evolution of the Medicare program.

New Paradigm for Conceptualizing Access

As alluded to in the previous discussions, the existing approaches for assessing access were developed in the context of an FFS system. These approaches may not adequately reflect the processes that influence care in the managed care environment. To respond to recent and ongoing changes in the Medicare program, reevaluation of the system used for monitoring beneficiary access to care is now required.

This reassessment will need to account for the growth of managed care, the growing emphasis on cost-effective delivery, and the wider range in health care delivery options likely to be made available in the Medicare program. First, the traditional access-monitoring approach must be modified to reflect features that are relevant to beneficiaries who use managed care arrangements. This will entail changes in the conceptual framework and along with it, changes in both the measures and the data used for measurement. Second, the traditional access-monitoring approach will need to be strengthened to better address growing concerns regarding efficiency and equity; this will entail more emphasis on the care provided to complement current emphasis on system entry, and will also require more refined techniques for identifying populations at risk. Third, there is a need for better risk adjusters in both cross-sectional and longitudinal analyses of access in the Medicare program.

Adapting the Framework

Existing frameworks for conceptualizing access generally fail to account for the fact that managed care plans are organized systems with both financing and delivery responsibilities. To revise the framework to represent the access issues that arise in managed care, it is necessary to account for the ways in which both of these responsibilities interact to affect access.

Obtaining access to care is a two-stage process in a managed care system. Individuals first select among the health plans available to them, with structural, financial, and personal characteristics influencing plan selection. People then seek care within the structure established by their plan. This structure may include unique care-delivery processes and rules for seeking care that, along with other factors not related to the specific health plan, may influence access for plan enrollees.

Given these differences, we have made preliminary modifications to the IOM conceptual framework in order to incorporate the influence of managed care on access (Figure 2).[5] Structural, financial, and personal variables labeled "barriers to access" in the IOM model are expanded and relabeled to account for the fact that they both determine plan selection and influence care received, and that they can have both positive and negative effects on access. The revisions also reflect the Medicare program's specific characteristics (e.g., supplemental coverage, needs associated with an elderly and disabled population).

The revised framework shows that a beneficiary's health plan selection situates him or her in a specific delivery system with its own attributes and procedures. These, as well as the more traditional financial and personal variables, influence the use of services. Mediating processes between use and outcomes are broadened from the IOM framework to include other mediators such as timeliness of initial treatment. The framework shows more directly that these processes are influenced not just by the use of services but also by features of the plan. Outcomes are generally similar to the original model, but issues of equity are expanded to include enrollment.

The framework also explicitly accounts for disenrollment and the reasons it occurs. This is useful in differentiating types of disenrollment behavior, particularly when disenrollment can be voluntary or involuntary and can occur at the end of any month. The framework assumes that mediating processes determine beneficiary satisfaction, which influences continued enrollment. Provider turnover influences this, as studies have shown that patient behavior is heavily influenced by a desire to retain provider relationships. In addition, any changes in the choices available influence whether enrollees stay in the plan. Disenrollment may also result from changes in patient needs and health status. Such disenrollment, from a policy perspective, may be desirable, neutral, or problematic, depending on the circumstances and the effects of disenrollment on access to care.

In contrast to voluntary disenrollment, involuntary disenrollment is presumed to occur when plans drop out of the program or change their service areas, or when beneficiaries move or die. In either case, beneficiaries who disenroll may return to traditional Medicare or join another Medicare managed care plan. As with voluntary disenrollment, involuntary disenrollment may affect access to care, particularly insofar

Figure 2 Revised Framework for Access Accounting for Managed Care Systems

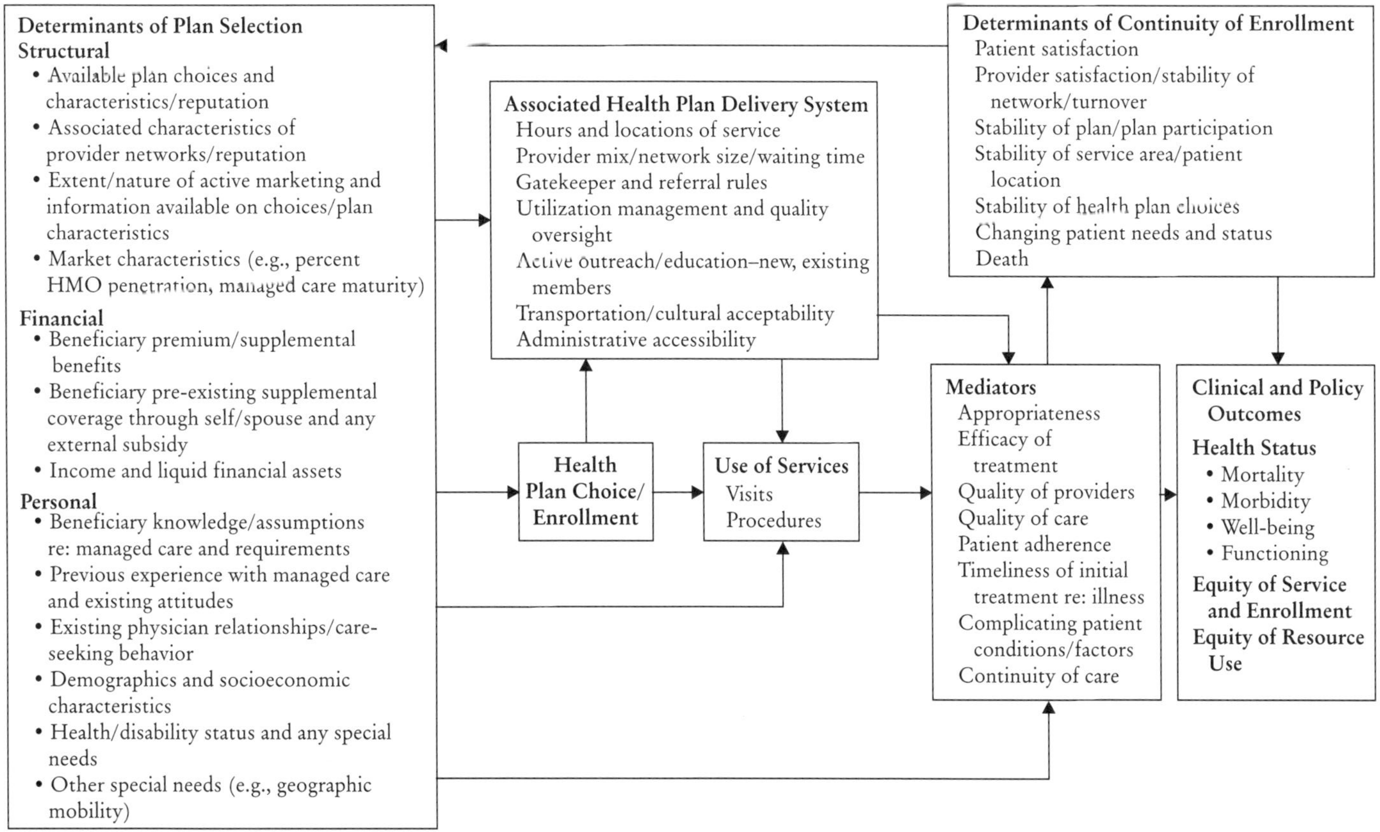

Source: (Gold, 1995).

as continuity of care is disrupted or the ability to obtain supplemental insurance is constrained.

Access Measures for Managed Care

Revisions in the conceptual framework for access will need to be supported by the development of new measures for monitoring access in the Medicare managed care program. Some traditional measures of access are not applicable, and those that are applicable may be insufficient to provide a complete picture of access to care in a more complex health care financing and delivery system. Therefore, additional measures are needed to assess the influence of various managed care plan processes and characteristics on access.

Traditional Measures of Access

Certain types of measures used in access monitoring in the traditional FFS Medicare program become obsolete in the managed care environment. Most importantly, many measures of service utilization, which have figured prominently in traditional access-monitoring efforts, appear to be of limited value in managed care monitoring. Because service use is expected to be lower in a system where care is effectively managed, comparing levels of utilization in the traditional Medicare program and the risk program would not provide much insight into differences in access. Similarly, monitoring aggregate trends in utilization and the use of specific services in the risk program is not likely to yield valuable information.

On the other hand, several types of traditional access measures are applicable to Medicare beneficiaries in both the FFS and the managed care programs. Measures of satisfaction with care and with the ability to obtain care, for example, can provide information for evaluating the access of all beneficiaries. Similarly, measures of the extent to which care is delayed or not obtained when believed to be needed and the rates at which beneficiaries experience trouble obtaining care are also universally relevant, as are measures of perceived barriers to care. Information on beneficiaries' waiting times for appointments and distance traveled to obtain care remains a consideration in assessing managed care access.

As noted previously, both the shift to managed care and the related emphasis on cost-effectiveness increase the value of focusing on measures of access that reflect quality and outcomes of care as well as system entry. Under the traditional framework, the major barriers to access were viewed as stemming from financial and structural (e.g., provider supply and participation) factors that limited system entry. Thus, access and quality were considered relatively independently.

With philosophies and cost constraints changing, the emphasis in access monitoring needs to be shifted to reflect the broader range of factors that determine access under a managed care model. Measures of access also will need to be more closely linked and broadened to include measures that take into account efficacy and cost-effectiveness of care as measured through process of care and outcomes indicators. Balancing these two perspectives—ease of obtaining care and quality of care—is not easy and may be among the more controversial elements of a refined access-monitoring system. This may be true particularly in the transition from the current conceptualization of access, which may be biased toward the features of the FFA environment in which it was conceived.

The use of clinically based measures of access appears particularly promising as a way to monitor access in all types of health care financing and delivery models in which information on service use and enrollment demographics is available. These types of measures can be used to determine whether appropriate care is provided and when avoidable outcomes occur. These indicators have been tested in the traditional Medicare program using claims data and could be applied to Medicare managed care access monitoring if encounter data were to be developed.[6]

New Access Measures

Access measures that account for relevant aspects of the Medicare managed care program and the participating plans will be needed to supplement applicable measures used in traditional FFS access monitoring. Many types of access measures reflect beneficiaries' experiences and perceptions. Use of these measures will require development of beneficiary survey data. Other measures draw on administrative data to provide objective assessments of access to care.

A new area in which access measures are needed is beneficiaries' understanding of managed care. Because a direct determinant of managed care enrollees' access to care is their ability to comply with the processes established by the plan, measures of ability to do so could provide important information on determinants of access. Measures in this category could include those to assess beneficiaries' understanding of their plans' primary-care gatekeeper arrangements and restrictions on use of non-network providers, and of their rights to appeal plan decisions not to provide or pay for a medical service. One challenge in developing such measures is to account for ways in which managed care plans might legitimately differ, such as in the offering of a point-of-service option that covers beneficiary use of non-network providers under some circumstances. As the types of health plans available to beneficiaries expand, these measures might become more difficult to interpret.

Process-of-care measures are also needed for understanding access in managed care systems. Because the processes developed by a managed care plan for the provision of health care will directly determine beneficiaries' access, measures of these processes and their perceived effects can be used in evaluating access. Processes of interest include those for selecting a primary-care provider, making an appointment, obtaining a referral to a specialist, and obtaining care when travelling outside of a plan's service area. The new-enrollee orientation process and the process for appealing a plan decision could also affect access. Finally, managed care plans may develop activities to promote access, such as new-enrollee risk assessment, case management, or distribution of materials promoting preventive care. Specific measures to address these processes include the extent to which they are perceived to facilitate or impede a beneficiary's ability to obtain care and the nature of any problems experienced. These types of measures may be very useful from a policy perspective in that the access problems they are designed to identify could be addressed through targeted interventions.

Another type of beneficiary-oriented measure used in access measurement is the satisfaction measure. Traditionally used measures of satisfaction will need to be supplemented for evaluating access in Medicare managed care. Beyond issues of satisfaction with care and with the ability to obtain care, measures of a beneficiary's satisfaction with the health plan and its features can also serve to assess access indirectly. For example, measures of beneficiary satisfaction with choice of primary-care providers and specialists could provide useful information, as could measures of satisfaction with the value of the benefits received, given the premium charged. These types of measures may be particularly useful in identifying the source of any access problems indicated by other measures.

In addition to these beneficiary-oriented access measures, some types of measures may be used to characterize the managed care plans participating in the Medicare program. In terms of access to providers, traditional provider participation rates may need to be replaced with measures of the geographical proximity of the provider panel, their willingness to take on new Medicare patients, and provider turnover rates.[7] New access measures may need to be created to reflect the plan's role in influencing access. For example, measures of plans' telephone arrangements, such as average time waiting on the telephone to make an appointment, and the rates at which enrollees terminate their telephone calls to their plans because of delays in plan response could be calculated. Other measures could also be developed to assess a health plan's capacity to ensure access for enrollees. Research on plan characteristics or practices that influence access to care for enrollees in general or for vulnerable groups in particular may provide the insight needed to develop such measures.

As shown in our revised conceptual framework, the opportunity for Medicare beneficiaries to change health care financing and delivery modes presents a new type of access consideration. A number of measures will be needed to capture the effects of managed care enrollment, disenrollment, and plan-switching on access to care. First, the rates at which each type of change occurs within groups of beneficiaries and over time are of interest, as such rates could provide an indication of changes in access to care. Distinction between voluntary and involuntary disenrollments must be made and information on the reasons underlying beneficiaries' decisions to change their enrollment status will be needed.[8] In addition, analysts will need to examine the effects of changing enrollment on access. For example, measures of changes in usual source of care or primary-care provider that are associated with the change in enrollment status could be important, as could measures of disenrolling beneficiaries' ability to obtain supplemental insurance coverage.

Data for Monitoring Purposes

Data for monitoring access in Medicare managed care are currently limited. Most notable is the lack of systematic, national-level data on managed care enrollees' use of services and their satisfaction with the ability to obtain care through their plans. As previously discussed, claims data and beneficiary survey data have served as the foundation for most efforts to monitor access; therefore, their lack in the Medicare managed care program has implications for the current ability to monitor the access of these enrollees. Other types of data are available that pertain exclusively to Medicare managed care enrollees, however, that could serve in an access-monitoring system geared toward these beneficiaries.

Utilization Data

The Medicare program does not now collect information on the use of services by enrollees in the risk-contracting plans. Unlike FFS providers under the traditional Medicare program, the risk-contracting plans are paid a fixed amount regardless of service use by their enrollees. Therefore, any information on utilization, costs of care, and patient case mix is developed by the plans only as in-house management tools or in response to purchasers' demands for information about costs and performance. Plans vary not only in whether they develop such data but also in the completeness and accuracy of their data-collection efforts.

Previous attempts at collecting such encounter data have been disappointing. Of 27 health maintenance organizations and competitive medical plans that participated in a Medicare risk-contracting demonstration lasting from 1980 to 1985, only two could provide even partial encounter data for ambulatory services (Langwell and Hadley, 1990). Eight years after the creation of the Arizona Health Care Cost Containment System, only one-half of the managed care organizations could satisfy HCFA's standards for encounter data (McCall et al., 1993).

Data on Medicare managed care enrollees' utilization may be available in the future, however. Through various demonstration projects, HCFA will be testing plans' ability to provide encounter data to support program monitoring efforts.

Survey Data

Survey data that document enrollees' access-related experiences and satisfaction with their managed care plans are also now limited. Although some Medicare managed care enrollee survey data are available, these are not ideal for use in measuring the access to care of these beneficiaries. The MCBS, for example, includes only a small number of Medicare managed care enrollees in its sample, which limits the ability to analyze access issues by subgroups of enrolled population.[9] More importantly, the items used in the MCBS were not developed specifically for evaluating the access of beneficiaries in managed care settings. Although some traditional survey measures of access can be used for beneficiaries across all delivery models, other items are less meaningful for beneficiaries enrolled in managed care plans. In response to changes in the Medicare program, HCFA at present plans to supplement the MCBS sample and questionnaire beginning with the fall 1996 round. These changes are designed to facilitate comparisons of Medicare FFS and managed care enrollees.

To test the feasibility of using a beneficiary survey for monitoring access in the Medicare managed care program, PPRC has contracted with MPR to develop and field a survey of Medicare risk-contract plan enrollees and disenrollees. Four groups were distinguished for survey sampling and questionnaire design purposes: new enrollees, continuous enrollees, disenrollees (who returned to FFS Medicare), and plan switchers (who disenrolled from one risk plan and joined another). The project entails both the examination of sampling issues and the development and testing of measures that reflect the influence of Medicare managed care on beneficiary access. Insight gained in these areas may inform future efforts to supplement or revise the MCBS.

Other Data for Access Monitoring

A system for monitoring access will need to rely on data from a variety of sources in order to obtain a multidimensional perspective. Additional types of data that are not applicable to the traditional Medicare FFS program are available or could be developed.

Information on the characteristics and processes of the private health plans that serve Medicare beneficiaries could be used in an access monitoring system. Data on health plan premiums, enrollment size, service area, and benefits are now available. Descriptive information on the comparison of plan networks could also be analyzed and monitored over time, although analyses would be complicated by factors such as group contracting arrangements. Such information could be supplemented by plan-level survey data on activities, practices, or characteristics that may influence enrollees' access to care.

Administrative data on plan enrollment and disenrollment could be used as a component of an access-monitoring system. Available information about enrollees and disenrollees includes demographic variables, Medicaid status, and Medicare managed care plan history. These data permit monitoring of trends in rates of enrollment and disenrollment by subgroups of the beneficiary population and by subgroups of the Medicare managed care plan population. The value of using plan-level beneficiary survey data for evaluating access to care has been demonstrated in a study by the Office of Inspector General of the U.S. Department of Health and Human Services (1995).

Data on beneficiary appeals of plan decisions might also serve as a component of a Medicare managed care access monitoring approach.[10] Changes in the rates of appeals or the types of appeals filed by beneficiaries could indicate changes in access to care generally or for specific services.

Vulnerable Groups

As is true in traditional monitoring, identification of vulnerable groups for targeted monitoring efforts will continue to be important. Certain groups of beneficiaries may, on average, be more susceptible to difficulties obtaining access to care in the managed care environment.

Some of the same groups that have been identified as vulnerable in FFS Medicare may also be at risk for access problems in Medicare managed care. As already discussed, these groups include black beneficiaries and those who live in urban Health Professional Shortage Areas or urban poverty areas. Beneficiaries in these groups could continue to be at risk to the extent that the underlying reasons for their vulnerability are unaffected by the managed care delivery system; for example, where access problems stem from a lack of transportation. On the other hand, access for beneficiaries in these vulnerable groups may in some cases be improved. This would be true, for instance, where vulnerability stemmed from financial barriers to access that could be reduced in managed care plans, depending on the premium and cost-sharing arrangements.

In addition to the groups already identified, two general categories of beneficiaries may be particularly at risk for access problems under managed care delivery systems. The first group is those who may not receive adequate care from health plans responding inappropriately to cost-containment incentives. Beneficiaries with a chronic medical condition who need resource-intensive care on an ongoing basis could be included in this category, as could beneficiaries with certain medical conditions that require specialized care. The second group is those who have difficulty navigating systems of care, whether because of medical, psychological, economic, sociological, or other factors. Beneficiaries who already have difficulties obtaining care under the FFS system may find that managed care systems pose additional challenges.

Because beneficiaries in the groups that may be particularly vulnerable under managed care may be difficult to identify in advance, proxies for beneficiaries in these categories will need to be identified for targeted monitoring efforts. For example, the study of access in Medicare risk-contracting plans being conducted by MPR for PPRC will analyze the access to care of disabled beneficiaries and those over age 85 as proxy categories for beneficiaries in these vulnerable groups.

Issues for Monitoring Access

Beyond the fundamental question of how best to monitor access for beneficiaries in managed care plans, the growth in managed care enrollment raises a number of additional issues that will need to be addressed in designing a monitoring approach.

Implications for Traditional Access Monitoring

The increasing availability and use of managed care arrangements in the Medicare program must be taken into account in traditional program-monitoring approaches. The majority of beneficiaries obtain their health care through Medicare's traditional FFS program and are expected to continue to do so for the near future. But the fact that most beneficiaries have the option to use other arrangements and that an increasing number choose to do so has implications for the ability to interpret the traditional measures and trends in utilization now used in monitoring access.

Beneficiaries' selection among alternative health plans may result in differences in the demographic and health-status characteristics of the underlying enrollment populations. These differences are likely to be reflected in any access-measurement efforts unless adequate adjustments that reflect underlying population differences can be made. Identification of appropriate risk adjusters will be important for interpreting trends in access as the pool of enrolled beneficiaries changes over time. Development of adjusters for outcomes and other types of measures is still at an early stage, however, and specific adjusters are not widely agreed upon. (For a discussion of the methodological issues, see Iezzoni [1994].) It is likely that the importance of making adjustments to measures will vary for different measures, assuming that some types are more sensitive to underlying characteristics of the population.

Implications of Expanding Plan Options

Policy proposals to expand the range of health-plan options that are available to Medicare beneficiaries also would have implications for access-monitoring approaches. Medicare restructuring proposals developed by Congress and by the Administration would open up the Medicare program to a wider variety of health plans. The Seven-Year Balanced Budget Reconciliation Act (passed by Congress in November 1995 and vetoed by the President), for example, would have expanded options under Medicare to include medical savings accounts, provider-sponsored organizations, preferred provider organizations, and so-called unrestricted FFS health plans, which would place no constraints on utilization or provider choice. These options could range widely in terms of benefits provided (beyond the basic Medicare benefits package), cost-sharing arrangements, lock-in requirements, provide incentives, and care-management strategies. Wide variation would be expected both across plan types and within categories of plans.

Monitoring access to care under a restructured program would be challenged by limitations in both measures and data. Increased diversity in health-plan options would mean that only those access measures that are unbiased for health care delivery models would be useful for monitoring at the program level. For example, measure of the extent to which beneficiaries fail to obtain or delay obtaining necessary medical care could continue to serve as an indicator of access problems. Access measures dependent on the delivery model or plan characteristics, such as those designed to assess the effects of cost-sharing arrangements, out-of-network restrictions, or the specialist referral process, on the other hand, would not be universally applicable or interpretable at the program level. Such indicators might instead be used selectively at the level of plan-specific monitoring.

The availability of data that are of uniform type and quality will greatly determine the ability to undertake access-monitoring efforts. Under a Medicare program restructured to provide a wider variety of health-plan options to beneficiaries, baseline access-monitoring efforts may need to rely primarily on beneficiary survey data in the absence of uniform information on service utilization. As more beneficiaries use alternatives to traditional FFS Medicare, the question of whether the program's ability to protect beneficiaries' access to appropriate care is compromised by the absence of these data will need to be resolved.

Conclusion

Our examination of the issues to be addressed in devising an access-monitoring system for Medicare managed care has shown that significant challenges remain to be addressed. Further work will be needed to identify access measures, data, and groups for targeted monitoring efforts.

Even as steps are taken toward developing the framework and methods for monitoring access in Medicare managed care, the program continues its evolution and rapid growth. Because of the need to use measures unbiased for health care delivery mode in programwide monitoring, identifying the source of access problems and potential policy solutions could become increasingly difficult in a program of diverse plan options. As diversification occurs, more analytic work will be needed to develop access measures that are universally relevant, and increased efforts to ensure the comparability of data will be necessary.

Notes

1. At the end of 1995, 8.8 percent of beneficiaries were enrolled in a Medicare managed care plan under a risk contract, and 1.9 percent were enrolled in a plan paid on a reasonable-cost basis.
2. For example, the Congressional Budget Office (O'Neill, 1995) projects that under the Medicare Preservation Act passed in November 1995, 17.5 percent of beneficiaries would use alternative delivery systems by 1998, and 25.3 percent would do so by 2002.
3. Many of these empirical studies had normative underpinnings to their approaches. For a discussion of normative approaches to access, see the President's Commission for the Study of Ethical Problems in Medicine and Biomedical and Behavioral Research (1983).
4. In the context of Medicare access monitoring, provider participation describes the number or portion of providers actually serving Medicare beneficiaries, not merely the number who sign participating provider agreements.

5. This framework was originally developed by Gold (1995).
6. Indicators of this type have been used in the Medicare managed care program in several studies using data collected for research purposes. Examples of such studies include Retchin and Brown (1990) and Riley et al. (1994).
7. The most recent version (2.5) of the Health Plan Employer Data and Information Set (National Committee for Quality Assurance, 1995), commonly known as HEDIS, includes the number and percent of primary-care physicians accepting new patients among its measures of access and satisfaction.
8. For example, some beneficiaries may change their health plan to retain their usual source of care in cases where their primary-care physician leaves a plan.
9. The tenth round of the MCBS, administered in 1994, contained approximately 860 managed care enrollees.
10. These data are collected and have been analyzed by HCFA's contractor, Network Design Group, Inc. (Richardson, Phillips, and Conley, 1993).

References

Aday, L.: *At Risk in America. The Health and Health Care Needs of Vulnerable Populations in the United States.* San Francisco. Jossey-Bass Publishers, 1993.

Aday, L., and Andersen, R.: Equity of Access to Medical Care: A Conceptual and Empirical Overview. *Medical Care* 19 (12): 4–27, Supplement 1981.

Adler, G.: A Profile of the Medicare Current Beneficiary Survey. *Health Care Financing Review* 15 (4): 153–63, Summer 1994.

Anderson, R., and Aday, L.: Access to Medical Care in the U.S.: Realized and Potential. *Medical Care* 16 (7): 533–46, July 1978.

Berki, S. E., and Ashcraft, M. L.: On the Analysis of Ambulatory Utilization: An Investigation of the Roles of Need, Access and Price as Predictors of Illness and Preventive Services. *Medical Care* 17 (12): 1163–81, December 1979.

Bindman, A. B., Grumbach, K., Osmond, D., et al.: Preventable Hospitalizations and Access to Health Care. *Journal of the American Medical Association* 274 (4): 305–11, July 26, 1995.

Escarce, J. J., Epstein, K. R., Colby, D. C., and Schwartz, J. S.: Racial Differences in the Use of Medical Procedures and Diagnostic Tests by Elderly Medicare Enrollees. *American Journal of Public Health* 83 (7): 948–54, July 1993.

Gold, M.: Unpublished working paper. Washington, DC. Mathematica Policy Research, Inc., 1995.

Health Care Financing Administration: *1994 Influenza Immunizations Paid for by Medicare.* Washington. U.S. Government Printing Office, 1995a.

Health Care Financing Administration: *Monitoring the Impact of Medicare Physician Payment Reform on Utilization and Access.* Washington. U.S. Government Printing Office, 1995b.

Iezzoni, L., ed.: *Risk Adjustment for Measuring Health Outcomes.* Ann Arbor, MI. Health Administration Press, 1994.

Langwell, K. M., and Hadley, J. P.: Insights from the Medicare HMO Demonstrations. *Health Affairs* 9 (1): 75–84, Spring 1990.

McCall, N., Korb, J., Cran, M., et al.: *Evaluation of Arizona's Health Care Cost Containment System Demonstration—Third Implementation and Operation Report.* San Francisco. Laguna Research Associates, 1993.

Millman, M., ed.: *Access to Health Care in America.* Washington, DC. National Academy Press, 1993.

Moy, E., and Hogan, C.: Access to Needed Follow-Up Services: Variations Among Different Medicare Populations. *Archives of Internal Medicine* 153: 1815–23, August 9, 1993.

National Committee for Quality Assurance: *HEDIS 2.5: Updated Specifications for HEDIS 2.0.* Washington, DC. January 1995.

O'Neill, J.: Letter to the Committee on Ways and Means, U.S. House of Representatives. Washington, DC. Congressional Budget Office, November 22, 1995.

Palmer, R., Clark, L., and Lawthers, A.: *DEMPAQ: A Project to Develop and Evaluate Methods to Promote Ambulatory Care Quality: Final Report.* Easton, MD. Delmarva Foundation for Medical Care, Inc., 1994.

Penchansky, R., and Thomas, J. W.: The Concept of Access: Definition and Relationship to Consumer Satisfaction. *Medical Care* 19 (2): 127–40, February 1981.

Physician Payment Review Commission: *Annual Report to Congress 1996.* Washington, DC. 1996.

Physician Payment Review Commission: *Monitoring Access of Medicare Beneficiaries.* Report No. 94-2. Washington, DC. 1994.

Physician Payment Review Commission: *Monitoring Access of Medicare Beneficiaries.* Report No. 95-1. Washington, DC. 1995.

President's Commission for the Study of Ethical Problems in Medicine and Biomedical and Behavioral Research: *Securing Access to Health Care.* Washington. U.S. Government Printing Office, 1983.

Retchin, S. M., and Brown, B.: Management of Colorectal Cancer in Medicare Health Maintenance Organizations. *Journal of General Internal Medicine* 5 (2): 110–14, March/April 1990.

Richardson, D., Phillips, J., and Conley, D.: *A Study of Coverage Denial Disputes Between Medicare Beneficiaries and HMOs.* Pittsford, NY. Network Design Group, Inc., September 1993.

Riley, G. F., Potosky, A. L., Libitz, J. D., and Brown, M. L.: Stage of Cancer at Diagnosis for Medicare HMO and Fee-for-Service Enrollees. *American Journal of Public Health* 84 (10): 1598–1604, October 1994.

U.S. Department of Health and Human Services: *Medicare Risk HMO Performance Indicators.* Office of Inspector General. Washington. U.S. Government Printing Office, October 1995.

Weissman, J. S., Gatsonis, C., and Epstein, A. M.: Rates of Avoidable Hospitalization by Insurance Status in Massachusetts and Maryland. *Journal of the American Medical Association* 268 (17): 2388–94, November 4, 1992.

CHAPTER

18

USING CONSUMER SATISFACTION SURVEYS TO ASSESS QUALITY OF CARE: CURRENT PRACTICE AND ISSUES

Marsha Gold and Judith Wooldridge[1]

Introduction

Managed care plans are a substantial and growing share of the market for health insurance (Gabel et al. 1994). Because managed care integrates financing with service delivery, measuring and overseeing quality and access to health care within individual plans is very important (Kongstvedt 1993). Some of this can be done by formal assessment of clinical quality using medical records, administrative systems, or similar information. However, these sources are not well suited to measuring the perceptions of the customers of health plans, for example. For identifying consumer perspectives, surveys are a very useful tool, providing more systematic data to complement information from grievance systems and other sources of consumer feedback. Surveys are receiving increased attention (AHCPR 1995) as a component of Total Quality Management and Continuous Quality Improvement to enhance quality of care and service (James 1994, Press et al. 1992, Inguanzo 1992, Kritchevsky and Simmons 1991, Berwick 1989). Though some controversy exists about

Adapted from *Health Care Financing Review* 16 (4): 155–173.

the role of consumer information in monitoring quality (Goldfield, Pine, and Pine 1991), most researchers, policymakers, and managers agree that consumer satisfaction is an important measure of quality and hence, of system and health plan performance (Cleary and McNeil 1988, Davies and Ware 1988a, Press 1994). However, because many of these applications are operational, they are poorly documented in the published literature, a shortcoming we aim to remedy with this chapter.

Focus and Approach

This chapter discusses the nature and use of consumer surveys as a means of generating information on satisfaction with individual health plans, including health maintenance organizations (HMOs), other managed care products such as preferred provider organizations (PPOs) and point-of-service (POS) arrangements, and traditional indemnity insurance. We summarize current knowledge about how widely surveys are used or encouraged by diverse parties such as individual managed care plans, government and voluntary oversight agencies, community and consumer groups, and public and private purchasers of care. We review the different kinds of surveys (for example, all enrollees, system users, users of particular services), survey content, and survey methods. Next, we consider outstanding issues relevant to using consumer surveys to assess plan quality and particularly to compare health plans. We end with brief conclusions on the use of surveys as a tool for assessing care and recommend three types of activities to better support such efforts.

Our approach to analyzing surveys on consumer satisfaction with healthcare plans was shaped largely by the data available to us. Information about surveys of consumer satisfaction with managed care plans is evolving rapidly, and it is not part of the formal literature. Furthermore, most surveys are intended to address operational needs rather than research objectives. As a result, this chapter relies heavily on information from the "trade press" and unpublished materials. These were obtained by reviewing materials we had, making calls to a selection of large plans known or thought to be involved in survey efforts to obtain information on their use of surveys, and referencing bibliographies and collections maintained in the Group Health Association of America (GHAA) library.

Our methods generated information on the most publicized and broad-based surveys as of mid-1994. This chapter is not intended to provide a complete inventory of surveys. In addition, it contains only limited information on the nationwide prevalence of the approaches illustrated. These are not major constraints, as the focus of the chapter is conceptual, stressing methodology, purpose, and illustrative applications rather than empirical results.

Nature and Uses of Consumer Surveys by Diverse Parties

Use by Managed Care Plans for Internal Management

While consumer surveys are used more widely today by managed care plans than in the past, the more established HMOs have long used such surveys. These surveys were generally initiated to support internal plan activities related to marketing and quality assurance (Kongstvedt 1993). Although most plans developed their approaches independently, there are now several examples of collective efforts by plans similar in management or philosophy.

A recently completed national survey of managed care plans documents the widespread use of consumer surveys by managed care plans. Virtually all HMOs (over 95 percent) and about half (55 percent) of the PPOs surveyed report that they conduct consumer surveys to monitor care (Gold et al. 1995b). Survey data are used to measure enrollee satisfaction and support such functions as strategic planning and marketing; improving quality; provider profiling and payment; and responding to employer requests. The more sophisticated plans use consistent survey methods over time to monitor trends and issues requiring management attention.

Surveys of new enrollees and of disenrollees are most likely to be conducted to support strategic planning and marketing. Some plans also survey area residents not enrolled in the plan to establish external benchmarks and identify opportunities for or barriers to growth. Plans will occasionally target special groups such as smokers or pregnant women to assess their special needs and their satisfaction with services.

Surveys of consumer satisfaction with various aspects of healthcare and health insurance are important input into efforts to improve quality and retain plan members (Packer-Tursman 1994). Such surveys capture information on users and nonusers of care and therefore are valuable sources of information on barriers to access. Plans vary in whether they ask individuals to answer questions about satisfaction with services they may not have used but about which they may have an opinion. To elicit information on how users of services perceive that care, plans may survey a sample of people using specific services (most often physician visits or specific hospitalizations, but also ancillary services) on their satisfaction with that specific service encounter. The success of using surveys to support quality improvement depends both on creating a structure through which results are reviewed, changes are identified, and improvements are charted, and on a commitment by staff to these activities (Kritchevsky and Simmons 1991).

In recent years, more surveys have been conducted to assess performance of individual providers or provider groups (as opposed to the plan as a whole). These techniques have been pioneered by network and independent practitioner association (IPA) models, which because of more dispersed physician practices, have a greater desire for information that promotes socialization to the norms of care management and assists in network management. Provider-specific surveys are being used to profile physician practices and compare peer profiles, to modify payment rates or provide bonuses, and to identify outliers—on the high and low ends—for closer review and potential exclusion from the network. The Group Health Association of America (GHAA 1993) reports that in 1992, 60 of the 326 plans responding to its Annual HMO Industry Survey used consumer satisfaction measures to adjust primary care physician payments, mostly on an annual basis. Among larger plans, the use of such techniques is even more common, with survey results serving as adjusters to physician compensation and also as input to decisions on physician contract renewals (Gold et al. 1995b). The most well-known applications of surveys involve sampling panel members of each physician or provider group to assess patient satisfaction, and using the results in provider payment calculations (Morain 1992).

Plans are also using surveys of individual provider performance to develop provider report cards. U.S. Healthcare, for example, develops report cards for individual practices by surveying members' use of primary care, specialists, and hospitals. These surveys focus on specific encounters or practices. At least one Kaiser plan uses its member surveys to develop quantitative ratings of physician and nonphysician providers, which are provided to facilities and physicians. Physicians are given comments written in on the surveys as part of their performance development system.

Some managed care plans enhance their ability to use survey data by participating in consortium survey efforts, typically involving other plans affiliated in some way. For example, Blue Cross and Blue Shield Association has done annual national benchmarking of consumer satisfaction since 1989, which member plans can use to aid in interpreting their performance. United HealthCare through its Center for HealthCare Policy and Evaluation has similarly developed a system to generate a performance measure that plans can use to benchmark themselves vis-à-vis others in the system, as well as to respond to external interests. The HMO Group, which consists of thirty member prepaid group practices, supports the regular exchange of data and information used to measure, report, and improve performance. They have sponsored a consumer survey biennially since 1988, again primarily as a benchmarking tool that can be used to identify quality improvement initiatives and opportunities at the plan level. Kaiser Central (headquarters) develops member and nonmember surveys that can be used to establish benchmarks and to compare the Kaiser plans with each other.

Use by Managed Care Plans for External Purposes

Though consumer surveys had their origin in internal operations, they are increasingly being applied for external uses. In particular, purchasers are requesting information from consumer surveys to help monitor plan performance, select plans to be offered, and facilitate employee choice. In 1991, 88 percent of the HMOs in the Group Health Association of America (GHAA) Annual HMO Industry Survey reported receiving requests for consumer satisfaction information from employers (GHAA 1992). Some HMOs probably meet these requests using data already collected for internal use purposes, but sometimes plans may initiate new studies to fill in the gaps or tailor information to employer specifications.

More recently, several plans have developed plan report cards, which have an external audience including both purchasers and enrollees or potential enrollees as well as a more broad-based national audience. These report cards typically include measures from administrative data, special studies, and consumer surveys. United HealthCare, U.S. Healthcare, and Kaiser Health Plan of Northern California are producing report cards (Zablocki 1994).

The issue of consistency in data definitions and measures, both across plans and across the kinds of requests made by purchasers, has created an interest in developing standardized tools that plans can use to respond to employer requests. The most prominent current effort was recently completed under the sponsorship of the National Committee for Quality Assurance (NCQA), which is the main accrediting body for HMOs.

NCQA's effort was based on version 2.0 of the Health Plan Employer Data and Information Set (HEDIS) (NCQA 1993). HEDIS 2.0 is a standardized list of about 60 measures of quality, access and patient satisfaction, membership and utilization, and finance. It does not mandate a standardized measure of consumer satisfaction, though its appendix provides as examples both the second edition of the Group Health Association of America's Consumer Satisfaction Survey and the

Employee Health Care Value Survey, which includes most of the GHAA instrument along with other batteries.

NCQA's pilot project involved 21 health plans from across the country selected for diversity of model-type, size, geographic location, and type of information system (NCQA 1995). The goal was to develop a report card based on a subset of HEDIS performance measures consistently defined across plans and audited by NCQA, with the experience serving to refine HEDIS 2.0. The pilot moved beyond HEDIS 2.0 in the area of consumer satisfaction, sponsoring a survey using the GHAA Consumer Satisfaction Survey instrument (second edition) with the intention of identifying a subset of the items that will be meaningful to consumers. While HEDIS 2.0 was developed chiefly to serve the needs of commercial insurers, NCQA (with support from HCFA and states) has a grant from the Packard Foundation to develop an adaptation suitable for measuring care received from publicly supported Medicaid enrollees in managed care.

Use by External Parties to Address Public Accountability, Oversight, and Community Assessment

The chief mechanisms for ensuring public accountability and oversight of health plans are state licensure, voluntary certification as a federally qualified HMO, and accreditation by voluntary organizations. Rarely do the regulatory entities or their agents conduct plan-based consumer surveys. However, they sometimes require or encourage plans to conduct surveys, and they verify that this and other requirements are met. These verification activities vary in nature and extent.

Accreditation programs for managed care plans have become much more established over the past few years. NCQA currently is the principal body accrediting HMOs (Gold et al. 1995b). NCQA requires that plans have mechanisms to protect and enhance membership satisfaction with plan services, including membership satisfaction surveys, studies of reasons for disenrollment, and evidence that the organization uses this information to improve the quality of its service. Relevant documentation (i.e., results of member satisfaction and disenrollment surveys) is reviewed by an NCQA team during the on-site review for accreditation. NCQA also requires, as part of a managed care organization credentialing system, a periodic performance appraisal of providers. This appraisal includes information from quality assurance activity, risk and utilization management, member complaints, and member satisfaction surveys. Current NCQA accreditation requirements do not require plans to be capable of producing HEDIS 2.0. However, we have been told that plans believe they will ultimately need to provide HEDIS 2.0 for accreditation and thus are gearing up for it as part of their accreditation activities.

As managed care grows, oversight likely will as well and with it the use of surveys. The last round of health reform deliberations emphasized oversight of managed care plans and proposals, mostly not implemented at this point, for the central collection of satisfaction data. The Clinton Administration's Health Security Act, for example, called for the AHCPR to administer a consumer survey on access, use of services, health outcomes, and patient satisfaction by plan and by state (Title V.A Section 5004). Consumer satisfaction surveys have been built into some state reform efforts as well. Two states leading the reform effort—Minnesota and Washington—are working through public-private partnerships to find ways to disseminate information on quality of care, including information from consumer surveys. A 1994 survey of senior state officials sponsored by The Robert Wood Johnson Foundation found that fewer than ten were currently involved in developing consumer satisfaction data by health plan, and that most such efforts were at an early stage. However, 73 percent of those responding perceived that data on health system and health plan performance were very important for health reform (Gold, Burnbauer, and Chu 1995).

Some plan-based consumer surveys have been sponsored independently by consumer and community organizations, occasionally with external funding. Two examples are the plan-specific consumer satisfaction survey information on 46 plans that was included as part of a detailed report on HMOs and other managed care products in *Consumer Reports* magazine (Consumer's Union 1992), and the Central Iowa Health Survey, funded by the John A. Hartford Foundation. The latter was a pilot study for the population-provided data component of the patient-centered Community Health Management Information System (CHMIS), which forms the core of the John A. Hartford Foundation's Community Health Management Initiative launched in 1991 (Allen 1993). CHMIS is intended to develop a blended data set incorporating claims, survey, and other kinds of data from competing organizations at multiple levels, including health plans, hospitals, and doctors' offices.

Use by Purchasers in Commercial, Medicare and Medicaid Markets

Purchaser-sponsored surveys represent a relatively new trend, and sponsors are, for the most part, the largest purchasers. Some surveys are sponsored by a single purchaser, while others involve groups of purchasers. The broader the purchaser coalition, the less distinction there is between this approach and community-based approaches. Most of these surveys are sponsored by employers, while fewer have been sponsored by Medicare or Medicaid so far (though this could change).[2]

The distinguishing feature of these surveys is that they involve estimates of satisfaction specific to the purchaser's population relative to the health plan overall. Leading examples include the Bank of America/Bay Area Business Group on Health (personal communication August 1994);[3] the Minnesota State Employees (State of Minnesota Joint Labor-Management Committee on Health Plans 1993a and 1993b); the Federal Employees Health Benefits Program (Francis 1994); and the employer consortium of Xerox, GTE, and Digital Equipment Corporation (Allen 1994). These employer-sponsored surveys represent three private employers, one state government employer, and the federal government.

In addition to corporate sponsors, management consultants and survey research firms are the other major sponsor of surveys aimed at the employer market. Potentially the largest such effort, the approach developed by the National Research Corporation (NRC) (1994), rests on a methodology that involves an ongoing panel drawing on 200,000 volunteer households. NRC also conducts customized surveys for a number of managed care plans (for example, CIGNA and Family Health Plan), and markets plan-specific results by geographic areas. Other firms such as Novalis (Ribner and Stewart 1993) and Towers Perrin (HMO Manager's Letter 1992a; 1992b; 1994) have conducted surveys on employee satisfaction with health plans, but the results are rarely plan-specific.

Externally sponsored consumer surveys are used less extensively in publicly financed programs such as Medicare and Medicaid though this is changing as managed care enrollment in these programs grows. Medicare does not routinely generate plan-based consumer information for use in monitoring managed care plans. Medicare mounts a continuing Current Beneficiary Survey. Periodic surveys that do not involve plan-specific estimates have been used in sponsored evaluations (e.g., Brown et al. 1993) and to address specific programmatic issues like disenrollment (Porrell et al. 1992). A recent HCFA initiative recommended using validated surveys to evaluate the quality of care and patient satisfaction with various aspects of the health care received by managed care plans (Delmarva Foundation for Medical Care, Inc. 1994).

Consumer surveys generating plan-specific estimates also are not common among Medicaid programs currently, though their use is growing. Because of the shared federal-state structure of Medicaid, states are more likely than the federal government to sponsor consumer surveys that are plan-specific, though federal interest in this area has expanded, particularly for demonstration projects involved in broad-based reforms. An early example of state use of surveys for the Medicaid population comes from California, which sponsored a 13-plan survey for 3 years (in the mid-1970s) to monitor prepaid health plan quality in response to highly publicized problems (Ware et al. 1981). Consumer information has been used in some national evaluations (for example, the Arizona Health Care Cost-Containment System) and will be used to support evaluations of 1115 waiver programs now being implemented. Some state Medicaid programs include consumer surveys as part of their quality monitoring activity. As of September 1992, 8 of 25 Medicaid agencies surveyed required HMOs to conduct patient satisfaction surveys; 7 conduct their own surveys, to assess recipient satisfaction (USDHHS 1992). More recent efforts include a survey of Medicaid recipients in Maryland that the state is fielding with Robert Wood Johnson Foundation funding, as well as consumer surveys conducted by states participating in a demonstration of the Medicaid Quality Assurance Reform Initiative (Felt 1995). We know of no efforts to use plan-based estimates from these surveys to support beneficiary choice and Medicaid has no parallel to the existing Medicare Current Beneficiary Survey. However, the Physician Payment Review Commission (1994) recommended that Congress fund such a survey based on research showing its feasibility for generating state-based estimates (Gold et al. 1995a). This work also highlighted the special issues that apply to surveying low-income and Medicaid populations, including limitations of the Medicaid eligibility files as a sampling frame, biases created by families not having telephones, and eligibility turnover.

Medicare and Medicaid may become more involved in sponsoring plan-based surveys to generate consumer information. HCFA contracted in 1994 for a study in which prototypes of consumer information materials will be developed. The data-based approaches are likely to involve the use of surveys (Research Triangle Institute 1994).

Survey Focus, Instrument Content, and Methods

Variations in Survey Focus

Surveys of consumer satisfaction with health plans vary in several ways, the most important of which are illustrated in Figure 1. First, surveys differ in terms of the population they are intended to represent. That population may be in a given geographic area, in a particular plan, or in the specific purchaser's share of the plan. The Novalis survey is an example of a geographically based survey that provides estimates of how satisfaction varies by type of plan, though it is not market-specific. Community-based efforts, like the Central Iowa Health Survey, and plan-based surveys provide plan-specific estimates. Most purchaser surveys focus on the employer-specific population in a plan.

Surveys differ according to whether they focus on all those eligible for the plan or on healthcare users only. Within each of the three types of populations (geographic, plan-specific, and employer-specific), we find surveys that focus on either all eligibles or users. The focus may have important implications for the results and how they are interpreted. The distinction is particularly important for surveys involving PPOs, because use in itself may be an important measure of satisfaction. Even for HMOs, surveys with the same questions may yield dissimilar estimates depending on whether all enrollees or only users respond. The two focuses persist largely because there are strong opinions, but no consensus, among survey developers about how information on satisfaction with use should

Figure 1 Varying Features of Samples for Consumer Satisfaction Surveys of Managed Care Plans

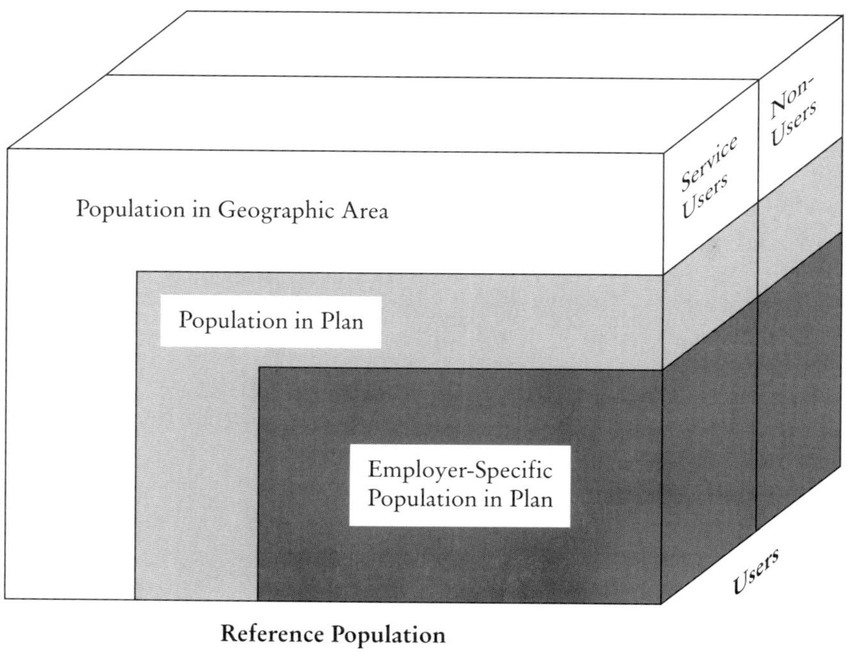

be collected. It is possible that this occurs in part because developers have different goals for the survey, for example, marketing or performance evaluation and quality improvement.

Although Figure 1 helps to create a basic understanding of survey population and focus, it simplifies reality. First, people move from one category to another over time, so changes in satisfaction may reflect changes in population composition as much as changes in plan quality or access. In addition, moves across categories vary across plans and types of populations (for example, Medicaid versus commercial enrollees), creating a potential source of bias in trend estimates. Second, the unit of analysis may not always be the person but may be a user of a particular service or provider, two "targets" common among internal surveys designed to support plan management efforts. Finally, "population" may be variously defined. Estimates may be based on a sample of all individuals in one of the three categories or only on those of a particular type (for example, only insured individuals, only commercial group enrollees). In addition, items may be framed to capture information on the household, the insurance unit, the subscriber, the respondent, or a child.

Item Content

Research studies since 1980 on consumer satisfaction and other performance measures were recently summarized by Miller and Luft (1994). Their analysis highlights the importance of item content, because the studies found that satisfaction varies for different dimensions of care.

Many of today's surveys designed to develop plan-based measures of satisfaction are based on the GHAA Consumer Satisfaction Survey instrument. This instrument was based on others, beginning with satisfaction measures developed in the 1970s with grants from the National Center for Health Services Research and Development (Ware and Snyder 1975; Ware et al. 1983) that were adapted for the Health Insurance Experiment (Davies et al. 1986) and later for the Medical Outcomes Study (Marshall et al. 1993). Table 1 summarizes the evolution of these related satisfaction measures.

This GHAA battery has subsequently been used by the Health Institute at the New England Medical Center in the Iowa Health Survey and other projects. In addition to batteries from the GHAA Consumer Satisfaction Survey, the Iowa Survey Instrument included a modified version of the inpatient hospital quality trends (HQT) which measures satisfaction with the most recent hospitalization (if within three months) (Meterko et al. 1990) and the visit satisfaction questionnaire (VSQ), which captures satisfaction with the last physician visit (if within four

Table 1 Evolution of Consumer Satisfaction Surveys

Battery	Development	Items	Sources	Content	Response Scale	Major Changes from Source	Primary Use
PSQ-I	1972–75	80	Literature reviews, content review of earlier instruments, and item generation studies produced pool of 2,300 items.[1–3]	Accessibility and convenience; availability of services; continuity of care; finances; interpersonal aspects; technical quality; facilities; and general satisfaction	Strongly agree; Agree; Not sure; Disagree; Strongly disagree	NA	Multiple tests to identify dimensions of care and services; test-scaling assumptions, score reliability; response bias; and validity
PSQ-II	1972–75	68	Same as PSQ-I and results of PSQ-I studies. Items were revised to emphasize or clarify object of measurement; improve score distributions, and reduce ambiguity.[2]	Same as PSQ-I	Strongly agree; Agree; Not sure; Disagree; Strongly disagree	Shorter than PSQ-I; more focused on empirically confirmed dimensions of care	Multiple field tests to replicate methodological studies; describe healthcare attitudes of adults across practices, cities, counties, and states
PSQ-43	1971–77	43	42 PSQ-II items and "crisis in health care" item from CHAS-NORC[2,3,8–10]	Same as PSQ-I; additional item does not assess attitudes toward own medical care and services	Strongly agree; Agree; Not sure; Disagree; Strongly disagree	Shorter than PSQ-II; retains fundamental concepts	Support assessments of health care (along with other batteries) in omnibus surveys; used in this way to compare health insurance plans in the HIE; develop norms for U.S. population in CHAS-NORC survey
PSQ-III	1984–85	50	PSQ-II items; pilot tests of new items written to distinguish financial and physical access[11,12]	Interpersonal manner; communication; technical quality; financial security; time spent with physician; access to care; and general satisfaction	Strongly agree; Agree; Not sure; Disagree; Strongly disagree	New items on financial security	Medical Outcomes Study
VSQ	1985–86	9	PSQ-III[13–15]	Physical access; telephone access; office wait; appointment wait; time spent with physician; communication; interpersonal aspects; technical quality; and overall care	Excellent; Very good; Good; Fair; Poor	Reduced in length to one item per concept; uses EVGFP response scale	Medical Outcomes Study

continued

Table 1 *Continued*

Battery	Development	Items	Sources	Content	Response Scale	Major Changes from Source	Primary Use
GHAA CSS (First Edition)	1987–88	35	Based on PSQ-III items, rewritten to be used with EVGFP response scale. (Satisfaction battery represents 1 of 3 included in entire survey; others capture prior use/experience with plan and sociodemographics.)[16]	Access; finances; technical quality; communication; choice; continuity; interpersonal care; outcomes; overall care; and general satisfaction	Excellent; Very good; Good; Fair; Poor	Uses EVGFP response scale; collapsed PSQ-III items to yield survey while retaining content; added outcomes	Made available to GHAA member plans and employers for use in producing plan-level estimates for employers
GHAA CSS (Second Edition)	1991	35 Care Services 14 Plan	Same care and services battery as GHAA CSS (first edition). Content of new satisfaction battery based on review of literature, individual plan surveys, and focus groups.[14]	As in GHAA CSS (first edition), but with the following additional items: services covered; information from plan; paperwork; costs of care; and overall plan	Excellent; Very good; Good; Fair; Poor	Addition of battery to yield ratings of selected managed care plan features in response to requests from plans and employers	Same as GHAA CSS (first edition)

Source: Davies, A.: Personal communication, 1994.

Notes: PSQ is Patient Satisfaction Questionnaire. VSQ is Visit Satisfaction Questionnaire. GHAA is Group Health Association of America. CSS is Consumer Satisfaction Survey. CHAS-NORC is Center for Health Administration Studies–National Opinion Research Center. HIE is Health Insurance Experiment. EVGFP is excellent, very good, good, fair, or poor.

[1](Ware and Snyder, 1975).

[2]Ware, J. E., Snyder, M. K., and Wright, W. R.: *Development and Validation of Scales to Measure Patient Satisfaction With Health Care Services*: Volume I of a Final Report. Part A: Review of Literature, Overview of Methods, and Results Regarding Construction of Scales. Pub. No. PB-288-329. Springfield, VA. National Technical Information Service, 1976a.

[3]Ware, J. E., Snyder, M. K., and Wright, W. R.: *Development and Validation of Scales to Measure Patient Satisfaction With Health Care Services*: Volume I of a Final Report. Part B: Results Regarding Scales Constructed From the Patient Satisfaction Questionnaire and Measures of Other Health Care Perceptions. Pub. No. PB-288-330. Springfield, VA. National Technical Information Service, 1976b.

[4]Ware, J. E., Wright, W. R., Synder, M. K., and Chu, G. C.: Consumer Perceptions of Health Care Services: Implications for the Academic Medical Community. *Journal of Medical Education* 50 (9): 839–848, 1975.

[5]Doyle, B. J., and Ware, J. E.: Physician Conduct and Other Factors That Influence Patient Satisfaction. *Journal of Medical Education* 52 (10): 793–801, 1977.

[6]Ware, J. E.: Effects of Acquiescent Response Set on Patient Satisfaction Ratings. *Medical Care* 16 (4): 327–336, 1978.

[7](Ware et al., 1983).

[8]Aday, L. A., Andersen, R., and Fleming, G. V.: *Health Care in the United States: Equitable for Whom?* Beverly Hills. Sage Publications, 1980.

[9]Marquis, M. R., Davies, A. R., and Ware, J. E.: Patient Satisfaction and Change in Medical Care Provider. *Medical Care* 21 (8): 821–829, 1983.

[10]Davies, A. R., Ware, J. E., Brook, R. H., and Peterson, J.: Consumer Acceptance of Prepaid and Fee-for-Service Medical Care: Results From a Randomized Control Trial. *Health Services Research* 21 (3): 429–452, 1986.

[11]Safran, D., Tarlov, A. R., and Rogers, W.: Primary Care Performance in Fee-for-Service and Prepaid Health Care Systems: Results From the Medical Outcomes Study. *Journal of the American Medical Association* 271 (20): 1579–1586, 1994.

[12](Marshall et al., 1993).

[13]Hays, R. D., and Ware, J. E.: Methods for Measuring Patient Satisfaction With Specific Medical Encounters. *Medical Care* 26 (4): 393–402, 1988.

[14](Davies and Ware, 1991).

[15](Rubin et al., 1993).

[16](Davies and Ware, 1988b).

months) (Rubin et al. 1993).[4] In addition to consumer satisfaction, the Iowa survey also measures health status through the SF-36 (Ware and Sherbourne 1992; Ware et al. 1993) and also included a pilot test of enrollees' ratings of management of care and coverage. The package of instruments is intended to be a reference set of batteries to be used individually or together for different purposes. This set of batteries has since been followed by the Employer Health Care Value Survey (EHCVS). The EHCVS satisfaction battery includes most items in the second edition of the GHAA Consumer Satisfaction Survey, augmented by a set of questions on the management of care and coverage (partially pilot tested in the Iowa survey). The EHCVS also includes the SF-36 and items on health risk behavior drawn from previous survey instruments.

Though GHAA's interest in sponsoring Davies and Ware to develop the Consumer Satisfaction Survey instrument was to promote consistency across surveys, most users have modified the instrument by adding and dropping items, adapting them to specific encounters or providers, and modifying the satisfaction categories. For example, the HMO Group survey instrument incorporates questions from the GHAA Consumer Satisfaction Survey but includes additional questions, for example, on prescriptions, lab tests, ease of choosing a primary care physician, and hospital care. There is also a module on out-of-plan visits. Many of these modifications reflect differences in philosophy and opinion about how certain methodological issues should be handled. The shortening of the instrument by omitting items may be intended to reduce respondent burden. It may also reflect a narrower set of purposes and individual user views on what is most valuable. While these adaptations, particularly the omission of items, make it impossible to compare plans on the nine scales, plans can be compared on matching retained items.

Adaptations of the GHAA instrument also illustrate differences in opinion about whether individuals should be asked to rate features of care they have not used, the relative emphasis on ratings of aspects of care versus reports on actual experiences; for whom the respondent should answer (for example, self versus family); and whether satisfaction should be requested, by proxy, for children.

There are other bodies of work on consumer satisfaction or related measures of health plans. For example, the Bank of America survey instrument includes satisfaction ratings and factual reports on process and outcomes of care (for example, Does this plan offer all the health services you need? How would you categorize the attitudes of doctors, nurses, and support staff serving you under this medical plan? In the past year have you had any illness or bad reaction caused by medicine your physician prescribed?). The instrument also has items that solicit information on health behaviors that may serve as markers of adverse selection based on incidence of health risks (for example, smoking, stress). It is distinguished mainly by its emphasis on the reporting of events rather than ratings of satisfaction, though both are included. The former have intuitive appeal to some purchasers, consumers, and health plan members. Current work is under way to identify better how surveys, particularly those with consumers as the intended audience, can be better grounded in an understanding of what information consumers really use to make decisions. For example, some say that knowing which providers are affiliated with a plan is more important to consumers than satisfaction information (Winslow 1994).

Because survey instruments have evolved independently, plans vary considerably in the instruments they use (Table 2). However, the availability of the GHAA survey has contributed to some consistency in use of instruments among plans that have recently initiated surveys. Of the 21 survey instruments we obtained from managed care plans, 10 of them draw on the GHAA satisfaction battery in whole or part, though 3 had modified the rating system (either using the response categories "satisfied" to "dissatisfied" or inventing new rating systems, such as 1 to 10 representing "unacceptable" to "excellent"). Some of them added items, for example, covering access to specialist care in greater detail and satisfaction with the facility appearance, staff demeanor and dress, and ease of parking. The length of these instruments varied from the 47-item GHAA survey (for a first-time baseline survey of plan satisfaction) to 9 items for a survey of satisfaction with specialist care.

Methodological Practices and Issues

Frequency, Mode of Administration, and Response Rates

Of the plans for which we have information, many reported using key surveys on a continual basis or at least annually. Plans were mixed between telephone, mail, and combined approaches. The extent to which plans are using surveys appears to be growing, particularly as more aim for NCQA accreditation, as survey models become more available, and as examples of applications become more publicized. However, the range of sophistication, uses, and methods vary considerably across plans, for example, we identified instances of quota sampling rather than random sampling.

Although in-person studies of satisfaction are sometimes conducted—mostly in focus groups—the predominant modes of administering plan-based surveys are telephone, mail, and mail with telephone follow-up. Of 21 surveys for which we have information on mode, 12

Table 2 Summary of Content of Plan-Based Consumer Surveys

Satisfaction with Aspect of Care or Service	Number of Plan-Based Surveys Included
Overall Quality and Satisfaction	21
Interpersonal Aspects	18
Communication or Information	18
Timeliness of Services	16
Intention to Recommend Organization	16
Technical Aspects	14
Time Spent with Providers	14
Access and Availability of Services	13
Intention to Use Organization Again	11
Satisfaction with Outcomes of Care	8
Choice or Continuity	8
Financial Aspects and Billing	8
Physical Environment	6

Note: Derived from 21 plan-based survey instruments collected from managed care organizations.

were administered by mail or mixed mode, and 9 were administered by telephone.

The advantages of mail surveys are lower expense and greater anonymity. Press, Ganey, and Malone (1992) insist on the importance of anonymity in collecting objective measures of satisfaction with hospital stays, citing differences in satisfaction level between the two modes (personal communication). The disadvantage of mail surveys is that they generally yield lower response rates (often less than 50 percent, though rates increase with follow-up mailings). Plans reported mail survey response rates to single-mailing surveys ranging from 30 percent to 60 percent.

Plans use telephone surveys almost as often as mail surveys to collect information on satisfaction, and many of them use computer-assisted interviewing, which reduces cost. Telephone response rates can be higher than response rates to single-mailing surveys, achieved through repeat calls to those not answering the first time. The lowest response rate to a plan telephone survey we identified was 60 percent. We found that some of the external surveys had response rates of 70 percent or more by telephone. However, the estimates frequently involve sampling with replacement to obtain a target sample size. Hence, the response rates for telephone surveys cannot readily be compared directly with mail surveys in which such techniques are not used.

Selection of Respondents

Respondents are typically members of the plan, though they can sometimes be the spouse of a member. They are usually asked about their own health care, but in some instances they are asked to respond in a general way, which implies they are answering for the family, or they are asked to respond specifically about their children's care.

Cultural and Ethnic Diversity

We were unable to identify from the materials collected how surveys account for cultural and ethnic diversity of members. This includes non-English speakers, the possibility of low levels of literacy (particularly for mail surveys), and any cultural differences in response sets, all of which might bias the results. One plan's approach to language on a mail survey is to express each item on the same instrument in English and Spanish. This issue is important, particularly as managed care penetration grows among low income populations, some of whom speak little English.

Sample Selection

We have very little information about sampling methods for the plan-based surveys, although most plans reference random samples. Having drawn a random sample, however, some plans appear to use quota sampling to collect a specified number of responses, while others describe fielding procedures that suggest attempts to complete all of the sample initially drawn. Packer-Tursman (1994) describes the increasingly targeted sampling methods being used by Kaiser Permanente. Satisfaction data across plans that use different sampling and fielding procedures will not be comparable. In addition, the quality and utility of the data obtained by individual plans obviously depends on whether the methods minimize potential bias and provide for generalizable estimates.

Type of Measurement

Existing surveys reflect at least three kinds of differences in how measures are developed. The first involves the emphasis on ratings versus reports, that is, whether consumers are asked to rate features of care and service or to report on actual events as they experience them. Ratings are more common, but interest in reports has grown because they are viewed by some as providing both the basis for more "objective" or "normative" performance standards, and potential substitutes for or complements to other sources of direct quality measurement.

The second difference involves the form of the scale. Historically, it had been most common to ask respondents to rate their care on some form of satisfied-dissatisfied scale or agree-disagree scale. Based on research on survey design (Ware and Hays 1988), some use a four-point scale running from "excellent" to "poor," which makes it easier to compare ratings across different features of care. It is also common to add a fifth category, "very good," making this a five-point scale. While such an approach may superficially appear imbalanced, this five-point part scale discriminates better among the large majority of respondents who typically cite care as either excellent or good.

The third difference in how measures are developed involves whether the emphasis is on composite scales constructed from multiple measures or individual items. For cross-plan comparisons of complex features of care that involve several dimensions of performance, scales are likely to provide more useful measures and more stable estimates. However, individual items may be more intuitively appealing and more useful for identifying specific aspects of performance that need improvement. In practice, it is not a matter of choosing one or another as both can be readily calculated.

Generating Comparable Plan-Based Measures

While there is considerable experience with using plan-based consumer surveys for internal management needs, the use of such data outside the plan is relatively recent. The use of survey data for cross-plan comparisons or other external purposes raises several operational issues that are otherwise nonexistent or less critical.[5] These issues are important to address if tools such as report cards are to be practical and relevant.

Developing a Sampling Frame

Health plans typically know their membership (or at least their users in the case of PPOs or indemnity products), and employers know their employees. However, lists that can be used to generate representative samples for the target population may not be available to other external survey sponsors (such as a community group). Such sponsors must therefore rely either on participating plans to voluntarily generate enrollment lists or samples or on population-based survey techniques. Plans may be hesitant to provide such lists, and they may be even precluded from participating because of confidentiality issues. Population-based sampling techniques are potentially feasible when enrollment is high in an area or can be predicted by known factors (for example, zip code). However, such techniques are generally not feasible for developing estimates for a large number of individual plans, many of which may represent only a small share of the population. This can be a particular problem in using surveys to compare health plans used by vulnerable populations like those on Medicaid, particularly since the heightened concerns for confidentiality often preclude sharing names with potential survey sponsors.

Ensuring Consistent Methods and Valid Results

There are two options for developing comparative information from consumers across health plans: collect it centrally or compile plan results individually. Central collection by a purchaser (or its agent) or other body allows for consistency in method across plans. If the central body is regarded as objective, this option is also likely to generate more credible data. Compiling individual plan reports (for example, from internal plan surveys) is less burdensome on the external entity and takes advantage of ongoing surveys. However, methods and results may not be comparable, and there may be incentives that introduce bias. A compromise is for the purchaser to provide or to agree, in conjunction with health plans, on a standardized methodology and to develop a mechanism for validating a sample of the data each plan then submits.

Developing Plan-, Purchaser-, or Purchaser Group–Specific Data

Individual purchasers (or groups of purchasers) may find plan-based data specific to their enrollees of greatest interest or value. However, only the largest employers are likely to be able to conduct surveys to collect such information. In any case, administrative costs may be high systemwide for a group-specific approach. Unfortunately, we know of little research comparing satisfaction across diverse purchasers, particularly those from a similar market segment (for example, comparing scores within commercial accounts rather than between commercial group accounts and Medicaid). Research is lacking on alternative ways of sampling or stratifying the analysis and on how these practices affect results and costs.

Market Segmentation and Risk Adjustment

Health plans serve differing market segments; hence, the characteristics of their enrollees vary. Some differences may be correlated with consumer responses to surveys, reflecting both objective differences (such as health risk or compliance) or response (for example, relative importance attributed to different characteristics or expectations). Differences of opinion exist about whether adjusting consumer responses for risk factors is appropriate, some arguing that consumer responses reflect the prevailing market and should not be adjusted. Among others who wish to compare across plans or markets, the issue is how to adjust for risk rather than whether to adjust. Unless these differences are accounted for in the measures developed from surveys, proponents of risk adjustment argue that the results may be misleading and biased in the plan comparisons they provide. For those wishing to adjust for risk, the issue can be addressed by separately reporting measures for different segments (such as group versus individual enrollees, commercial accounts versus Medicaid) or by standardizing the data to represent a standardized population across plans. However, the latter approach may not be feasible if some plans do not serve key segments of the population (in which case there are no performance data to apply to the standardized population mix). It may also imply that different standards of performance are acceptable across the population. For different purposes, it is important to present both unadjusted and adjusted data. Again, these issues are particularly germane to public purchasers.

Disenrollment Bias

The same degree of dissatisfaction may generate different disenrollment behavior across plans depending on the scope of the network. At one extreme, those dissatisfied with care under indemnity coverage retain the same health insurance but switch providers. At the other extreme, those dissatisfied under a tight network-based managed care plan with no point-of-service option may be much more likely to switch plans. Surveying only current users will overstate satisfaction and may lead to biased comparisons across plans and delivery systems with distinctly different designs.

Conclusions and Recommendations

There is a growing interest in plan-based measures of consumer satisfaction with access and quality. While there is no consensus on survey content or approach, there is a growing body of work and experience that can inform future developments. The content of instruments appears to be better developed than do the methods for using them. In addition, work on rating-type approaches is more advanced than work on report-type approaches. Yet, there are enough examples to conclude that methodologically sound surveys with high response rates are achievable. The two key constraints on this effort are likely to be resources and the sophistication of users, particularly given the large number of potential sponsors and estimates desired. Current experience also suggests that item content for consumer surveys needs to be based on an understanding of the varying objectives of the surveys and that no one instrument or survey methodology can meet all needs.

Our review and analysis suggest that research and policy support can strengthen considerably the ability to develop effective plan-based surveys. Our work suggests that both increasing the availability of information on consumer satisfaction survey methods and furthering the development of these methods is important.

Existing experience with plan-based surveys is decentralized. Communication about what is being done and how is ad hoc. Proprietary interests and concerns contribute to this situation because public disclosure could limit marketing opportunities or remove competitive advantages. Yet the content of many survey instruments is readily available. In addition, there are many ongoing efforts where disclosure would not appear to create disadvantages and a little effort would make it easier for individuals and organizations to find out about those efforts. These include, for example, publicly available and current compilations of existing survey instruments and documentation of their application; and guidance to help potential users understand the strengths, weaknesses, and potential applications of alternative survey purposes, the batteries appropriate for each, and what "best practices" may exist for specific purposes.

Our review also suggests that there are several areas that need methodological study if plan-based surveys become more common. Three particularly important areas for research are:

1. **Development of methods for risk adjusting plan-based survey results.** The socio-demographic mix in managed care plans varies, often considerably. To the extent these characteristics are correlated with survey response, they may lead to biased comparisons among health plans. From a public policy perspective, such biases are of particular concern since they can create incentives diametrically opposed to desirable social responses—for example, service to the poor, the chronically ill, and those with special social or medical needs. Research is needed to assess whether risk-adjustment makes a difference to consumer responses, and, if it does, to extend current risk adjustment work from medical to social risk adjustment and to adjusters suitable to survey data. In addition, alternative forms of adjustment and correction need review.
2. **Short-form batteries for diverse needs.** Many surveys are constrained in the number of items they can include, leading users to develop various "short forms" of items from larger batteries. Often these are developed in an ad hoc manner and are not well validated. The use of diverse surveys also reduces the ability to compare across plans. A systematic study comparing the validity of existing approaches and testing alternative new "short forms" would be a valuable contribution. While such forms exist for visit

and hospital services, they are much less developed for general enrollee surveys.

3. **Concordance between employer-specific, group enrollment, and plan-wide estimates of satisfaction.** Current trends will contribute to a proliferation of surveys for diverse populations. This can enhance consumer information but could add to administrative cost and burden. Yet there is little research to show how well more general measures predict sub-group responses and whether plan-wide measures are just as effective in discriminating among health plans based on performance.

A final note of caution: The healthcare system is sufficiently complex that diverse information could potentially be analyzed and distributed to consumers to help them assess access to health care provided in different health plans (see, for example, the review in Sofaer 1993). To provide it all could be expensive, could create overload, and could risk not communicating the most essential information. Moreover, consumers may not find satisfaction ratings particularly helpful.

Acknowledgments

This chapter draws substantially on work originally commissioned by the Agency for Health Care Policy and Research for use at a conference on "Consumer Survey Information in a Reformed Health Care System," September 28–29, 1994, Vienna, Virginia, jointly sponsored by the Agency for Health Care Policy and Research and The Robert Wood Johnson Foundation. The full report is included in the proceedings (AHCPR 1995) from that conference. Allyson Ross Davies provided advice on sources of information, reviewed and commented on drafts of the AHCPR work, and assisted in identifying the evolution of survey content. We also benefited from the advice of Jill Bernstein, Terry Shannon, and Sandy Robinson on the staff at AHCPR. At Mathematica, Barbara Foot, Rachel Thompson, and Sabrina Perrault provided research support. Daryl Hall edited the chapter. Ann Miles, Marjorie Mitchell, and Kathleen Donaldson provided secretarial support.

Notes

1. The authors are, respectively, Senior Fellow and Vice President with Mathematica Policy Research, Inc. This chapter is based to a considerable extent upon work commissioned by the Agency for Health Care Policy and Research under contract # 282-91-0027. The opinions are solely those of the authors.
2. This may reflect (1) a lesser extent of penetration by managed care in Medicare and (2) the fact that there are more employers than states.

3. The results were reported in *Bay Area Consumers' Checkbook* (1991), making this survey an early example of efforts to identify individual HMOs by name.
4. The VSQ is included as a model in the appendix of the second edition of the GHAA Consumer Satisfaction Survey) (Davies and Ware 1991).
5. Some of the same issues arise, however, when comparing subunits within plans (for example, centers, physicians, regions).

References

Agency for Health Care Policy and Research (AHCPR). 1995. *Conference Summary: Consumer Survey Information in a Reforming Health Care System*, AHCPR Pub. No. 95-0083. Rockville, MD: U.S. Department of Health and Human Services, Public Health Service.

Allen, H. M. 1993. "Consumer Assessment of Health and Health Care: The Central Iowa Pilot Study." Boston, MA: The Health Institute, New England Medical Center.

Allen, H., H. Darling, D. McNeill, et al. 1994. "The Employee Health Care Value Survey: Round One." Boston, MA: The Health Institute, New England Medical Center.

Bay Area Consumers' Checkbook. 1991. "Health Maintenance Organizations: Results of an Innovative Survey of Enrollees Conducted by the Bay Area Business Group on Health."

Berwick, D. M. 1989. "Continuous Improvement as an Ideal in Health Care." *New England Journal of Medicine*, 320 (1): 53–56.

Brown, R. S., J. W. Bergeron, D. G. Clement, et al. 1993. "The Medicare Risk Program for HMOs—Final Summary Report on Findings from the Evaluation." Princeton, NJ: Mathematica Policy Research, Inc.

Cleary, P., and B. J. McNeil. 1988. "Patient Satisfaction as an Indicator of Quality of Care." *Inquiry* (Spring): 25–36.

Consumers Union. 1992. "Health Care in Crisis: Are HMOs the Answer?" *Consumer Reports* (August): 519–31.

Davies, A., and J. E. Ware, Jr. 1988. "Involving Consumers in Quality of Care Assessment." *Health Affairs* (Spring): 33–48.

———. 1988b. *GHAA's Consumer Satisfaction Survey and User's Manual*, 1st ed. Washington, DC: GHAA.

———. 1991. *GHAA's Consumer Satisfaction Survey and User's Manual*, 2nd ed. Washington, DC: GHAA.

Davies, A., J. E. Ware, Jr., R. H. Brook, et al. 1986. "Consumer Acceptance of Prepaid and Fee-for-Service Medical Care: Results from a Randomized Controlled Trial." *HSR: Health Services Research* 21 (3): 429–52.

Delmarva Foundation for Medical Care, Inc. 1994. "External Review Performance Measurement of Medicare HMOs/CMPs." Easton, MD: The Foundation.

Felt, S. 1995. "The First Twenty Months of the Quality Assurance Reform Initiative (QARI) Demonstration for Medicaid Managed Care: Interim Evaluation Report." Washington, DC: Mathematica Policy Research.

Francis, W., and the Center for the Study of Services. 1994. *Checkbook's Guide to 1995 Plans for Federal Employees*. Washington, DC.

Gabel, J., D. Liston, G. Jensen, and J. Marsteller. 1994. "The Health Insurance Picture in 1993: Some Rare Good News." *Health Affairs* 13 (1): 327–36.

Gold, M., L. Burnbauer, and K. Chu. 1995. "Half Empty or Half Full: The Capacity of State Data to Support Health Reform." Washington, DC: Mathematica Policy Research.

Gold, M., R. Hurley, T. Lake, T. Ensor, and R. Berenson. 1995b. *Arrangements Between Managed Care Plans and Physicians: Results from a 1994 Survey of Managed Care Plans*. Selected External Research Series Number 3, Washington, DC: Physician Payment Review Commission.

Gold, M., J. Hadley, D. Eisenhower, et al. 1995a. "Design and Feasibility of a National Medicaid Access Survey with State Specific Estimates." Washington, DC: Mathematica Policy Research.

Goldfield, N., M. Pine, and J. Pine. 1991. *Measuring and Managing Health Care Quality: Procedures, Techniques, and Protocols*. Gaithersburg, MD: Aspen Publishers.

Group Health Association of America. 1992. *HMO Industry Profile*. Washington, DC: The Association.

———. 1993. *HMO Industry Profile*. Washington, DC: The Association.

HMO Managers Letter. 1992a. "BCBSA/Gallup Survey: HMO Member Satisfaction Tops 90 Percent for 3rd Straight Year." *HMO Managers Letter* (May 26): 5.

———. 1992b. "Recent Surveys Find Managed Care's Popularity with Employers on the Rise." *HMO Managers Letter* (July 27): 5.

———. 1994. "Towers Perrin Survey Shows HMO Members as Satisfied as Members of Other Health Plans." *HMO Managers Letter* (April 4): 4.

Inguanzo, J. M. 1992. "Taking a Serious Look at Patient Expectations." *Hospitals* (September 5).

Intergovernmental Health Policy Project. 1993. "Expanding Access to Health Care: An Overview of 1992 State Legislation." IHPP.

James, V. 1994. "Quality Assurance: The Cornerstone of Managed Care." Presented at the conference, "Understanding Managed Care: An Introductory Program for New Managers in HMOs." Washington, DC: GHAA.

Kongstvedt, P. R. 1993. "Member Services and Consumer Affairs." In *The Managed Health Care Handbook*, 2nd ed., edited by P. R. Kongstvedt. Gaithersburg, MD: Aspen Publishers, Inc.

Kritchevsky, S. B., and B. P. Simmons. 1991. "Continuous Quality Improvement: Concepts and Applications for Physician Care." *Journal of the American Medical Association* 266 (13): 1817–23.

Marshall, G. N., R. D. Hays, C. D. Sherbourne, and K. B. Wells. 1993. "The Structure of Patient Satisfaction with Outpatient Medical Care." *Psychological Assessment* 5 (4): 477–83.

Meterko, M., E. C. Nelson, and H. R. Rubin. 1990. "Patient Judgments of Hospital Quality: A Taxonomy." *Medical Care* 28 (9) Supplement: S10–S14.

Miller, R. H., and H. S. Luft. 1994. "Managed Care Plan Performance Since 1980: A Literature Analysis." *Journal of the American Medical Association* 271 (19): 1512–19.

Morain, C. 1992. "HMOs Try to Measure (and Reward) 'Doctor Quality.'" *Medical Economics* 69 (7): 206–15.

National Committee for Quality Assurance. 1993. *Health Plan Employee Data and Information Set, HEDIS 2.0*. Washington, DC: NCQA.

———. 1995. *Report Care Pilot Project, Technical Report*. Washington, DC.

National Research Corporation. 1994. *Satisfaction Report Card: National Results*. Lincoln, NE: National Research Corporation.

Packer-Tursman, J. 1994. "Keeping Members." *HMO Magazine* 35 (2): 39–43.

Physician Payment Review Commission. 1994. *Annual Report to Congress*. Washington, DC: PPRC.

Pine, M., and P. R. Kongstvedt. 1993. "Quality Management." In *The Managed Care Handbook*, edited by Peter R. Kongstvedt. Gaithersburg, MD: Aspen Publishers.

Porell, F. W., C. Cocotas, P. J. Perales, et al. 1992. "Factors Associated with Disenrollment from Medicare HMOs: Findings from a Survey of Disenrollees." Waltham, MA: Brandeis University.

Press, I. 1994. "The Last Word." *Hospitals and Health Networks* (March 5).

Press, I., and M. P. Malone. 1993. "Patient Satisfaction and the Cost/Quality Equation." *Journal of Health Care Benefits* 3 (2): 40–43.

Press, I., R. Ganey, and M. Malone. 1992. "Patient Satisfaction: Where Does It Fit in the Quality Picture?" *Trustee* (April).

Research Triangle Institute. 1994. *Information Needs for Consumer Choice*. Prepared for the Health Care Financing Administration under Contract Number 55-94-0047. Research Triangle Park, NC: The Institute.

Ribner, S., and J. Stewart. 1993. *1993 Novalis National Health Care Survey: Consumer Ratings of Managed Care, A Special Report*. Albany, NY: Novalis Corporation.

Rubin, H. R., B. Gandek, W. H. Rogers, et al. 1993. "Patients' Ratings of Outpatient Visits in Different Practice Settings: Results from the Medical Outcomes Study." *Journal of the American Medical Association* 270 (7): 835–40.

Sofaer, S. 1993. "Informing and Protecting Consumers Under Managed Competition." *Health Affairs* 12 (Supplement): 76–86.

State of Minnesota Joint Labor-Management Committee on Health Plans. 1993a. "1993 Survey of Employees on Health Plans and Medical Care."

———. 1993b. *Health Plans and Medical Care: What Employees Think*.

U.S. Department of Health and Human Services, Office of the Inspector General. 1992. *A Review of HMO Quality Assurance Standards Required by Medicaid Agencies*. Washington, DC: DHHS.

Ware, J. E., Jr., B. Curbow, A. R. Davies, and B. Robbins. 1981. *Medicaid Satisfaction Surveys Research (1977–1980): A Report of the Prepaid Health Research, Evaluation, and Development Project*. Sacramento, CA: California State Department of Health Services.

Ware, J. E., Jr., and R. D. Hays. 1988. "Methods for Measuring Patient Satisfaction with Specific Medical Encounters." *Medical Care* 26 (4): 393–402.

Ware, J. E., Jr., and C. D. Sherbourne. 1992. "The MOS 36-Item Short-Form Health Survey (SF-36): I. Conceptual Framework and Item Selection." *Medical Care* 30 (6): 473–83.

Ware, J. E., Jr., K. K. Snow, M. Kosinski, and B. Gaudek. 1993. *SF-36 Survey Manual and Interpretation Guide*. Boston, MA: The Health Institute, New England Medical Center.

Ware, J. E., Jr., and M. K. Snyder. 1975. "Dimensions of Patient Attitudes Regarding Doctors and Medical Care Services." *Medical Care* 13 (8): 669–82.

Ware, J. E., Jr., M. K. Snyder, W. R. Wright, and A. R. Davies. 1983. "Defining and Measuring Patient Satisfaction with Medical Care." *Evaluation and Program Planning* 6: 247–63.

Winslow, R. 1994. "Health-Care Report Cards Are Getting Low Grades from Some Focus Groups." *Wall Street Journal* May 19: B1.

Zablocki, E. 1994. "Employer Report Cards." *HMO Magazine* (March/April): 26–32.

CHAPTER

19

THE DESIGN OF THE COMMUNITY TRACKING STUDY: A LONGITUDINAL STUDY OF HEALTH SYSTEM CHANGE AND ITS EFFECTS ON PEOPLE

Peter Kemper, David Blumenthal, Janet M. Corrigan, Peter J. Cunningham, Suzanne M. Felt, Joy M. Grossman, Linda T. Kohn, Charles E. Metcalf, Robert F. St. Peter, Richard C. Strouse, Paul B. Ginsburg, and Peter J. Cunningham

THE HEALTH care system in the United States is evolving at an unprecedented rate. Purchasers' drive to control rising health care costs, development of new technologies for managing care, and anticipation of modified policies from the Clinton health reform effort have stimulated significant changes in the health care market. Consolidation, vertical integration, and growth of managed care are central features. These organizational and market changes can be expected to alter the delivery of care and ultimately to affect patients. Yet, little systematic information exists about the market changes or their effects on people.

From *Inquiry* 33 (Summer): 195–206.

The Community Tracking Study is being undertaken to provide information on these fundamental changes. The study, which is being conducted by the Center for Studying Health System Change and funded by the Robert Wood Johnson Foundation, is designed to track changes in the health care system and their effects on care delivery and people. As its name suggests, the two key elements of the study are its focus on communities and on tracking them longitudinally. The study establishes a longitudinal cohort of *communities* for the long-term study of health systems analogous to the Framingham cohort of *individuals* for long-term epidemiological studies. This paper describes the design of the Community Tracking Study.

Objectives of the Study

The major changes in the health system that have been reported include: consolidation of the health market at all levels (medical groups, hospitals, insurers, and health plans); vertical integration of providers (e.g., hospitals and physicians) and of insurers and providers; increased risk sharing by providers; growth of large, national, for-profit health care enterprises; and adoption of the newly developed techniques for clinical care management (e.g., clinical information systems, quality improvement techniques, utilization management, etc.). "Health system change" as used here refers generally to these types of changes in health care organizations and markets, and the employer and government policies that are driving them.

A key feature of recent health system change has been the growth of managed care. Managed care products' share of the insurance market has been increasing rapidly at the expense of traditional indemnity insurance.[1] Study of managed care products and the organizations that provide them is, therefore, central to the study of current health system change. The growth of managed care, however, is not synonymous with health system change, and we will study change more broadly, including other changes brought about by market competition or public policy.

The overall goal of the Community Tracking Study is to provide an information and analytic base to monitor and understand changes in the health system and their effects. The study has three objectives within that broad goal.

Tracking changes in health systems. The first objective of the study is to document health system changes through intensive study of a selected number of communities. The study will address the following questions: What are the organizational relationships among insurers and health plans, hospitals, physicians, safety net providers, and other providers, and how are they changing? How is the behavior of these various organizations affecting the health system and how are they responding to the changing market? What role do employers, consumers, and government play in driving changes in the health care system?

Tracking changes in outcomes. Health system change could have important favorable or unfavorable consequences for individuals. It may alter their insurance coverage, access to care, service use and delivery, cost, and quality of care—which are referred to here as "outcomes." The second objective of the study is to monitor the effects on people by tracking indicators of these health system outcomes.

Understanding the effect of health system change on outcomes. Given the absence of systematic local or national information on these issues, documenting changes in health systems and outcomes is of great interest in its own right, and it lays the foundation for accomplishing the third objective of study: to understand how differences in health systems are related to differences in outcomes. This will be done by analyzing—qualitatively and quantitatively—the relationship between health systems and insurance coverage, access, service delivery, cost, and quality.

Overview of the Study Design

Central to the design of the Community Tracking Study is its focus on communities. The study will track changes in health systems in a sample of communities using data collected at two-year intervals beginning in 1996. This community design has been adopted because health care delivery is primarily local and differs due to history, culture, and state policy. Therefore, information at the local market level is needed to analyze and understand institutional changes in delivery system and their effects on people. For example, the implications for people of being uninsured depend in part on the safety net available in the community.

The study design exploits the combination of data from a variety of sources in the same communities. Site visits are designed to provide an understanding of health systems and the dynamics of change through interviews with key actors in the system. Surveys of health care organizations (insurers and health plans, hospitals, and physician organizations) will obtain information about their structure and characteristics of the health system in each community. Surveys of households, physicians, and employers, and hospital discharge records will provide information on outcomes. By combining data on health systems and outcomes in the same communities, the study is designed to relate differences in outcomes to differences in health systems.

Another important design feature is reliance on a combination of qualitative and quantitative data. By interviewing key players in the study communities, it is possible to understand the health system and benefit from insights of knowledgeable people working in it. By combining this qualitative information with quantitative data obtained from surveys and hospital discharge records, we will gain a better understanding and obtain more insights than would be possible using either type of information alone.

The study will be conducted in 60 randomly selected communities, or "sites." The 60 sites form the first stage of sampling for the surveys of households, physicians, employers, and health care organizations which also will be nationally representative.

A random subset of 12 sites will be studied intensively. Selected according to the methodology described subsequently, they are: Boston, Cleveland, Greenville, S.C., Indianapolis, Lansing, Mich., Little Rock, Miami, Newark, N.J., Orange County, Calif., Phoenix, Seattle, and Syracuse (see the figure). Case studies of the subset will be based primarily on site visits. In addition, survey samples are designed to permit site-specific estimates of market characteristics and outcomes. Specifically, samples of 1,225 households, 450 physicians, and 450 employers will be interviewed at each of the 12 sites.

The other 48 sites will be studied less intensively, with smaller survey samples and without site visits. The 12 high-intensity sites will let us track and understand changes in the health systems in depth; the 48 low-intensity sites will ensure that our findings are not the result of

Figure 1 Community Tracking Study Sites

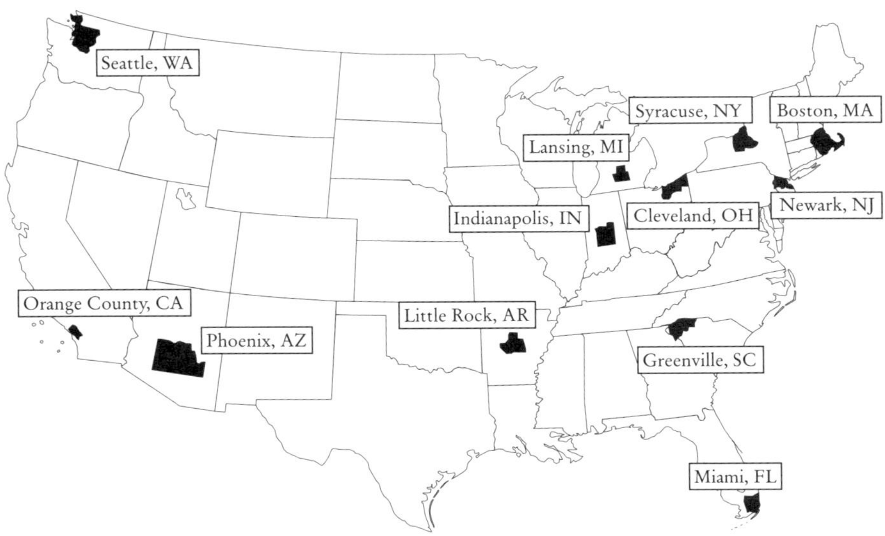

idiosyncrasies of the high-intensity sites and will permit generalization to the nation. (The sample design is described more fully following the discussion of methodology.)

Methodology for Tracking Changes in Health Systems

To track and understand changes in health systems, the study will rely heavily on a case study methodology. Interviews will be conducted in each of the 12 high-intensity sites by teams of four knowledgeable analysts, who will be on-site for approximately a week every two years. Team members will interview representatives of employers, government, consumer groups, hospitals, physician groups, health plans and insurers, integrated health delivery systems, and safety net providers (hospitals of last resort, community health centers). The focus of the interviews will be on understanding how various functions are organized and changing in the system as a whole, rather than on the respondent's particular organization. Between the biennial visits, the sites will be monitored through review of local press coverage of health news and telephone interviews with key informants identified during the visits.

Case studies resulting from the first round of site visits will provide a baseline description of the health systems in the communities and the dynamics of change, with retrospective information on change and the reasons for it. The completed baseline studies, as well as the underlying interview database, will allow comparison of the health systems across the 12 sites. The purposes of the cross-site analyses are to document the commonalities and the range of variation in the characteristics of the health care systems, the dynamics of change they experience, and the assessments of respondents concerning the likely effects of the changes on people. Subsequent rounds of site visits and cross-site analyses will use the same case study methodology but will focus on change during the intervening period.

A challenge of analyzing qualitative information involving multiple researchers is how to use the full information objectively, and avoid having the researchers disproportionately influenced by the particular sites they visit or interviews they conduct. To ensure objectivity and comparability across sites, data collection will be systematized by using a standard interview protocol, selecting similar types of organizations and respondents for interviews at all sites, and covering a consistent set of topics in all case studies. Qualitative information collected will be organized by topic, respondent, and site in a relational database for subsequent analysis. Cross-site analyses will rely on tables of qualitative information constructed from this database. These tabular presentations arrayed by site enable systematic review of relevant interview responses and permit analyses of the extent to which the health systems differ across sites. Having senior researchers involved in the site visits and analysis will ensure that the interpretation is insightful and goes beyond the simple reporting of differences in site characteristics. To encourage objectivity in our interpretation of causes of various health systems changes in a community, we will distinguish between inferences drawn by researchers and assessments made by respondents in the site visits.

In addition to the qualitative information from site visits, the cross-site analyses will draw on secondary data on, for example, demographics, hospitals, state policy, Medicaid and Medicare costs, and HMO penetration. Surveys of physicians, households, employers, and health care organizations also will be used to develop quantitative measures characterizing the health system. Examples of characteristics to be constructed include the percentage of households with various types of insurance coverage, the percentage uninsured, the percentage of workers in firms offering insurance, the types of choices offered, and the average share of primary care physicians' revenue that is capitated.

These data will be used to place the case study sites in the context of the nation. The 60 high- and low-intensity sites together provide a substantially larger sample for tracking health system change using measures from the survey data than is possible for the case studies alone. In addition, high-intensity sites can be compared with this national sample to validate the representativeness of the sites where case studies are performed with respect to the measures of system characteristics obtained from the surveys.

Methodology for Tracking Changes in Outcomes

To track changes in insurance coverage, access, service delivery, cost, and quality, measures of each will be obtained from telephone surveys of households, physicians, and employers and from hospital discharge records. We chose to rely primarily on surveys for two reasons. First, they permit tracking of outcomes for the entire population and, therefore, are not subject to bias due to changes in insurance coverage. Most computerized record systems have data only for the insured or for a particular type of insurance. (The exception is hospital discharge records, which we do plan to use.) Second, survey data are available across sites and over time—an important requirement given the analytic comparisons planned. We chose telephone over in-person interviews because of the substantial difference in cost.

Technically, tracking will be achieved by estimating population means of various outcome indicators for each time period and comparing them. Changes in these means will be tracked individually for the 12 high-intensity sites and for the nation. Differences over time in site means will be required to be significantly different from zero statistically to be considered a change. Although conceptually straightforward, the implementation of the statistical tests will require nonresponse adjustments, imputation of missing data, and estimation of standard errors that account for the complex sample design (particularly for national estimates). The table provides an overview of the type of outcome indicators to be tracked and their sources.

Insurance coverage. To track insurance coverage, household survey respondents will be asked whether they are covered by insurance and, if covered, about the attributes of the insurance product, such as whether the policy has a defined list of doctors, whether using doctors outside the list entails an additional charge, etc. From the responses, the percentages of the population who are uninsured and covered by insurance products with particular attributes can be estimated and tracked over time. Given the importance of understanding changes in insurance products purchased and the questionable ability of household respondents to report on insurance attributes, a followback from households to insurers is being pilot tested. The goal of the pilot test is to determine the feasibility of confirming household responses from insurers and obtaining additional insurance product attributes for people in the household sample (e.g., how the plan pays physicians, whether physicians are required to serve enrollees in the plan exclusively, etc.). Finally, the employer survey will provide information on whether employers offer insurance and the types of products offered.

Access. To track access to care, traditional indicators such as difficulty obtaining needed care, ease and convenience of obtaining care, and whether individuals have a person or place where they usually go for care, will be obtained from the household survey. In addition, indicators of physicians' ability to obtain services for their patients (such as referrals to specialists), whether they accept Medicaid patients, and the amount of charity care they provide will be obtained through the physician survey. Finally, rates of hospitalizations for conditions that are sensitive to the availability of ambulatory care will be constructed from hospital discharge records. For example, a high rate of hospital admission for asthma will be used as an indicator of poor access to primary care.

Service delivery. It is primarily through the delivery of care that health system change is likely to have its effect on people. Measures of use of different types of services obtained from the household survey will allow basic tracking of changes in the type of services used. In addition,

Table 1 Outcome Variables and Data Sources

Variables	Household Survey	Physician Survey	Employer Survey	Discharge Records
Insurance coverage	Rates of coverage Product attributes[a] Changes in insurance coverage Insurance offered at work Choice of plans		Insurance offered Choice of plans	
Access to care	Ease of using health care Perceived changes in access Barriers to care Usual source of care	Amount of charity care Accepting Medicaid patients Ability to obtain services		Avoidable hospitalization
Service delivery	Receipt of services Hospital days Physician visits Patient trust	Practice styles Physician autonomy Scope of care Effect of care management		Surgical procedure rates
Cost[b]	Out-of-pocket cost		Private insurance premiums Employee share of premiums	
Quality	Consumer satisfaction Preventive service use Health status Tobacco use	Ability to provide quality care		Mortality rates Adverse outcomes

[a]Information on insurance product attributes will be obtained from the insurance followback interview.
[b]Medicaid and Medicare expenditures also will be obtained from state Medicaid offices and the Health Care Financing Administration.

the physician survey will provide important indicators of changes in the way medicine is practiced. For example, clinical vignettes—short clinical descriptions of a patient followed by a choice of treatment options—will provide information on primary care physicians' propensities to use various diagnostic and therapeutic services. The physician survey also will cover physicians' perceptions about their clinical autonomy, scope of care provided, and the effect of various care management techniques on doctors' practice of medicine. Finally, hospital discharge records will be used to construct surgical procedure rates for conditions known to exhibit unexplained geographic variability.

Cost. Cost tracking will measure expenditures primarily from the payer's perspectives. Premiums for private insurance obtained from the employer survey, together with government data on per capita Medicaid and Medicare expenditures, employer data on employees' share of premiums, and households' responses to a question about out-of-pocket expenses will provide the primary indicators of changes in health care expenditures. Premiums also will be tracked by type of insurance, permitting an assessment of how much of the changes in overall premiums are due to shifts among types of insurance.

Quality. To track quality of care, the household survey will obtain a variety of indicators of quality: consumers' satisfaction with care, preventive service use, tobacco use and whether a physician advised stopping smoking, and health status. These will be supplemented by quality indicators constructed from hospital discharge records, such as fetal death rates, rates of newborns with serious health conditions, and rates of post-surgical complications. Finally, the physician survey will collect physicians' perceptions of their ability to provide quality care.

Methodology for Inferring the Effects of Health Systems on Outcomes

Tracking changes in health systems and outcomes will be of greatest value if differences in outcomes can be related to differences in health systems. Using both qualitative and quantitative methods, we will use the natural variation across communities and over time to infer the effects of health systems on people.

Qualitative Analysis

This analysis is straightforward in concept. Means of outcome indicators (and when longitudinal data are available, changes in outcomes) will be compared across sites. When significant differences are observed across sites, we will make analytic judgments about what may account for the observed differences—informed by the understanding of health systems acquired from the case studies.

Based on only the high-intensity sites where case studies are conducted, it will not be possible to attribute the cause of differences in outcomes unambiguously to potential explanatory factors, such as health system characteristics, state policy, and local economic changes, which often vary together. Nonetheless, having an in-depth understanding of the health system and assessments from key informants of likely effects of the system on outcomes means that this qualitative analysis will generate hypotheses and lay a strong foundation for the interpretation of quantitative analyses.

Quantitative Analysis of the Effect of Health Systems on Outcomes

Our second approach to inference will be multivariate analysis relating outcomes to health system characteristics in the 60 sites. For individual outcomes, such as access to care, the unit of analysis is the individual; for physician outcomes, such as practice patterns, the unit of analysis is the physician; and for outcomes obtained from employers, such as insurance offerings, the unit of analysis is the establishment.[2] At baseline, the analysis is cross-sectional; when follow-up data become available, the analysis will exploit variation over time as well as variation across sites. Formally, the reduced form model to be estimated for individuals is given by:

$$Y_{ist} = \alpha_o + \alpha_H H_{st} + \alpha_X X_{ist} + \varepsilon_{ist} \qquad (1)$$

where Y_{ist} is the outcome of interest for individual i in site s at time t; H_{st} is a vector of health system characteristics; X_{ist} is a vector of individual characteristics such as health status, income, and demographic characteristics; ε_{ist} is the error term; and α_o, α_H and α_X are the coefficients to be estimated. Because some of the variation across individuals will be due to unobserved site-level effects, fixed effects models or error component models will be needed to ensure that standard errors are estimated correctly. (For the analysis of baseline data, error component models are the only option for accounting for this correlation because H_{st} would be perfectly collinear with the binary site variables.) Models for physicians and employers are direct extensions of this basic model.

This methodology treats the variation in health systems across the 60 sites as a natural experiment in health system change. However, unlike a social experiment where the intervention is well-defined at the outset and usually univariate, health system change is not well-defined.

Indeed, one of the objectives of this study is to understand health system change and to define those changes. Specification of the health system characteristics in the model, therefore, is central to the analysis. Some characteristics, such as measures of HMO penetration, have been used in earlier cross-market analyses. Others, such as the generosity of the state's Medicaid benefit and concentration in the service delivery market, appear straightforward. Considerable work remains to be done defining the measures, however, and we expect them to evolve as we gain an in-depth, systematic understanding of health systems through our site visits and analysis. We also expect that different health system characteristics will be important for different outcomes.

Quantitative Analysis of the Effect of Type of Insurance

In addition to analyzing the relation between health systems and outcomes, we also will analyze the effect of type of insurance coverage (e.g., HMO vs. other insurance) on access, service use, and satisfaction. As indicated, we do not view growth in managed care as equivalent to health system change, but it is—at least at present—the most important component of health system change. This is reflected at the individual level by changes in the type of insurance or health plan held, which motivates us to conduct this analysis.

It is reasonable to expect that we will continue to observe changes in the type of health insurance choices individuals face and increases in the proportion of the population enrolled in managed care in the future. An obvious question is: Does the type of insurance product individuals have affect their access, service use, and satisfaction? Here the unit of analysis is the individual and the estimation methodology includes correction for favorable and adverse selection into different types of insurance products. A simple model of effect of type of insurance on outcomes is given by:

$$Y_{ist} = \beta_o + \beta_I I_{ist} + \beta_X X_{ist} + \eta_{ist} \tag{2}$$

where I_{ist} is a variable indicating type of insurance coverage and η_{ist} is the error term.

Because individuals may play a role in selecting the type of insurance coverage they have and because their decision may depend on their propensity to use health care, the choice of insurance is not independent of service use and the other outcomes of interest. Equation 3 gives a simple model of insurance choice.

$$I_{ist} = \alpha_o + \alpha_X X_{ist} + \alpha_Z Z_{ist} + \xi_{ist} \tag{3}$$

where Z_{ist} is a vector of measures of preferences that affect insurance choice but not outcomes, and ξ_{ist} is the error term. Because selection of insurance can bias estimates of the effect of insurance type on outcomes (due to the correlation of errors between equations 2 and 3), the outcome model (equation 2), will be estimated using a standard selection bias model.

The success of this modeling effort certainly is not guaranteed. Measures of preferences to be collected in the household survey, such as a person's propensity to take above average risks and willingness to pay more to retain choice of physician without restriction, may not predict insurance coverage and identify the selection bias model. Given the great likelihood of selection into different types of insurance, however, it will be important to investigate this issue and control for selection bias in the best way feasible.

As with the analysis of effects of health system differences, the baseline analysis of the effect of insurance type will rely on the cross-sectional data. However, as discussed later, part of the sample in the subsequent round of data collection will be longitudinal observations of individuals included in the baseline sample. (The other half is a new representative cross-section that will be followed in the next round of data collection.) For purposes of estimating equations 2 and 3, the longitudinal observations are particularly valuable because individual differences are controlled for substantially by observing the same individuals. Indeed, the data provide the opportunity for special studies that estimate the model on the longitudinal sample only or focus on those who have changed insurance.

Sample Design

The sample design—the number and type of communities studied; the number and type of households, physicians, employers, and health care organizations surveyed; and the method of selection—is central to the validity and ultimate defensibility of the study findings. The samples are designed with the objectives of: 1) tracking change at the community level and 2) generalizing to the nation.

Sites

An unusual feature of the design of the Community Tracking Study is the random selection of sites, including the 12 selected for case studies. Although random selection requires additional design work, it has a number of important advantages:

1. It protects against researcher bias in site selection due, for example, to a preference (perhaps inadvertent) to study sites that are known to the researcher, experiencing particular types of market changes, perceived at present to be the most "interesting," or particularly desirable to visit.
2. It increases confidence that the communities reflect changes representative of the nation.
3. It increases the face validity of the sample of sites to be studied.
4. It ensures that the household, physician, employer, and organization survey samples, which are nested within the sample of sites, are representative of the nation.
5. It protects against the perception that sites have been chosen to support a particular agenda, such as an approach to health reform.

Because an important objective of the study is to determine effects on people, sites have been sampled with a probability of selection that is proportional to population. This ensures that the study sites represent health systems in the communities where people in the United States tend to live. The sample was stratified to ensure its geographic diversity.[3]

The high-intensity sites were chosen from metropolitan areas[4] with populations over 200,000, thus restricting case studies to large and medium-sized metropolitan areas. Because small metropolitan and rural areas are extremely diverse, one or two case studies of these areas would be likely to be dominated by unique features of that community, with limited generalizability.

We also considered whether to oversample cities with high HMO penetration, but decided against it. Unlike large surveys where weights can be used to adjust for oversampling, case study data cannot be adjusted by reweighting. Because case study results typically are presented as separate observations, interpretation is based on readers' implicit weighting of the sites. Readers are likely to weight case studies roughly equally, regardless of any warnings to the contrary from the author. Because our sample of study sites is approximately self-weighting, except for sampling variability, the case studies can be expected to be representative of health systems experienced by people living in large and medium-sized metropolitan areas throughout the nation—without reweighting.

Household Survey

The primary purpose of the household survey is to track people's insurance coverage, access to care, service use, satisfaction with care, and health status. Because of the priority placed on tracking these changes at the site level, the household sample size is relatively large (n = 36,200).

This sample is designed to permit us to test hypotheses about change in each of the high-intensity sites. Specifically, the sample at high-intensity sites ($n = 1{,}225$) is sufficient to detect (with 70% power) a .05 difference between two time periods in an outcome measure with a mean of .50. For attributes with means of more or less than .50, smaller percentage point differences can be detected with equal power. For example, with a mean of .10 a difference of .03 can be detected.

Samples at the low-intensity sites ($n = 375$) are too small to detect changes at this level of precision for individual sites. However, if low-intensity sites are grouped by a common characteristic that is of analytic interest, then changes can be detected for a group of at least three sites. These smaller samples are also large enough to construct site-specific measures of health system characteristics, such as percentage of the population uninsured, measured precisely enough to be used as explanatory variables in multivariate analysis.

To ensure that households without telephones are represented in the sample, interviews for approximately 4% of the sample in high-intensity sites will be conducted in person. Area probability sampling methods will be used to select interviewing areas with probability proportional to the prevalence of nontelephone households. Households then will be screened to identify families without working telephones.

Because the 60 sites are selected randomly, the combined sample is nationally representative and therefore permits tracking at a national level. However, because of the clustering of the sample (that is, the concentration of the sample in 60 sites without any sample in the many other sites in the nation), the effective sample size for national estimates from these sites alone is relatively small—equivalent to a simple random national sample of less than 2,800. To permit national tracking with greater precision, therefore, we have added a national sample that is not confined to the 60 sites in the site-specific sample ($n = 3{,}500$). The combined sample, which is equivalent to a random national sample of perhaps as many as 7,000, is large enough to detect changes over time for subgroups constituting roughly 20% of the population, depending on the specific subgroup and variable being tracked (using the same criterion of detecting a .05 difference).[5]

The sample design employs a strategy that takes advantage of the strengths of repeated cross-section and longitudinal designs. Roughly 45% of the sample will be a longitudinal cohort and the other 55% a new cross-section each round. (This is the split between the longitudinal and cross-section samples that yields the largest longitudinal sample subject to the constraint that the split can be replicated in subsequent rounds.) On the one hand, a repeated cross-section design is far simpler analytically and avoids bias due to sample attrition, aging of the sample, and migration. On the other hand, a longitudinal design permits analyses of change at the individual level and, hence, some analyses that cannot be addressed with repeated cross sections (e.g., analysis of the choice of insurance type using data on individuals who switch insurance). A longitudinal design also improves the ability to draw causal inferences by making it easier to control for unmeasured individual characteristics. A longitudinal design is also more powerful, requiring smaller sample sizes because the individual correlation in outcomes over time reduces the variance of differences in means over time. Because each design has important strengths and limitations, we have adopted a combined strategy that gains some of the benefits of each.

Physician Survey

The physician survey will be used to track changes in service delivery, access, and perceived ability to provide quality care, and to collect health system characteristics, such as the proportion of physician revenue that is capitated. The sample design parallels that of the household survey, but with a smaller total sample (n = 12,600). Primary care physicians will be oversampled at approximately a 2.5 : 1 rate to expand the sample for analysis of their practice of medicine. The capacity to analyze primary care in this way comes at a price in ability to track change for all physicians combined—all physicians can be traced with the same statistical precision as primary care physicians alone. Specifically, the sample at high-intensity sites (n = 450) will permit testing hypotheses about change concerning primary care physicians and all physicians (but not specialists separately). When combined with that of low-intensity sites (n = 125) and a small national supplement (n = 1,200), the sample is sufficient to test for changes nationally for primary care physicians and specialists separately.

Employer Survey

The main objective of the employer survey is to track changes in employers' offering of insurance, the types of insurance offered, premiums, and employees' share of premiums.[6] In addition, limited information on employers' purchasing behavior with respect to health benefits will be collected. The sample design again parallels the design of the household survey. The sample for high-intensity sites (n = 450) is designed to test hypotheses about change in premiums at the site level. At the low-intensity sites, the sample (n = 85) is designed to test for change in premiums for groups of six to seven sites and to measure market characteristics, such as the percentage of establishments offering insurance, with sufficient precision at the site level to be used as explanatory variables in multivariate analysis. Establishments will be sampled with probability approximately proportional to employment using a mixed cross-section, longitudinal design. Like the household survey design, the 60-site sample will be augmented with a national sample (n = 1,600) to improve the capacity to track insurance offerings and premiums at the national level.

Hospital Discharge Records

Hospital discharge records will be used to track and analyze changes in access, service delivery, and quality. Many states have hospital discharge data files, although these files are not equally easy to obtain and use and are available only with a substantial time lag. They consist of claims data or uniform hospital discharge data, both of which include a standard set of core elements, such as diagnoses, procedures, admission and discharge status, age, gender, and zip code. These files will be obtained for the subset of sites where they are available. Because their availability will be limited, quality indicators obtained from hospital discharge records cannot be tracked at the national level. However, we will be able to document the extent to which those sites where discharge records are available are representative of the nation.

Surveys of Health Care Organizations

Surveys of health care organizations (i.e., insurers and health plans, hospitals, and physician organizations) are designed to describe the market structure and organization of the health system at high- and low-intensity sites. These surveys will be designed after the first round of site visits so that we can build on the knowledge obtained from the visits and have a better basis for estimating the number of organizations in each site. Our current plan calls for censuses of insurers and health plans and physician organizations at high- and low-intensity sites. Because they are censuses, sample size is not a consideration. In practice, of course, less than a census will be achieved due to nonresponse, which will introduce some error in site-specific estimates. For hospitals, plans call for a census at high-intensity sites and a 50% sample (on average) at low-intensity sites. The (near) censuses of the various organizations in the 60 sites will provide a sufficient sample to test hypotheses about change in the nation.

Conclusion

It is appropriate at the outset of the Community Tracking Study to reflect on whether we can expect to achieve the study's objectives and overcome the challenges it faces.

The first objective, tracking change in health systems, can be expected to be achieved. Using case studies to document variation and change in the 12 high-intensity sites will provide a rich understanding of changes in those sites. The study promises information on health systems that is systematic across a representative sample of communities, allowing an assessment of the magnitude of change. Moreover, it is reasonable to anticipate that organizational change will be great enough to produce findings of interest.

We also can expect to achieve the second objective, tracking changes in outcomes. Surveys of households, physicians, and employers, as well as hospital discharge records, are in place with sufficient samples to detect reasonable size changes if they occur. However, achieving this objective is subject to two major risks.

First, although we have consulted experts and sought to use the best measures available and to construct new ones when good measures did not exist, the measures of insurance coverage, access, service delivery, cost and quality are limited necessarily by the methodology used to collect them—primarily telephone surveys. The limitations are most apparent in the area of cost, where comprehensive measures are unavailable, and quality, where (except for hospital discharge records at selected sites) data necessary to construct clinical outcome measures—medical records for large samples of people with specific diagnoses—will not be collected.

Second, changes may not occur or may not be large enough to detect over relatively short intervals. Changes in the health systems, as indicated, are likely to be observable over a two-year interval because of the rapid pace of organizational change. Real changes in the delivery of care that affect people, however, are likely to take longer. In addition, not all outcomes are equally prone to be affected by health system change. Type of insurance, service delivery, and cost, for example, are likely to be affected. Access and satisfaction may be affected, but the direction is ambiguous. And health status is not likely to be affected enough that change could be detected at the population level using a telephone survey.

The third objective, understanding how health systems affect outcomes, is the objective of ultimate interest. It is also the most difficult to achieve. As indicated, this objective is approached in three ways, each of which has some risks associated with it. Qualitative analysis of differences across the 12 high-intensity sites benefits from rich understanding of institutions and insights of actors in the delivery system, but is inherently limited by the small number of sites. Quantitative analysis of health system differences across sites exploits variation among the larger sample of 60 sites. However, it depends on the development of adequate measures of health system characteristics from surveys and on there being sufficient variation across sites and over time to constitute a natural experiment. Quantitative analysis of the effect of type of insurance coverage on outcomes exploits the strength of individual level data to address a well-defined question, but runs the risk of invalidation due to selection bias that cannot be corrected for econometrically.

By approaching this objective with these three analytic methods, the likelihood of understanding the effect of health system change on people is enhanced. If all three approaches come to similar conclusions, that will substantially increase the confidence in the results. Nonetheless, it is this third objective, which requires drawing causal inferences, that runs the greatest risk of not being fully achieved.

The study faces a number of broader challenges that often are not confronted in research projects. One is integrating large amounts of data from multiple sources, both quantitative and qualitative. Our plan is for all Center researchers to conduct site visits and contribute to the design of survey instruments and to analyze both qualitative and quantitative data. Despite the study's commitment to integrating qualitative and quantitative information, we recognize that doing so is a challenge.

Also a challenge is producing information quickly—the rapid pace of change makes timely information of great interest and increases the risk that results will be outdated before they are produced. We have pushed to complete the design of the surveys and site visit protocols so that data collection can begin this summer and be completed next winter. Case studies and cross-site analyses based on the site visits are planned for the spring and summer of 1997, respectively. After development of survey weights, imputation of missing data, and other database development work, Center staff will begin analysis of the survey data, with initial baseline descriptive analysis scheduled for fall 1997. This is an ambitious schedule for a data collection and analysis effort of this scale, but we believe it is important to provide findings in time to be useful.

Finally, we must balance the need for dissemination of data to other researchers with the need to ensure confidentiality. The survey data collected as part of the Community Tracking Study will be made available to researchers outside the Center subject to confidentiality limitations so that its full potential can be exploited. Developing a plan is difficult because the concentration of the sample in named sites makes identification of respondents much easier than in a simple random sample. Our current plan is to release data to researchers who submit requests that indicate a bona fide research purpose and who sign a strict confidentiality contract. We also are exploring whether public use files without site identifiers could be released without confidentiality risks.

The design presented here represents our initial plan. It provides for a solid baseline, a representative sample of communities, and a skeleton for a long-term tracking study with the flexibility to adapt over time. We intend for the study to evolve as health systems and policies change and results stimulate new questions. This evolution may involve revision of the data collection methods, new data collection, analysis of planned data in ways not now foreseen, special follow-up efforts in selected sites, and more intense study of low-intensity sites. Now and over the course of the tracking effort, we welcome comments and suggestions from researchers and public and private decision makers with an interest in systematic information on the changing health care system and its effects on people.

Notes

This paper was presented at the annual meetings of the Association for Health Services Research in Atlanta, June 9–11, 1996. The authors are grateful to: the Robert Wood Johnson Foundation for its support of the Center; Robert Hughes and James Knickman for the original conception of a longitudinal community study to track change; Barbara Carlson, Embry Howell, and Ed Hoke for development of the database and hospital discharge records collection plan; Randy Brown, Jon Christianson, Lynn Etheredge, Marsha Gold, Debra Lipson, Hal Luft, Steve Long, Bob Miller, Pam Short, Bruce Steinwachs, Judith Woolridge and members of the Foundation staff for helpful comments on the design during its initial development; the many other researchers who have generously contributed their advice since the initial development; and Cheryl Feeling for assistance in producing the manuscript.

1. "Managed care" products, as used here, incorporate restrictions or incentives designed to encourage use of a defined set of providers. Managed care products can include a variety of features to promote efficiency—payment mechanisms ranging from discounts to capitation and care management ranging from utilization review to sophisticated profiling and performance evaluation—and typically provide a broad range of services with minimal copayments.
2. Note, however, that some components of expenditures (Medicaid and Medicare) are collected as an aggregate at the site level and, therefore, cannot be analyzed using a model like equation 1. These expenditures and total expenditures will be analyzed at the site level only.
3. We also had hoped originally to stratify by city size and HMO market penetration as a proxy for extent of market activity, but the small number of sites severely limited the extent of stratification possible. Only in the Northeast, where metropolitan areas are geographically concentrated, was it also possible to stratify by city size.
4. Urban sites are defined based on the census's definition of economic areas, metropolitan statistical areas (MSAs), which are based on commuting patterns. (In the case of the largest areas, "consolidated metropolitan statistical areas," sites are defined as the smaller component "primary metropolitan statistical areas" [PMSAs] except when their population is less than 350,000, in which case they have been combined with contiguous PMSAs.) This economic definition of sites was used because: insurance most often is obtained through employers, making it more likely that an economic definition of the market will approximate insurance markets; they constitute generally recognizable urban areas; and they are aggregates of counties, for which secondary data are available. It also represents a compromise among market sizes, which is necessary because some parts of health care, such as tertiary

care, have larger markets than a metropolitan area, while others, such as primary care physicians, are more localized. Nonmetropolitan sites are defined as groups of counties within a state that are part of the same Bureau of Economic Analysis Economic Areas, an extension of the definition of economic area to rural areas.

5. We considered oversampling various groups, such as the uninsured and poor, but decided against it because we are interested in tracking the entire population. One group we would like to oversample is persons with high need for care, because they are most likely to experience changes in the health system and be most affected, favorably or unfavorably. Unfortunately, a simple telephone screening question that identifies persons with high need does not exist, and complex screening is not cost effective in a telephone survey. Consequently, between the first and second round, we will consider using the first-round interview to identify the high-need subgroup to be oversampled in the longitudinal sample.
6. The employer survey is part of a joint effort with RAND, which will design and oversee the employer survey. The Community Tracking Study sample described here will be integrated with the RAND State Initiatives project sample.

Index

F

G

I

J

N

O

R

S

T

ABOUT THE EDITOR

Marsha Gold, Sc.D., is a senior fellow in the Washington office of Mathematica Policy Research, an employee-owned public policy research firm whose primary clients are agencies of federal and state government, foundations, and Congress. At Mathematica, Dr. Gold's research has focused on managed care and its effects on access and the healthcare system. She is particularly interested in work addressing the complexities of today's healthcare system in a timely and policy-relevant way that will be respected and will contribute to the ongoing debate nationally, in states, and in localities about the healthcare system.

Dr. Gold brings to her research both practical and academic experience. Before joining Mathematica in 1992, she served as research director with what then was the Group Health Association of America from 1987 until 1991. From 1981 until 1986, Dr. Gold served as director of policy analysis and program evaluation in the Maryland Department of Health and Mental Hygiene. Dr. Gold has been on the faculty of the Department of Health Policy and Administration at the University of North Carolina at Chapel Hill, as well as serving as a guest lecturer at a number of leading universities and an active participant in national meetings of researchers, public policymakers, and healthcare executives and managers. She is currently active as an adjunct associate on the faculty of the School of Public Health at Johns Hopkins University, where she has been teaching graduate courses on contemporary issues of managed care.